$125.00

W9-AHS-072

History of Cognitive Neuroscience

History of Cognitive Neuroscience

M. R. Bennett and P. M. S. Hacker

WILEY-
BLACKWELL

This edition first published 2008

© 2008 by M. R. Bennett and P. M. S. Hacker

Blackwell Publishing was acquired by John Wiley & Sons in February 2007. Blackwell's publishing program has been merged with Wiley's global Scientific, Technical, and Medical business to form Wiley-Blackwell.

Registered Office

John Wiley & Sons Ltd, The Atrium, Southern Gate, Chichester, West Sussex, PO19 8SQ, United Kingdom

Editorial Offices

350 Main Street, Malden, MA 02148-5020, USA

9600 Garsington Road, Oxford, OX4 2DQ, UK

The Atrium, Southern Gate, Chichester, West Sussex, PO19 8SQ, UK

For details of our global editorial offices, for customer services, and for information about how to apply for permission to reuse the copyright material in this book please see our website at www.wiley.com/wiley-blackwell.

The right of M. R. Bennett and P. M. S. Hacker to be identified as the authors of this work has been asserted in accordance with the Copyright, Designs and Patents Act 1988.

Library of Congress Cataloging-in-Publication Data

Bennett, M. R.
 History of cognitive neuroscience / M.R. Bennett and P.M.S. Hacker.
  p. ; cm.
 Includes bibliographical references and index.
 ISBN 978-1-4051-8182-2 (hardback : alk. paper)   1. Cognitive neuroscience–History.   I. Hacker, P. M. S. (Peter Michael Stephan)   II. Title.
 [DNLM: 1. Cognitive Science–history.   2. Neuropsychology–history.   3. Brain–physiology.
 4. Cognition–physiology. WL 11.1 B472h 2008]
  QP360.5.B463 2008
  612.8'233–dc22

                                                                                           2008018526

A catalogue record for this book is available from the British Library.

Set in 10 on 12 pt Bembo by SNP Best-set Typesetter Ltd., Hong Kong
Printed in Singapore by Utopia Press Pte Ltd

1   2008

For Adam and David

Contents

List of Figures

List of Plates

Foreword

Anthony Kenny

Max Bennett and Peter Hacker's *Philosophical Foundations of Neuroscience* (Blackwell, 2003) was the most significant contribution to philosophy of mind in recent years. It examined thoroughly and carefully the pretensions of cognitive science to have superannuated philosophical psychology. It showed how the writings of some of the most prominent proponents of the new discipline are infected throughout with philosophical confusion. Those who scorn our ordinary concepts of thought, intention, and reasons as relics of a folk psychology, are engaged, as Bennett and Hacker showed, in sawing off the branches on which any scientist exploring the neurological basis of the mind must have to sit.

Since many a substantial reputation had been built upon the pretensions thus questioned, it was unsurprising that the book encountered hostile reaction, in particular from philosophers who had invested in cognitive science. Two of the best known, Daniel Dennett and John Searle, elaborated severe criticisms at a meeting of the American Philosophical Association in New York in 2005. The objections and responses from this session were published in 2007 by Columbia University Press as *Neuroscience and Philosophy,* a volume that enabled the world at large to see that Bennett and Hacker had more than held their own against their critics. But there remained in the minds of some readers a lingering suspicion that the two authors were not as close as they should have been to the technical work in cognitive neuroscience.

The present volume should set these doubts definitively at rest. Against a broad historical background it sets out in detail the research papers since Helmholtz in the nineteenth century that are considered to have established the discipline of cognitive neuroscience. In each section the authors first describe the relevant investigations, next subject to critical analysis the interpretations that the investigators placed on their findings, and finally restate the conclusions of the research in terms that have been purged of philosophical confusion.

Thus, to take one example, the authors describe the functional disorders consequent on commissurotomy, which led Gazzaniga and Le Doux to claim that each of the two hemispheres of the brain has a mind of its own. They object to this claim as an instance of the mereological fallacy: only a complete human being, not any part of one, can have a mind. They then restate the research results in neutral terms: the transmission of neural signals across the corpus callosum is a necessary condition for a person to know what is visually presented to him.

Another example: the examination of the memory abilities of patients with damaged temporal lobes led a number of investigators to conclude that memory involved the storage, in the hippocampus, of neural representations of past experiences. Bennett and Hacker show that this involves a misuse of the concept of *representation*. What the studies have shown, they claim, is simply that but for certain neural configurations or strengths of synaptic connections one would not be able, for example, to remember the date of the Battle of Hastings.

The reader's first reaction to Bennett and Hacker's restatement of research results like these may be that they take all the glamour out of them, presenting them in black and white, as it were, instead of in technicolour. But, in fact, these restatements are much more deflationary than that: they not only concern the presentation of the story of cognitive neuroscience but have a significant effect upon the plot itself.

According to Bennett and Hacker, the besetting sin of neurophysiological researchers has been the attribution to brain parts and brain processes of states and activities that are logically ascribable only to entire animals. It makes no sense, they insist, to ascribe to parts of a creature such psychological attributes as being conscious, thinking, believing, perceiving, hypothesising, knowing, or remembering.

Such attribution defeats the explanatory project in two different ways. On the one hand, it offers illusions of explanation when no explanation has been given. The idea that there is a stored representation available to a person that makes him able to remember presupposes memory and cannot explain it: for were such records available to us we would still have to remember how to read them. On the other hand, the mereological fallacy also throws up questions that are only pseudo-problems, such as how information carried by different neural pathways enables an animal to perceive a unified object ('the binding problem'). The critical stance of the present book presents no threat to neuroscientific research: it only averts futile questions that can have no answer, and deflates hype that goes beyond the empirical results.

In the background of this history of the relationships between philosophy and physiology two intellectual giants stand out: Aristotle and Descartes. In physiology Aristotle's influence was malign and Descartes' was benign; in philosophy the situation is reversed. Many of the functions of the brain were erroneously attributed by Aristotle to the heart; fortunately it was not long before the brain was given its rightful place by Galen. Descartes, however, made substantial contributions to neurophysiology and, if we are to believe Bennett, his insistence that biological explanation must be in terms of efficient causation was the foundation of all the advances in neurophysiology since the seventeenth century. On the other hand, Descartes' philosophical dualism threw philosophy of mind into utter darkness, and his shadow is so long that contemporary materialists still believe in a Cartesian ego, merely identifying it with the brain rather than with the mind. Bennett and Hacker constantly recall us to the Aristotelian concept of the unitary human being, recently given magisterial restatement by Wittgenstein.

In this book the findings of neurophysiological research are presented in an original and unfamiliar light. This is not because of fresh empirical investigation or new experimental work: it is the result of logico-linguistic analysis of the concepts involved in exploring the relationship between the mind and the brain. This style of inquiry will be unfamiliar to many physiologists, but it is a tool that is essential to the research project. 'The moral of our tale,' Bennett and Hacker say, 'is that neuroscientists need to devote as much care to ensure conceptual coherence and lucidity as they do to the experiments they undertake.'

Acknowledgements

Portions of chapters in this book have been published by us in the following journals and books:

Chapters 1 and 3: 'Perception and memory in neuroscience: a conceptual analysis'. *Progress in Neurobiology* 65 (2001), 499–543. Copyright (2001). Reprinted with permission of Elsevier Science.

Chapter 4: 'Language and cortical function: conceptual developments'. *Progress in Neurobiology* 80 (2006), 20–52. Copyright (2006). Reprinted with permission of Elsevier Science.

Chapter 5: 'Emotion and cortical-subcortical functions: conceptual developments'. *Progress in Neurobiology* 75 (2005), 29–52. Copyright (2005). Reprinted with permission of Elsevier Science.

Chapter 6: 'The motor system in neuroscience: a history and analysis of conceptual development'. *Progress in Neurobiology* 67 (2002), 1–52. Copyright (2002). Reprinted with permission of Elsevier Science.

Chapter 7: 'The conceptual presuppositions of cognitive neuroscience: a reply to critics', in *Neuroscience and Philosophy: Brain, Mind and Language* (2007) by Maxwell Bennett, Daniel Dennett, Peter Hacker and John Searle, pp. 127–62. Copyright (2007). Reprinted with permission of Columbia University Press.

Introduction

Neuroscience is concerned with understanding the workings of the nervous system, thereby helping in the design of strategies to relieve humanity of the dreadful burden of such diseases as dementia and schizophrenia. Cognitive neuroscientists, fulfilling this task, also illuminate those mechanisms in the brain that must function normally in order for us to be able to exercise our psychological faculties, such as perception and memory. Cellular and molecular neuroscientists study such mechanisms as those involved in the propagation of the action potential in neurons and their axons and investigate how this potential change releases transmitter substances from the axon terminal onto closely apposing neurons at the synapse. (For the development of this subject see Bennett 2001.) Cognitive neuroscientists are especially interested in how networks of synapses operate to fulfil their functions in the brain. Such networks, consisting of thousands to millions of neurons, each possessing up to 10,000 synapses, are found in parts of the brain that must function normally in order for us to be able, for example, to, remember a novel event for more than about one minute (the hippocampus) and to see (the retina and primary visual cortex V1).

For the last two decades, the mechanism of operation of the hippocampus has been a major focus of neuroscientific research. The neuron types to be found in the hippocampus, their spatial distribution and synaptic connections were first described by Ramon y Cajal (1904). A favourite approach to understanding hippocampal functioning is to develop what is taken to be a neural synaptic network representation, reflecting an engineering approach to the problem. Brindley (1967) suggested that some synapses in the hippocampus and therefore in its synaptic network representation should be considered modifiable. What he meant by this term is that the synapses are able permanently to change their properties following the arrival of an action potential in the axon terminal, so that in the hippocampus 'conditioning and memory mechanisms of the nervous system store information by means of modifiable synapses' (p. 361). Later, Marr (1971) suggested that 'the most important characteristic of archicortex (hippocampus) is its ability to perform a simple kind of memorizing task' (p. 23). He went on to show that the pattern of synaptic connections in certain parts of the hippocampus indicated that it could function as an autoassociative memory if the efficacy of the excitatory synapses were modifiable and if the membrane potentials of the large neurons were set by inhibitory interneurons that measure the total activity of the synaptic network. Marr's suggestions, framed in engineering terms, were very influential. For example, in one account of how such neural network representations of the hippocampus work, it was suggested that 'the recall of a memory begins with the firing of a set of pyramidal neurons that overlap with the memory to be recalled' and that 'the firing of different sets of pyramidal neurons then evolves by discrete synchronous steps' until the stored memory pattern of neurons is retrieved (Bennett et al., 1994, p. 167).

The reduction of parts of the brain to engineering devices such as neural networks in the past half century or so has been accompanied by a major movement in the cognitive neurosciences: namely, that of taking the psychological attributes that are normally ascribed to humans (and in some cases to other animals) and attributing them to neural synaptic networks, either before or after they have been reduced to engineering devices of varying degrees of complexity and modifiability. In this book, we examine the claims that particular synaptic networks or clusters of synaptic networks in the brain can see (chapter 1), attend (chapter 2), remember (chapter 3), understand, think and translate thought into speech (chapter 4), and have emotions (chapter 5). Our approach has been to illuminate the historical development of these ideas and how they have been incorporated into the accepted jargon of mainstream cognitive neuroscience by studying the experiments whose interpretation gave rise to them. By conceptual analysis we hope to have shown what is awry with the interpretations of eminent neuroscientists such as J. Z. Young (1978), who suggests that 'We can regard all seeing as a continual search for the answers to questions posed by the brain. The signals from the retina constitute "messages" conveying these answers (p. 119).' Blakemore (1977) contends that the visual cortex in the occipital pole possesses neurons that 'present arguments on which the brain constructs its hypotheses of perception' (p. 91). Zeki (1999, p. 2056) argues that 'the interpretation that the brain gives to the physical property of objects (their reflectance), an interpretation that allows it to acquire knowledge rapidly about the property of reflectance' is required for us to see colours. Gazzaniga and his colleagues (2002) postulate that 'The right hemisphere is capable of understanding language but not syntax' and that 'The capacity of the right hemisphere to make inferences is extremely limited' (p. 414). Critical scrutiny of the idea that synaptic networks in the brain possess psychological attributes is at the heart of the present work.

In our previous co-authored work, *Philosophical Foundations of Neuroscience* (*PFN*), we identified conceptual problems in important current neuroscientific theories concerning, for example, perception, memory and emotion. Contemporary writing on the nature of consciousness by both neuroscientists and philosophers also received critical appraisal. The present work is distinguished from *PFN* in that we here present a study of experiments that have given rise to the various claims over the past century or so concerning the relationship between brain function and our psychological attributes (hence the large number of illustrations). In addition, the present work provides the opportunity for us to respond to philosophical critics of *PFN* such as Paul Churchland, Daniel Dennett and John Searle, especially on the subject of the brain and consciousness (chapter 7).

We hope that the present work, being much closer to the experimental activity of cognitive neuroscientists than was *PFN*, will engage their interest and critical response. In this way a dialogue might be generated amongst the neuroscientists in addition to philosophers concerning what cognitive neuroscience might hope to reveal about brain function in relation to the exercise of our psychological faculties. It is only through an ongoing critical, analytical appraisal of the experimental observations and their interpretation by both philosophers and cognitive neuroscientists that the subject, stripped of hyperbole, will truly prosper.

1

Perceptions, Sensations and Cortical Function: Helmholtz to Singer

1.1 Visual Illusions and their Interpretation by Cognitive Scientists

Helmholtz (fig. 1.1), in his *Treatise on Physiological Optics*, suggested that the formation of a perception involves the development of an unconscious hypothesis based on inductive inferences gained from sensations. For him perceptions are conclusions of unconscious inferences the premises of which are unconscious and (more or less) indescribable sensations and (unconscious) generalizations about the correlation between past sensations and objects perceived. The viewer shown in fig. 1.2 takes the strangely shaped object in the foreground, looked at with one eye, to be a cube because it has all the identifiable features along the line of sight that a cube has. On Helmholtz's hypothesis inductive inferences are made by the person in fig. 1.2 on the basis of the sensations due to the rays of light from the object, and these support the most likely hypothesis: namely, the perception of a cube.

A variety of illusions (e.g. The Ponzo illusion, Kanizsa's illusion, the Ames Room illusion) have been taken as explicable in terms of Helmholtz's theory (Glynn, 1999). That is, these illusions can be explained by reference to the brain's drawing inferences from its past experience to form hypotheses about the objects of its present experience. In the Kanizsa illusion (fig. 1.3a) a ghostly white triangle emerges as a consequence of our inferring that this is the obvious way of interpreting the missing sectors in the three black discs and the edges of the black triangle. In the Ponzo illusion (fig. 1.3b) the upper horizontal bar looks longer than the lower one because the near vertical converging lines are interpreted as railway tracks with parallel lines receding into the distance. Another example of this alleged process of inductive inference is provided by the Adelbert Ames distorting room which produces the experience of extraordinary variations in size of people placed at different positions in the room (fig. 1.4). This room is constructed so that when it is viewed through an eyehole with one eye, an image is produced on the retina identical with that of a rectangular room of uniform height, whereas actually the far wall recedes and both the floor and the ceiling slope, as shown in the small diagram. When people are placed in the far corners of the room, their size is judged in relation to the dimensions of the room on the assumption that this is rectangular. Yet another example which is taken to support Helmholtz's hypothesis

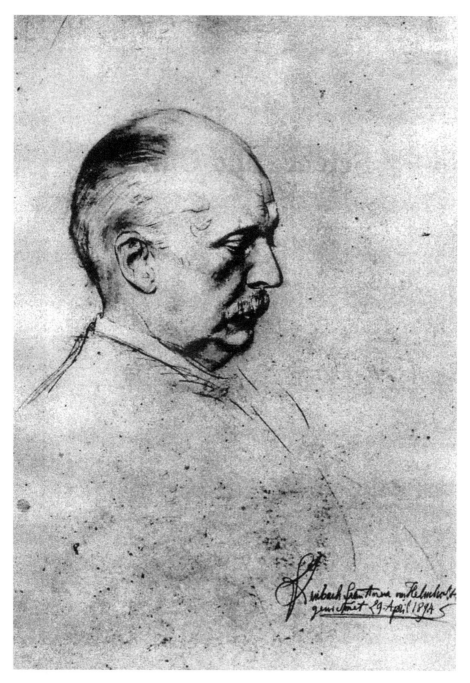

Fig. 1.1. Helmholtz. Sketch by Franz von Lenbach (1894). Courtesy of the Siemens-Forum, Munich.

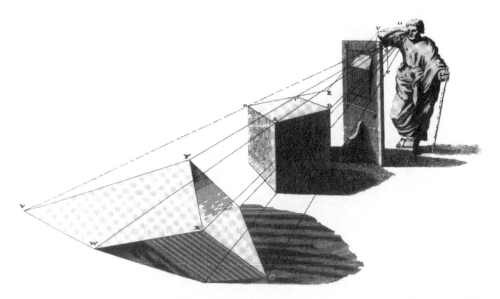

Fig. 1.2.   Drawing to illustrate Helmholtz's argument on how a perception is formed. (Glynn, 1999, p. 197.)

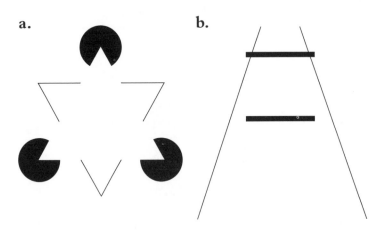

Fig. 1.3.   **a**: the Kanizsa illusion. **b**: the Ponzo illusion. (Glynn, 1999, p. 196.)

is provided by the Ramachandran photograph of fig. 1.5. This shows bumps and hollows that reverse on inversion of the photo. Whether it is interpreted as bumps or hollows is a function of the shading which is ambiguous, depending on the direction of the light. One interpretation of this is that we assume that the light comes from above rather than that the objects face one direction and the different shadings result from different light sources. In the Maurits Escher repeated pattern of fishes and birds (Plate 1.1), the same outline is

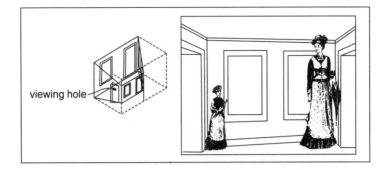

Fig. 1.4.   The Adelbert Ames distorting room. (Glynn, 1999, p. 196.)

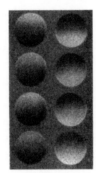

Fig. 1.5.   Ramachandran's bumps and hollows. (Glynn, 1999, p. 196.)

shared by the two different figures. As contours normally only outline an object against its background, Helmholtz's theory holds that the visual system selects either the fishes or the birds for attention, with the other becoming background.

Contemporary neuroscientists support Helmholtz's theory. Thus Glynn comments that 'explanations of this kind do not tell us how the brain manages to make the inferences though they provide a clue to the kind of information processing that may be involved' (Glynn, 1999, p. 195), and Kandel and his colleagues suggest that 'Illusions illustrate that perception is a creative construction based on unconscious conjecture about many of the assumptions the brain makes in interpreting visual data' (Kandel et al., 1991, p. 433). Furthermore, Damasio emphasizes that

When you and I look at an object outside ourselves, we form comparable images in our respective brains. . . . But that does not mean that the image we see is the copy of whatever the object outside is like. Whatever it is like, in absolute terms, we do not know. The image we see is based on changes which occurred in our organisms . . . when the physical structure of the object interacts with the body. . . . The object is real, the interactions are real, and the images are as real as anything can be. And yet, the structure and properties in the image we end up seeing are brain constructions prompted by the object. . . . There is . . . a set of correspondences between physical characteristics of the object and modes of reaction of the organism according to which an internally generated image is constructed. (Damasio, 1999, p. 320)

A phenomenon that is often used to provide what is taken to be a rather dramatic example of the extent to which the cortex makes inferences based on visual sensations to arrive at what we perceive is given by the phenomenon of 'filling in'. Fig. 1.6a presents a black cross and a circle on a white background, which should be viewed about 25 cm away with the left eye closed. Focus on the cross and slowly bring the figure towards your right eye; the circle will eventually disappear from your vision, as the image falls on the part of the retina where the optic nerve begins and there are no photoreceptors present. This is your 'blind spot'. Contemporary neuroscientists, following Helmholtz, suggest that the visual cortex fills in the gap in the blind spot to make it the same as the white background or surroundings. A more dramatic example of this 'filling in' is

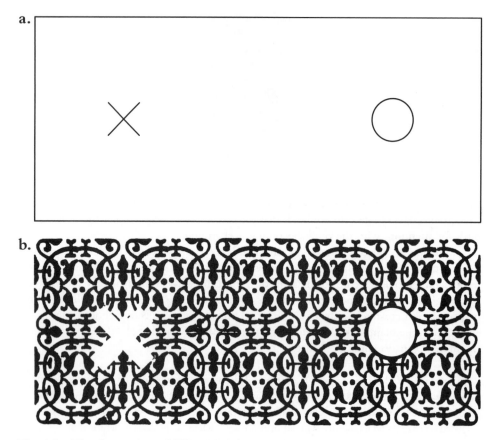

Fig. 1.6.   The phenomenon of 'filling in'. (Glynn, 1999, p. 199.)

given by repeating this kind of experiment but using instead fig. 1.6b, which instead has a white cross and a white disc on a patterned background. This time focus on the white cross and slowly bring the figure towards the right eye with the left eye closed as before. Again the disc disappears, but this time the pattern is continuous across the region previously occupied by the disc. Thus, it would seem, the blind spot does not normally give rise to a black area in one's visual field but is continually 'filled in' by an unconscious inference during normal vision.

1.1.1   Misdescription of visual illusions by cognitive scientists

Helmholtz and his contemporary followers interpret visual illusions in terms of the particular theory of perception, mentioned above: namely, that physical stimuli to the retina are transmitted to the brain, where they become sensations, which are conceived to be the raw material from which perceptions are synthesized by the unconscious mind. However, this theory is incorrect. For there are no visual 'sensations' in the brain, although pressure on the brain may produce a sensation: namely, a headache. There is no such thing as combining sensations to form a perception. Furthermore, perceptions cannot be conclusions of unconscious inferences the premises of which are unconscious and more or less indescribable sensations and (unconscious) generalizations about the correlations between past sensations and objects perceived. So illusions, such as the Ponzo illusion, Kanizsa's illusion, and the Ames room illusions, are not explicable in Helmholtz's terms.

   To perceive something is not to form a hypothesis. A hypothesis is an unconfirmed proposition or principle put forward as a provisional basis for reasoning or argument, a supposition or conjecture advanced to account for relevant facts. Only human beings, not their brains, can form hypotheses and make inferences. There is no such thing as a brain's putting forward a proposition as a basis for reasoning or argument or acting on a supposition. Hypotheses are formed on the basis of data which consist of information that is thought to provide evidential support for the hypothesis. However, the brain does not, and could not have, information in this sense. Only thinking creatures *with brains* can form hypotheses or conjectures on the basis of the information available to them.

   A perception – i.e. a person's perceiving something – is not a hypothesis, but an event or occurrence, and so cannot be the conclusion of an inference, which is a proposition, not an event or occurrence. Finally, inferences are neither conscious nor unconscious mental processes. For inferences are not processes at all. Rather, inferences are transformations of propositions in accordance with a rule, derivations of propositions from premises in conformity with a pattern of derivation. But perceiving something does not involve transformations of propositions by a perceiver (or his brain).

   Locke, and the British empiricist tradition that he originated, conceived of ideas and impressions as the result of the impact of the material world on our nerve endings. This misconception is the source of the thought that perceiving always involves sensations which are, on Helmholtzian theory, the premises of unconscious inferences. For Helmholtzian 'sensations' are, in effect, empiricist 'ideas' or 'impressions'. It is also the source of the equally misguided and far more widespread thought that what is seen (or heard, etc.) when we see (or hear, etc.) something is a picture or image (visual or auditory). This representationalist view is defended by Damasio above, but is confused. For what one perceives by the use of one's perceptual organs is an object or array of objects, sounds and smells, and the properties and relations of items in one's environment. It is a mistake to suppose that what we perceive is always, or even commonly, an image, or that to perceive an object is to have an image of the object perceived. One does not *perceive* images or representations of objects unless one perceives paintings or photographs of objects. (Of course, one may *have* after-images or conjure up mental images, but one does not *perceive* them.)

1.2   Gestalt Laws of Vision

After the First World War, Max Wertheimer (1924), Kurt Koffka (1935) and Wolfgang Köhler (1929), following Helmholtz, determined to find the laws that relate what we perceive to what we are actually looking at. In particular, they were concerned with how the overall configuration of a scene, rather than particular elements in it, informed the interpretation of the scene. The way in which the *Gestalt* or configuration of the scene provides us with an interpretation is dramatically illustrated by means of Edgar Rubin's vase or two faces (fig. 1.7a), depending on what is assumed to be background or figure, or by Jastrow's duck–rabbit (fig. 1.7b). The laws formulated by the Gestalt psychologists are illustrated by means of fig. 1.8. The 'law of proximity' is shown by the fact that the circles in fig. 1.8a are seen as arranged in horizontal or vertical lines rather than oblique lines, because they are further apart in the oblique lines. The 'law of similarity' is illustrated by fig. 1.8b, in which the dots are now seen as horizontal lines because those forming horizontal lines are more similar than those forming vertical lines. An example of the 'law of good continuation', which states that we perceive the organization that interrupts the fewest lines, is shown in fig. 1.8c, in which the small dots are seen to form a wavy line superimposed on a profile of battlements rather than as the succession of shapes shown at the bottom of the figure. Cognitive scientists believe that Gestalt psychology has shifted the fundamental empiricist's question 'What are the basic components of this

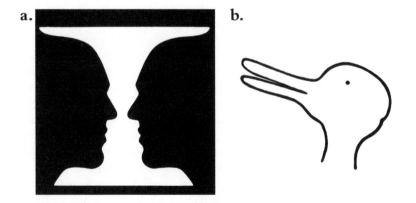

Fig. 1.7.   **a**: Edgar Rubin's vase or two faces. **b**: Jastrow's duck–rabbit. (Glynn, 1999, p. 199.)

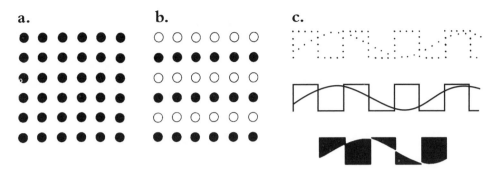

Fig. 1.8. Illustrations of the Gestalt 'Laws' of (**a**) 'proximity'; (**b**) 'similarity'; (**c**) 'good continuation'. (Glynn, 1999, p. 200.)

perception?' to 'What neural transformation produces this perception?', thus offering a common scheme for merging psychological and neurobiological investigations into the process of vision.

1.3   Split-Brain Commissurotomy; the Two Hemispheres may Operate Independently

Patients with intractable epilepsy often undergo surgery to relieve the condition. This involves cutting the corpus callosum that connects the two halves of the brain. In the early 1960s Michael Gazzaniga and Roger Sperry showed that the two hemispheres of such patients possess their own specializations, with the left hemisphere dominant for language and speech and the right being largely causally responsible for visual motor tasks (Gazzaniga and Sperry, 1967). If a visible object (or picture of an object) occurs in the right visual field (so that concomitant neuronal activity occurs only in the left hemisphere) of such split-brain patients, then they can describe what they see; but if the visible object occurs in the left visual field (with concomitant neuronal activity restricted to the right hemisphere), they cannot. In this case, the patients could point at a similar object to that presented in their left visual field if asked to, but they were not able to say what it was (Gazzaniga et al., 1965).

Similar results were found for the other sensory modalities of touch, sound and smell. In addition, the right hemisphere was shown to be causally responsible for the processes involved in controlling the left hand, whereas the left hemisphere was causally implicated in the control of the right hand. Gazzaniga and Sperry concluded that each hemisphere in humans is causally implicated in different aspects of thought and action. Fig. 1.9a shows the kind of experimental set-up used by Gazzaniga and Sperry to collect data in early split-brain studies (see Gazzaniga, 1995; Baynes and Gazzaniga, 2000). Presenting a written name for an object to the left visual field (involving the right hemisphere) of a

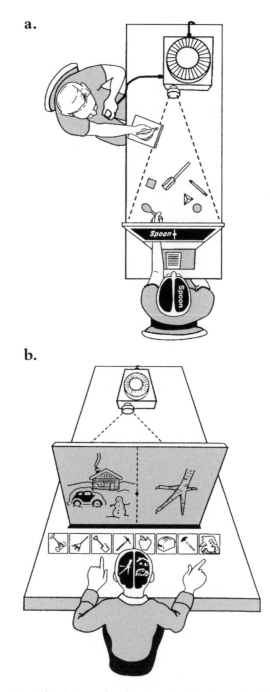

Fig. 1.9. **a**, **b**: experimental techniques for observing the behaviour of split-brain patients. (Baynes and Gazzaniga, 2000, p. 126.)

patient provides the condition for the patient to use his left hand to select the correct object by touch (in this case 'spoon'; Gazzaniga, 1983). In fig. 1.9b, when presented with *bilateral* picture displays, the patient confabulates about the choices he previously made with his left hand. As Gazzaniga describes the experiments, the right hand selects a rooster to match the claw seen when the left hemisphere is involved, but the patient states that the shovel selected by the left hand was needed to clean out the chicken house. According to Gazzaniga and Le Doux (1978), 'the left hemisphere Interpreter has no knowledge of the snow scene seen by the right hemisphere' in this test. These and other experiments led Gazzaniga (1997, p. 1392) to suggest that 'mind left dealt with the world differently than mind right seemed to be the major conclusion of studies during the era'.

Sidtis (1981) suggested that axons of the corpus callosum which carry information relating to the sensory dimensions of a stimulus are located in a different part of the callosum to those that carry semantic information. His experiment is illustrated in fig. 1.10. The patient underwent a staged callosal section in which the posterior half of the callosum alone was sectioned. This was taken by Siditis to show that the sectioning prevented the transfer of information relating to the sensory but not the semantic dimensions of the stimulus.

1.3.1   Misdescription of the results of commissurotomy

According to the above interpretation of the results of commissurotomy by Gazzaniga and Le Doux, the hemispheres of the brain may possess knowledge and can perceive. However, only human beings can know and perceive, not their brains – which can neither see nor hear, neither write nor speak, nor interpret anything or make inferences from information. The hemispheres of the brain cannot be said to be aware or unaware of anything; they cannot intelligibly be said to recognize or misrecognize anything. They do not make choices or judgements of grammaticality, and they are neither knowledgeable nor ignorant.

The additional claim that the forms of functional dissociation consequent upon commissurotomy produce two minds, one belonging to the left hemisphere, the other to the right, is also awry. The brain does not have a mind, and neither do the two hemispheres of the brain. It is human beings, not their brains, that are said to have minds. To ascribe a mind to a creature is to say that it is a creature with a distinctive range of capacities: in particular, capacities for concept-exercising thought, self-consciousness, memory and will.

1.3.2   Explaining the discoveries derived from commissurotomies

The general form of the explanation for the observations of Gazzaniga and his colleagues on the dissociation of functions following commissurotomy is that severing the corpus callosum deprives human beings of their capacity to exercise normally co-ordinated functions. And that in turn is to be explained in terms of the disconnection of neural groups that are causally implicated in the exercise of the relevant capacities. The transmission of

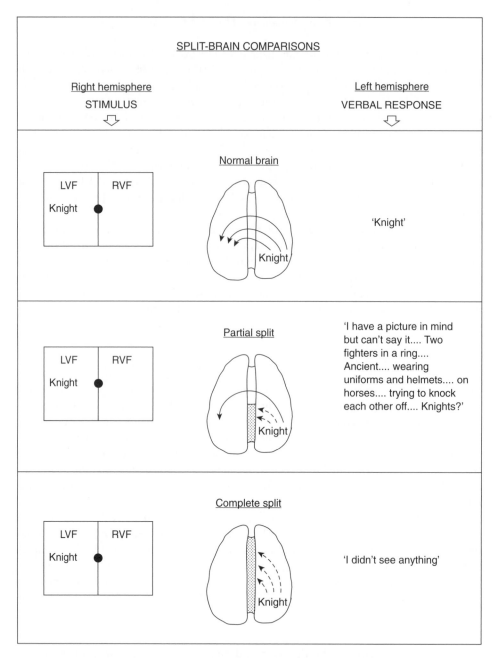

Fig. 1.10. Evidence that axons have different functions in different parts of the corpus callosum. (Gazzaniga, 1995, p. 222.)

neural signals across the corpus callosum is a necessary condition of a person knowing, and being able to say, what is visually presented to him (under the experimental conditions in question). It is this which is prevented by commissurotomy. Nevertheless, the patient is still able to respond to what is visually presented to him by making choices with his hands, even though he does not know why he thus points, and confabulates a tale to explain it.

1.4   Specificity of Cortical Neurons

David Hubel and Torsten Wiesel as well as Vernon Mountcastle discovered that the cortex contains neurons which are excited by very specific stimuli. These discoveries were founded on the notion of the receptive field of sensory neurons, such as the ganglion neurons in the retina which connect it to the brain. In this case 'the receptive field' refers to that region of the photoreceptor sheet which, when stimulated by a spot of light, changes the frequency of impulse firing in the ganglion neuron being studied. The receptive fields of retinal ganglion neurons consist of two concentric circles; when a spot of light shines on the inner circle, impulse firing in the neuron is increased for some ganglion neurons but decreased for others; if a spot of light shines in the surrounding region outside this, then a reciprocal change in firing is found to that in the centre of the field. There are, therefore, ganglion neurons with a central excitatory region and surround inhibitory region, and others with a central inhibitory region with surround excitation. Hubel and Wiesel, in the late 1950s and early 1960s, examined the receptive fields of neurons in the first relay-station between the retina and the cortex in cats: namely, the lateral geniculate nucleus, and found that they were similar to those of retinal ganglion neurons. Next they examined the receptive fields of neurons in a region of the cortex in cats and monkeys to which the principal neurons in the lateral geniculate nucleus project, called the primary visual cortex or area 17 (Hubel and Wiesel, 1959, 1962, 1968). The referring expression 'area 17' is a designation that dates back to the work of Brodmann (1909), who divided the cortex up into a number of distinctive areas based on differences in the arrangement and types of neurons as well as in the pattern of the myelinated fibers. Such a 'cytoarchitectural' map of the human cortex is shown in fig. 1.11 for both its convex surface (a) and its medial surface (b). There is evidence for a 'modular' organization of brain function that is more fine-grained than that suggested by the cytoarchitectural maps of Brodmann. In the case of the visual system many of these modules have been given 'V' numbers, such as V1 (which encompasses area 17) as well as V2, V3 and V4 (each of which encompass part of area 18). It is therefore more appropriate to adopt this nomenclature when referring to pathways in the visual cortex (see Plate 1.4b and c).

The receptive fields discovered by Hubel and Wiesel in V1 were often much more complex than those of retinal ganglion neurons. Some neurons could be stimulated by lines, bars, squares and rectangles of light, rather than by the spots of light used to characterize the receptive fields of retinal ganglion neurons and neurons in the lateral geniculate nucleus. Fig. 1.12 shows recordings from the receptive field of a neuron in the visual cortex made by Hubel and Wiesel in 1968; the field is indicated by the broken rectangles in the left

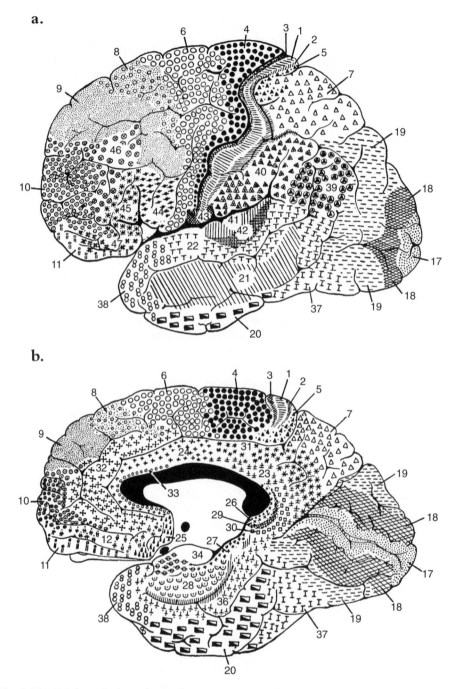

Fig. 1.11. Brodmann's chart of cortical areas: **a**, convex surface; **b**, medial surface. (After Brodmann, 1909; from Carpenter, 1976.)

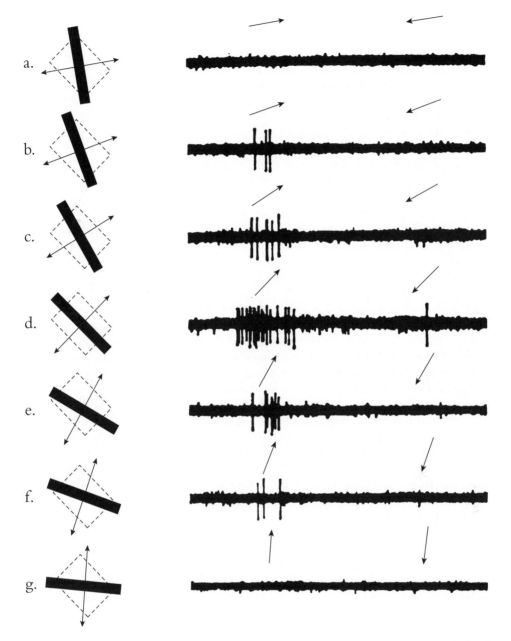

Fig. 1.12. Neuronal orientation selectivity in primary visual cortex (area 17 or V1). (Hubel and Wiesel, 1968, p. 219.)

column. In this case, the visual stimulus that was viewed by the monkey consisted of a bar of light that was moved back and forth through the receptive field of the cell in each of seven different orientations, indicated in rows a to g. The different directions of motion used for each orientation are indicated by the small arrows. Recorded traces of neuronal activity are shown at the right, in which the horizontal axis represents time, and each vertical line represents an action potential. This neuron responded most strongly to a bar of light oriented along the diagonal (stimulus d), particularly when the bar was moved through the receptive field from lower left to upper right. Neurons of this type were found by Hubel and Wiesel to be common in the visual cortex, and Hubel commented that

> The *map* of the receptive field of a cell is a powerful and convenient shorthand description of the cell's behaviour, and thus of its output. Understanding it can help us to understand why the cells in the intermediate stages are wired up as they are, and will help explain the purpose of the direct and indirect paths. If we know what ganglion cells are telling the brain, we will have gone far toward understanding the entire retina. (Hubel, 1988, p. 39)

The research of Hubel and Wiesel culminated in the discovery that neurons in the primary visual cortex with particular receptive field properties are organized in narrow 100–200 mm–wide vertical columns passing from the surface of the cortex to the white matter (Hubel and Wiesel, 1977). Such a columnar organization had previously been discovered for neurons with particular receptive field properties in the somatosensory cortex by Vernon Mountcastle (1957). In the case of the visual cortex there is also an arrangement by which the input from each eye is segregated into columns. Fig. 1.13 shows a beautiful anatomical representation of these ocular dominance columns. In order to display such columns, the right eye of a monkey was injected with radio-labelled proline and fucose, which is transported transneuronally to the cortex. Fig. 1.13a shows a dark field autoradiograph of a tangential section of area V1 of the right hemisphere obtained after 10 days' exposure. Radioactivity can be seen in the form of white stripes, which correspond to thalamic axon terminals in layer 4 of the cortex that relay input from the injected eye. The alternating dark stripes depict the position of the afferents from the geniculate axons subserving the uninjected eye (Hubel et al., 1977). Fig. 1.13b shows a reconstruction of the ocular dominance columns in area V1 of the right hemisphere, showing the regular layout of the columns. These discoveries for both the visual cortex and the somatosensory cortex were then taken to indicate that sensory cortex in general is organized along columnar lines in which neurons with similar receptive field properties are found in a particular column.

1.4.1   Cardinal cells

Hubel and Wiesel suggested that the complex properties of neurons in the primary visual cortex (i.e. area V1, see Plate 1.4b) could be thought of as arising from combinations of the 'simple' centre–surround receptive fields possessed by retinal ganglion neurons and neurons in the lateral geniculate nucleus. This idea indicated that there might be a hierarchical increase in complexity of neuronal receptive fields for neurons at progressively higher levels of the cortex – that is, at levels progressively further removed from the retinal input.

a. Normal

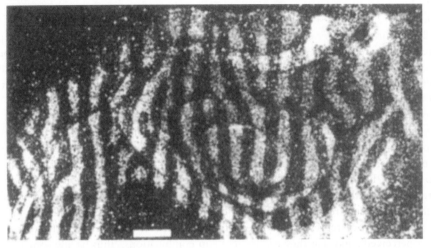

b. Reconstruction: normal ocular dominance columns

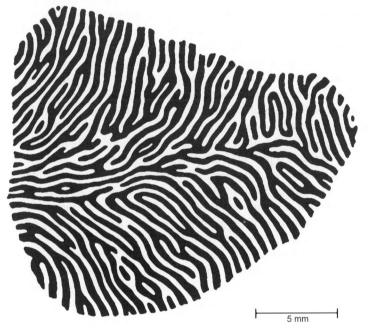

5 mm

Fig. 1.13. Anatomical representation of ocular dominance columns in primate visual cortex. (**a:** Hubel et al., 1975, p. 584; **b:** Hubel and Wiesel, 1977, p. 35, reproduced from LeVay, Hubel and Wiesel, 1980, reprinted with permission of Wiley–Liss, Inc., a subsidiary of John Wiley & Sons, Inc.)

Barlow (1972) gave these neurons with very complex receptive field properties the title 'cardinal neurons'. Such neurons might, for example, fire maximally when faces were presented in their receptive field, which could be quite large – that is, a large proportion of the entire visual field. The main function of cardinal neurons was not to respond to some specific characteristic of the retinal illumination (as in the primary visual cortex) but 'to continue responding invariantly to the same external pattern' (in this case to faces). The neuron doctrine in perception fostered the belief that the pathways that are active for a given sensory scene converge and produce activity in a single cell (named 'a cardinal cell' or sometimes 'a grandmother cell') or a group of cells (cardinal cells) 'whose role is to represent the scene'. This idea was motivated, at least in part, by the thought that if the animal is to see, the brain must combine the information derived from the retina to produce a representation of the visual scene. Horace Barlow suggested in 1972 that the hypothesized cardinal cells 'do not represent arbitrary or capricious features in the environment, but features useful for their representative role' – that is, 'their role as correlates of features of the object perceived', and that they can be active in combinations, 'thus having something of the descriptive power of words' (Barlow, 1997, pp. 421–2).

Gross and his colleagues (1969) discovered neurons in the inferior temporal cortex of monkeys (IT, see Plate 1.4b) which possessed just the properties which Barlow had predicted for a class of cardinal neurons. In the monkey's temporal lobe there are neurons that fire impulses at maximal rates when a monkey is viewing a specific object. Some of these neurons respond specifically to the presentation of faces; indeed, these neurons discharge specifically, depending on whether the faces are presented in profile or face on. Fig. 1.14 shows the relationship between a series of images presented and the rate of firing of a temporal lobe neuron. When the monkey is looking directly at the image of another monkey face on, there is maximal firing; but when the image of the head gradually turns around so that it appears only in profile, then the firing occurs at a much lower level. And although somewhat 'monkey like', if the picture of a toilet brush is presented, then the rate of firing of the neurons is much less than when the image of another monkey face is presented. In addition, if an image is presented consisting of the juxtaposition of different elements of the face in a bizarre geometry, again the firing rate is not nearly as high as it is when those elements are put together to make up a proper monkey face. Furthermore, it can be shown that if different elements of the monkey's face such as the mouth or the eyes are taken away, then the firing rate will drop. Finally, the pattern corresponding to the presentation of a monkey's face is different from that resulting from presentation of a human face. The work of Gross and his colleagues has therefore shown that that there are neurons in the temporal lobe that are of the 'cardinal' type as postulated by Barlow, inasmuch as they fire impulses vigorously only when a particular kind of object – in the case illustrated in fig. 1.14 a particular kind of face – is presented.

1.4.2   Misdescription of experiments leading to the conception of cardinal cells

The claim made by Barlow that cardinal neurons have a representative role and 'thus have something of the descriptive power of words' cannot be sustained. For the sense in which

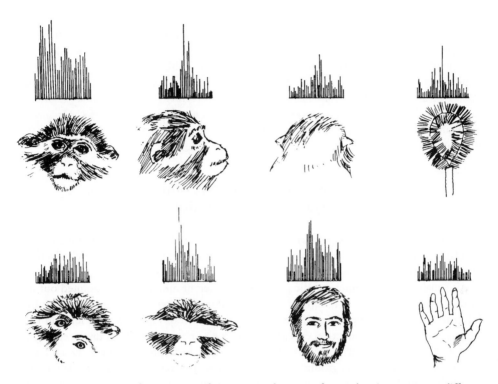

Fig. 1.14. Firing rate of neurons in inferior temporal cortex of a monkey in response to different images of a monkey face, brush, human face and a hand. (Bennett, 1997, fig. 1.5.)

the excitation of a group of cells represents a certain feature in the visual field is the sense in which a wide ring in a tree trunk represents a year with ample rainfall. That has nothing whatsoever to do with the lexical or semantic sense in which a sentence represents the state of affairs it describes, or with the iconic sense in which a picture represents what it depicts. Furthermore, neither in the iconic nor in the lexical sense could there be any representations of the external world in the brain. Representations, in the lexical sense, presuppose a rule-governed system of symbols and a practice of their employment in the lives of language-using, symbol-employing creatures. It is not intelligible to suppose that the brain has or uses *a language*, any more than it is intelligible that the brain should *draw pictures* and look at them or *make maps* and consult them. And even if we were to suppose that there is nevertheless some as yet unexplained sense in which the brain can be said to contain *maps* (as is commonly argued today) or *pictures* (on the pineal gland, as Descartes supposed), this will contribute nothing to an explanation of how animal vision occurs or is rendered possible. For one cannot explain what the neural processes of seeing items in the visual field consist in by referring us to the brain's *seeing* a picture or map of the objects in the visual field. For, first, we do not know what it would be for the brain to *see* anything (after all, it has no eyes!). Secondly, even if we could give sense to the brain's seeing things, how would the process of human sight have been explained? To claim that for a human being to see something, his brain must see a representation of the same thing explains the puzzling by reference to the unintelligible. What human beings (and other animals) see are, among other things, objects in their environment. How could representations in the brain, which they cannot see or read, help them to see what is in their environment? Certainly not by means of anything *symbolically* or *iconically* represented. For in whatever legitimate sense (if any) there is to the supposition that there is a representation of what is seen in the brain, that representation is neither what the owner of the brain sees nor anything that is communicated to him.

1.5   Multiple Pathways Connecting Visual Cortical Modules

The conception of the visual pathway construed in terms of different modules was advanced by David Marr in the 1970s as part of what he called the 'computational view' of sensory processing (Marr, 1982). According to this theory, the process of sensory perception can best be analysed by assigning specific processes to different modules. Marr pointed out that evidence for such modules is apparent in the random-dot stereograms produced by Bela Julesz in 1960. An example of such a stereogram is shown in Fig. 1.15. The left and right images in this figure are identical except for a central square region that is displaced slightly in one image. When fused binocularly, the images yield the impression of the central square floating in front of the background. Marr held that such percepts are caused solely by the stereo disparity between matching elements in the images presented to each eye, so that the analysis of stereoscopic information can proceed independently in the absence of other information. Marr put forward the idea that the study of perception can be subdivided into

Fig. 1.15.   Random-dot stereogram. (Marr, 1982, fig. 1.1.)

specialized parts, each of which can be treated separately. Such parts are 'independent modules of perception' (1982, p. 10).

Damasio and others have presented evidence that the human visual cortex possesses specialized modules like those found in other primates. Lesions in one or more of these modules due to disease or injury lead to the expected behavioural deficits corresponding to the visual experience of the patient. For instance, damage to the occipital and subcalcarine portions of the left and right lingual gyri (containing areas V2 and V4) gives rise to the condition of achromatopsia, i.e. loss of colour vision, so that such patients see the world only in shades of grey (Rizzo et al., 1993). Damasio and colleagues (1979, 1983) have also reported that patients with lesions in the temporal segment of the left lingual gyrus are afflicted with a condition called 'colour anomia'. In this case, they experience colours in the normal way, and are able to rank hues of different saturation, but they use colour names incorrectly. So, for example, they use the word 'blue' or 'red' when shown green or yellow; and, given a colour name, they will point to the wrong colour. Patients with lesions in the left posterior temporal and inferior parietal cortex lose the ability to produce appropriate word morphology. For example, they produce distorted colour names like 'buh' for 'blue'.

Following the discoveries of Hubel and Wiesel in the 1960s, Semir Zeki and others in the 1970s examined the receptive field properties of single neurons outside the primary visual cortex involving higher centres concerned with visual perception in primates. They showed that the properties of these receptive fields were very complex. Using the properties of these fields as the criterion, the visual cortex outside the primary area was shown to be compartmentalized into different regions or modules. Zeki's research has also been taken as supporting this idea of modules, particularly in showing that one area of visual cortex, designated the middle temporal area (MT or area V5; see Plate 1.4b and c) in primates, possesses neurons that are responsive to motion and to the particular direction of movement of an object. A spectacular example of the functioning of the middle temporal area in humans is shown in the phenomenon called the 'waterfall effect'. This name derives from the fact that if a subject looks for some time at water streaming downward in a waterfall and then turns away and looks, for example, at the opposite bank of the river, then the trees on the bank will appear to be momentarily moving in the opposite direction to the flow of the water in the waterfall. Thus the stationary objects (the trees) appear to move. The time course of this illusion can be described quantitatively using psychophysical experiments in conjunction with brain imaging. These show that the middle temporal area is involved (Tootell et al., 1995). Plate 1.2a shows a visual stimulus that consists of a series of concentric rings, either expanding or stationary. Plate 1.2b indicates that the middle temporal area is excited by the moving rings as determined by the non-invasive visual imaging technique, functional magnetic resonance imaging (fMRI; note that the brain is shown in normal and inflated format). The same increase in activity in the middle temporal area is observed when stationary concentric rings are viewed immediately after observing the rings expanding, but not when observing just stationary rings without prior exposure to moving rings, or after prior exposure to rings moving in one direction and then moving in the opposite direction. It is known that the subject experiences an after-effect of apparent visible motion in the first case but not in the latter two cases; that is, the stationary rings appear to move in the

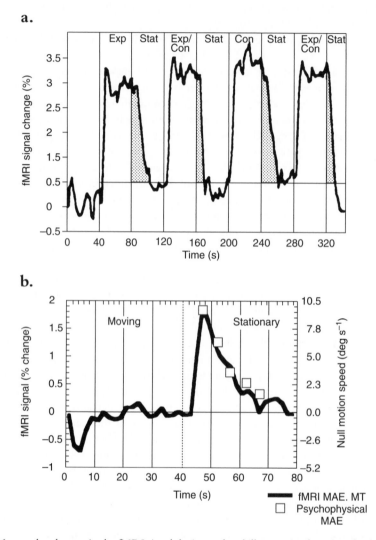

Fig. 1.16. **a:** the changes in the fMRI signal during real and illusory visual motion. **b:** the quantitative relationship between the visual after-effect and activity in the middle temporal area as measured by magnetic resonance imaging. (Tootell et al., 1995)

opposite direction to that used in the conditioning period (the period of contracting and expanding stimuli) for some time thereafter.

Fig. 1.16a depicts the changes in the magnetic resonance imaging signal during real and illusory visual motion. The strength of the signal in the middle temporal area is shown for the case of the moving concentric rings either continuously expanding (Exp), continuously contracting (Con), reversing direction (expanding then contracting, Exp/Con) or stationary

(Stat). Following the periods of continuous unidirectional local motion (the expanding or contracting stimuli), a visual motion after-effect is seen by the subject in the physically stationary rings. Following the period of reversing the direction, no motion after-effect was reported by the subject. The magnetic resonance imaging response during the period of expansion of the rings, contraction of the rings, or reverse direction expansion/contraction is about the same (between 3.0 and 3.5 per cent). The important point to notice is that the magnetic resonance imaging response immediately after the single-direction stimulus (i.e. when the motion after-effect was being experienced) remained high for a considerable period of about 20 seconds after the stimulus offset, much longer than that of the case when there is no after-effect, such as the case of reverse expansion/contraction in the stimulus, for which the magnetic resonance imaging signal returns to the no stimulus baseline in about 5 seconds. Thus the middle temporal area remains active during the period when there is no stimulus but the subject experiences the visual after-effect.

Fig. 1.16b shows the quantitative relationship between the visual after-effect and activity in the middle temporal area as measured by magnetic resonance imaging (compare with fig. 1.16a). The line gives the magnetic resonance imaging amplitudes during and after single-direction expansion of the concentric rings minus the amplitudes during and after reversing-direction conditions. During the first 40 seconds there was no difference between the activation produced by a single-direction versus reverse-direction stimulus (see fig. 1.16a). During the next 40 seconds, the magnetic resonance imaging results show that as the subjects observed stationary stimuli, the magnetic resonance imaging was elevated for about 20 seconds following the single-direction stimulus. These results may be compared with the psychophysical data indicated by the open squares. These measured the period as reported by the subject of the time course of the visual illusion which was experienced while observing the stationary rings in a related series of psychophysical experiments. There was very good agreement between the time course of the decline in the visual illusion given by the open squares and that of the activity in the middle temporal area as indicated by the magnetic resonance imaging. The results show that illusions are accompanied by neural activity in the brain, and in the case of the waterfall effect this is to be located in the middle temporal area.

Another area, designated V4 in the primate cortex, possesses neurons that are excited by particular wavelengths of light as well as, on occasion, responding to the orientation of lines. This indicates that they are concerned with colour and form. Still other adjacent areas, designated V3 and V3a, have been shown to be selective for form alone (Zeki, 1993). All this work led Zeki to speculate that the visual cortex of primates possesses modules: namely, separate areas that are functionally specialized for various properties of objects in the visual world such as motion, form and colour. Zeki (1999) expresses this modularity of the visual pathway in vivid terms, contrasting the modular system concerned with colour with that concerned with faces: 'Assuming that, through the operation of its logic, the brain makes an inference about certain physical properties of surfaces, interpreted as colour, it seems difficult not to believe that it uses the same inferential method to deduce, for example, the expression on a face or the appearance of an object' (p. 2058).

More than thirty of these modules have now being identified by Van Essen and his colleagues (Felleman and Van Essen, 1991). Plate 1.3a shows many different cortical areas on the right-hand side of the macaque's brain, with those colour-coded indicating the position of different cortical modules devoted to vision. The two smaller figures on the smaller scale on the left show the view of the right-hand side of the brain viewed from the outside (the upper one) and from the inside as if the brain were cut in half (the lower one). The folded macaque cortex has been unfolded using sections of the brain, so that the spatial relationships between the different cortical modules can be appreciated. The different names of these modules have in most cases been abbreviated to initials. The interconnections of these modules are shown in Plate 1.3b, with each line representing many axons (from a few hundred thousand to millions) passing in both directions (see also Plate 1.4c). The retinal ganglion cells at the bottom of the figure project to the lateral geniculate nucleus (LGN) in the thalamus, which in turn then projects to the first visual area in the cortex, V2 (which has four parts). At the very top, HC is for hippocampus, and ER for entorhinal cortex. Note that at the highest levels, module 46 receives a very large number of inputs. These can best be appreciated by reference to Plate 1.5, which shows the topological organization of the macaque cortical visual system. Reciprocal connections are coloured red; one-way projections going from left to right are coloured blue; and one-way projections going from right to left are green. A total of 301 connections is represented, of which 62 are one-way. This non-arbitrary structure is a best-fit representation in two dimensions of the connectional topology of this system, in which the positions of areas are specified by their positions, being ones that minimize the distance between connected areas and maximize the distance between areas that are not connected. The analysis represents in a spatial framework the organizational structure of the network of cortico-cortical connections between modules of the visual cortex.

1.6   Mental Images and Representations

Helmholtz's conception of perception as a matter of unconscious hypothesis formation was further developed in the late twentieth-century computational theory of visual perception. In its most sophisticated form, this conception was elaborated by David Marr, who 'adopted a point of view that regards visual perception as a problem in information processing' (Marr, 1980, p. 203). The informational input is conceived to be the light array (which he referred to as an 'image') falling upon the retina, and the output is held to be the construction of efficient and useful symbolic descriptions of objects in view. According to Marr, 'vision is the *process* of discovering from images what is present in the world and where it is' (Marr, 1980, p. 3). It is the process of transforming the information implicit in an image into an explicit description of what is seen. Marr conceived of the brain as operating a system of symbols that represent features of an image in order to construct descriptions. By a series of computational operations on the symbolism, the brain can, in the final stage of the visual process, produce a description of shapes of objects, their distance, orientation and identity. Marr suggested that 'if we are capable of knowing what is where in the world, our brains must somehow be capable of representing this information' (Marr, 1980, p. 3).

Marr suggested that a strong argument in favour of this representational process is provided by the experiments of Shepard and Metzler (1971), illustrated in fig. 1.17. This shows

a.   **b.**   **c.**

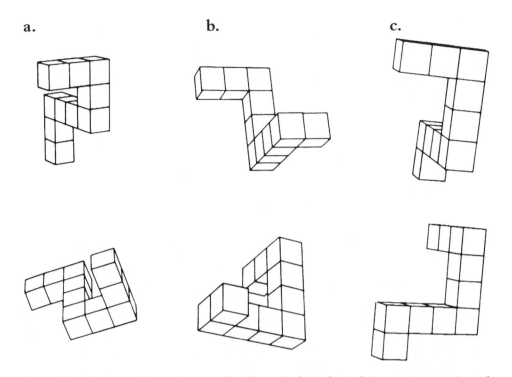

Fig. 1.17.   Drawings similar to those used by Shepard and Metzler in their experiments on 'mental rotation'. (Marr, 1982, fig. 1.2.)

line drawings of simple objects that differ from one another either by a three-dimensional rotation or by a rotation plus a reflection. Those in (a) are identical as a clockwise rotation of the page by 80° shows; those in (b) are also identical, and again the relative angle between the two is 80°, but a rotation in depth is required to make the first coincide with the second; those in (c) are not identical, as no rotation brings them into congruence. Shepard and Metzler showed that the time taken to decide whether a pair are congruent varied linearly with the angle through which one figure had to be rotated in order to be brought into correspondence with the other. This led them to the idea that mental representations of the shapes of the pair existed, that one of them is being rotated at constant volocity relative to the other in mental space until they match. Marr (1982) considered this kind of experiment to offer good evidence for the existence of mental representations involved in the normal recognition of objects in the visual field.

In the late 1970s Anne Treisman and her colleagues performed psychological experiments in order to develop models of feature perception and integration in a visual search task that could be tested by neurobiologists. Treisman and Gelade (1980) established that the search time for a unique item is faster when all items differ by one attribute than if all items differ by two or more attributes. If a subject is instructed to identify whether an item is present or not in an image such as that in Plate 1.6a, the unique stimulus 'pops out', and subjects take about the same time to find the stimulus regardless of how many items are present in the display, as shown in the graph of Plate 1.6c. Treisman took this to be consistent with a pre-attentive process in the display in which all attributes are scanned for the particular feature at once. If, however, the unique item differs by two attributes, as in Plate 1.6b, then it does not pop out. In this case of a conjunctive search, the more items present, the longer the search takes, as shown in the graph of Plate 1.6c. Treisman regarded this as being consistent with a serial search and successive shifts of attention (see Treisman et al., 1977).

In order to account for the differences in feature and conjunction searches Treisman (1986) suggested a hypothetical model of feature perception and integration, shown in Plate 1.7, taken to indicate how different types of visual information are processed separately and then combined into a coherent image. The elementary properties of objects in the visual field (such as colour, orientation, size and distance) are taken to be processed in separate parallel pathways, each of which generates a map that is tuned to a specific feature. Thus object perception is thought to begin with the parallel analysis of its component features, which does not involve attentional mechanisms. Stimuli automatically activate cells tuned to their features on these maps, which are representational structures that indicate the presence or absence of features. In the colour search of Plate 1.6a the subject would simply have to determine whether the feature blue was active in the colour maps. Conjunction searches, as in Plate 1.6b, are much more complicated, involving in this case the checking of activation on two different maps and their association with a particular location. Cognitive psychologists now take it that targets that give flat search functions, like that in Plate 1.6c, are dealing with visual primitives which are taken as the basic building blocks of perception, and are found by neurobiologists in the early parts of the visual pathway. As to the later parts of the visual pathway, as Crick comments:

> We can see how the visual parts of the brain take the picture (the visual field) apart, but we do not yet know how the brain puts it all together to provide our highly organized view of the world – that is, what we see. It seems as if the brain needs to impose some global unity on certain activities in its different parts so that the attributes of a single object – its shape, color, movement, location, and so on – are in some way brought together without at the same time confusing them with the attributes of other objects in the visual field. (Crick, 1994, p. 22)

1.6.1 Misconceptions about images and representations

Marr's suggestion that there can be symbolic descriptions of objects in view in the brain does not make sense. A description is a form of words or symbols, a sentence expressing a proposition that specifies an array of features of an object, event or state of affairs. It can be true or false, accurate or inaccurate, detailed or rough-and-ready. A symbolic description may be written down or spoken; it may be encoded for concealment or for transmission. But there is no such thing as a description in the brain. For something to be a (semantic) symbol, it must have a rule-governed use. There must be a correct and an incorrect way of using it. It must have a grammar determining its intelligible combinatorial possibilities with other symbols, which is elucidated by explanations of meaning that are used and accepted among a community of speakers. There can be no symbols in the brain; the brain cannot use symbols and cannot mean anything by a symbol. A symbol is used only if the user means something by it – but brains cannot mean anything. To mean something by a symbol is roughly to intend the symbol to signify such-and-such a thing – but brains can have no intentions.

Marr's idea that the output of the computational process is the production of a description of visible objects that is embodied in an internal representation which is made available as a basis for decisions is confused. The 'output' of the neuro-visual process, in so far as it can be said to have an 'output', is that the creature sees. But to see something is no more to construct or produce a description than it is to construct Helmholtzian hypotheses.

Shepard and Metzler's rotation experiments have also been misinterpreted. The fact that the time taken in all of these experiments is proportional to the angle of rotation of the figures visualized does not suggest that it takes longer to perform a greater rotation at constant velocity 'in mental space' than to perform a lesser rotation, since there is no such thing as rotating a mental image at constant (or variable) velocity – only such a thing as imagining an object rotating at constant (or variable) velocity. One can imagine a rotating object. But to imagine an object moving quickly does not mean that anything moved quickly in the imagination. The idea that it must take longer to imagine rotating a figure by 90° than to imagine rotating it by 45° is as misconceived as the thought that it must take longer to paint a slow-moving figure than it takes to paint a fast-moving one. There is no obvious reason why it should take longer to imagine a figure rotating through 90° than to imagine it rotating by 45° – for one is at liberty to imagine the first figure rotating fast and the second more slowly. To assume that it takes longer to match a figure rotated by 90° than to match one rotated by 45° because the figure is being rotated at constant velocity adds a further incoherent hypothesis to the misconception.

Treisman's interpretations of her experiments in terms of representational structures that indicate the presence or absence of features is also awry. One does not perceive representations of objects, unless one perceives paintings or photographs of the objects. To see a red apple is not to see an image or representation of a red apple. Nor is it to have an image in one's mind or brain, although one can conjure up images in one's mind, and sometimes images cross one's mind independently of one's wish or will. But the mental images we thus conjure up are not visible, either to others or to ourselves – they are 'had', but not seen.

Crick's assertion that 'the visual parts of the brain take the picture . . . apart' is likewise a misdescription. The visual scene is not a picture, although it may contain a picture if one is in an art gallery. The electrochemical reactions of the rods and cones of the retina to the light falling on them cause a multitude of responses in different parts of the 'visual' cortex, but that is not correctly characterized as 'taking the picture apart'. Nor does the brain have to 'put it all together' again in order to provide our view of the world. For our 'view of the world' is not a picture of the world (or of the visible scene), and the attributes of the visibilia in front of us do not have to, and cannot, be 'brought together'. For the colour, shape, location and movement of the red geraniums swaying in the wind cannot be taken apart (there is no such thing as separating these attributes from the objects of which they are attributes), and the colour, shape, location and movement of the geraniums cannot be brought together in the brain, since these attributes are not to be found in the brain, either together or separately.

The pattern of neural firing that is a causal response to a stimulus in the visual field can be described without resort to Marr's idea of 'symbolic descriptions'. There are no 'symbols in the brain', but there are neural events that are causally correlated with certain other phenomena, such as seeing. We use our sense-faculties, such as vision, for apprehending how things are in our environment. The sense-organs are not information-transmitters, although we acquire information by their use. The neural correlates of features in a visual scene are neither 'representations' nor 'symbols'.

The experiments of Shepard and Metzler suggest that it may take longer to work out how a certain figure will appear when rotated thus than to work out how the same or another figure will appear when rotated otherwise. For one needs to exercise one's imagination – that is, one's powers to think of possibilities, to work out where this part of the figure will lie in relation to that part if the whole figure is rotated by 90°. One needs to think about the rotation of a figure, not to rotate an imaginary figure (since there is no such thing). In so thinking, one may, but need not, imagine a rotating figure. (And it is important to remember that thinking about something does not imply saying anything to oneself.)

We have seen that Crick's concern that the activities of the differently located cells which respond severally to colour, shape, location and movement when one is viewing an object need to be united somehow in order to form an image is misplaced. For no image is or needs to be formed in order to see the object which is visible. It may well be, however, that the firing of certain neurons in the brain is a causal condition for being able to see an object in the visual field, and that some of these are required to fire in response to shape, others in response to colour, and yet others in response to motion, etc. It is plausible to suppose that these functionally related groups of cells must fire more or less simultaneously if the animal is to enjoy normal visual perception. What is not plausible, because not intelligible, is that these functionally related groups of cells must form an image of anything or enable the brain to form an image. Their normal functioning is what makes it possible for *an animal* (not *the brain*) to *see* (not to *form images*).

1.7   What and Where Pathways in Object Recognition and Maps

The modules that compose the visual pathway from the retina to higher visual centres follow two diverging streams in the cortex (see Plate 1.4a): one pathway extends dorsally to terminate within the parietal lobe, including the motion detection area MT and the visual areas of the posterior parietal cortex; the other pathway extends ventrally to terminate in the temporal lobe (including V4 and the inferior temporal cortex). The work of Mortimer Mishkin and his colleagues in the early 1980s suggested that these two pathways serve different functions: the dorsal pathway is concerned with *where* an object is in visual space (motion, distance); the ventral pathway is concerned with *what* an object is (form, colour, texture, all of which are involved in object recognition) (Ungerleider and Mishkin, 1982).

Plate 1.4a illustrates these pathways, showing lateral views of the rhesus monkey brain, indicating the two major pathways both originating from V1, with arrows indicating the dorsal 'where' cortical stream, which takes a dorsal route to the parietal cortex, as well as a ventral 'what' cortical stream, which takes a ventral route to the temporal cortex. A simplified version is given in Plate 1.4c of the modules that participate in these two streams, together with their interconnections, the lines indicating both forward- and backward-projecting axons. The ventral stream (the 'magnocellular' (M) for the large lateral geniculate nucleus (LGN) neuron stream) consists of modules in the striate cortex (V1) which project from there to the middle temporal (MT) modules that are concerned with movement, as mentioned above. Projections proceeding from these to modules that include the medial superior temporal cortex (MST), fundus superior temporal cortex (FST), ventral intraparietal cortex (VIP), and finally to the posterior parietal cortex (PP) and superior temporal polysensory cortex (STP). The dorsal stream (the 'parvocellular' (P) for the relatively small lateral geniculate nucleus neuron stream) consists of modules in the striate cortex (V1) which project from there to extrastriate cortex (V2) and to V4 and finally to modules in the inferior temporal cortex (IT). It is clear that the 'cardinal' cells of the inferior temporal cortex that are involved in face recognition, mentioned above, fit neatly into the idea that the inferior temporal cortex module is involved with the 'what', i.e. with identification of objects.

Gerald Edelman has sought explanations for why the modules in the lateral geniculate nucleus and cortex, illustrated in Plate 1.4c, receive at least as many connections in the backward direction as in the forward direction to the 'what' and 'where' final pathways. He refers to these backward projections as 'reentrant': that is, nerves which make connections in the reverse direction to those along the principal pathway. An example of a reentrant pathway is that made by nerves which project back from the primary visual cortex (V1) to the lateral geniculate nucleus (LGN) in the thalamus, which is the reverse of the forward pathway from the retina to the thalamus to the primary visual cortex. Referring to the modules in the visual pathway as maps, he comments that:

> The visual system of the monkey, for example, has over thirty different maps, each with a certain degree of functional segregation (for orientation, color, movement, and so forth), and linked to the others by parallel and reciprocal connections. Reentrant signalling occurs along these connections. This means that, as groups of neurons are selected in a map, other groups in reentrantly connected but different maps may also be selected at the same time. Correlation and coordination of such selection events are achieved by reentrant signaling and by the strengthening of interconnections between maps within a segment of time. (Edelman, 1992, p. 85)

1.8 Misuse of the Term 'Maps'

When certain features of the visual field can be mapped on to the firings of groups of cells in the cortex, then the idea of maps in the brain arises. Neuroscientists often take these 'maps' as playing 'an essential part in the representation and interpretation of the world by the brain, *just as the maps of an atlas do for the reader of them*' (Blakemore, 1990, p. 265; our italics). It is by no means evident what could be meant by the claim that the topographical relations between groups of cells that are systematically related to features of the perceptual field play an essential role in the brain's interpreting something. To interpret, literally speaking, is to explain the meaning of something, or to take something that is ambiguous to have one meaning rather than another. But it makes no sense to suppose that the brain explains anything or that it apprehends something as meaning one thing rather than another. The claim that 'brain maps' (which are not actually maps) play an essential part in the brain's 'representation and interpretation of the world' cannot be 'just as the maps of an atlas do for the reader of them'. For a map is a pictorial representation, made in accordance with conventions of mapping and rules of projection. Someone who reads an atlas must know and understand these conventions in order to read anything off from the maps at all. The brain is not akin to the reader of a map, since it cannot be said to know any conventions of representations or methods of projection or how to read anything off the topographical arrangement of firing of cells in accordance with a set of conventions. For the brain cannot follow rules or conventions – since that presupposes knowledge of the rules and an intention to comply with them. Furthermore, the cells are not arranged in accordance with conventions at all, and the correlation between their firing and features of the perceptual field is not a conventional but a causal one.

1.9   The Binding Problem and 40 Hz Oscillations

The binding problem has been taken to arise when considering how the neurons responsive to the distance, textures, colours, different orientations of lines and edges of say, a house are interrelated so that the animal will be able to perceive the house as a unified object. More generally, neuroscientists have been puzzled about how the modularization of cellular function in the neural processes involved in perception enables the perceiving animal to apprehend a unified object in the visual field. Eric Kandel and Robert Wurtz, in a discussion interestingly entitled 'Constructing the Visual Image' (Kandel et al., 2000, ch. 25), explain that 'information about' (i.e. presumably, electrochemical responses to) form, motion and colour is carried by parallel pathways. This, according to Kandel and Wurtz, creates the 'binding problem':

> How is information carried by separate pathways brought together into a coherent visual image? . . . How does the brain construct a perceived world from sensory information and how does it bring it into consciousness? . . . what the visual system really does [is] to create a three-dimensional perception of the world which is different from the two-dimensional image projected onto the retina. (Kandel and Wurtz, 2000)

> How is information about color, motion, depth and form, which are (*sic*) carried by separate neural pathways, organized into cohesive perceptions? When we see a square purple box we combine into one perception the properties of colour (purple), form (square), and dimensions in depth (box). We can equally well combine purple with a round box, a hat or a coat . . .

. . . visual images are typically built up from the inputs of parallel pathways that process different features – movement, depth, form and color. To express the specific combination of properties in the visual field at any given moment, independent groups of cells must temporarily be brought into *association*. As a result, there must be a mechanism by which the brain momentarily associates the information being processed independently by different cell populations in different cortical regions. This mechanism, as yet unspecified, is called the *binding mechanism* (Kandel et al., 2000, p. 502)

Kandel and Wurtz puzzled over the question of how, for example, adjacent houses and the trees in their gardens are each perceived, *with all their properties bound together*, as separate objects?

Francis Crick suggested that, at any given moment, any particular object in the visual field is 'represented by' (i.e. causally correlated with) the firing of a set of neurones, which are distributed in different 'visual' areas (for form, colour, motion, etc.). We perceive the object as a unity. 'One striking feature of our internal picture of the visual world is how well organized it is. . . . we seldom get things jumbled in space when seeing them under ordinary conditions' (Crick, 1994, p. 232).

In the late 1980s, Singer and his colleagues offered a solution to the binding problem conceived as described above (Singer, 1991). They obtained what they took to be experimental evidence for the proposal that temporal synchrony of neuronal firing patterns may underlie binding (Gray and Singer, 1989), and suggested that 'synchrony of oscillatory responses in spatially separate regions of the cortex may be used to establish a transient relationship between common but spatially distributed features of a pattern' (Gray et al. 1990). They discovered that when some components of a visual scene were perceived by an observer as properties of a single object there was synchrony of the temporal impulses in the neurons that subserved each of the different components.

Consider, for example, two vertically oriented light bars moving at the same speed in the same direction past the eyes. Despite the fact that the bars are sufficiently far apart to register on two quite different parts of the retina which project to two distinct neuronal groups in the visual cortex (V1), there is a tendency for these bars to appear as a single object. The photomicrograph in fig. 1.18 shows the position of two such neuronal groups in area V1 of a cat. The bars are sufficiently far apart to be registered by two quite different parts of the retina which project to two neuronal groups in the visual cortex that are 7 mm apart (as indicated on the photomicrograph of the surface of the visual cortex by the white arrows). The black areas in this flat mount of the surface of the cortex indicate columns of neuronal groups, of which only the tops are shown, that are particularly responsive to vertical light contours. Microelectrodes are placed in the vicinity of these two neuronal groups, and the recordings made are shown in fig. 1.18a. The average impulse firing of the neurons in each of the groups (as shown by the field potentials) is oscillatory. Fig. 1.18b shows on an expanded time scale that the oscillation of both of the groups is at 40 Hz, and that they are in phase, despite the fact that they are 7 mm apart. No such coupled firing would be expected for neuronal groups at such a distance, and because of this coupling Singer and his colleagues took it that these two light bars would appear as a single object to the cat. The experience that the two light bars are one object is correlated with the fact that the

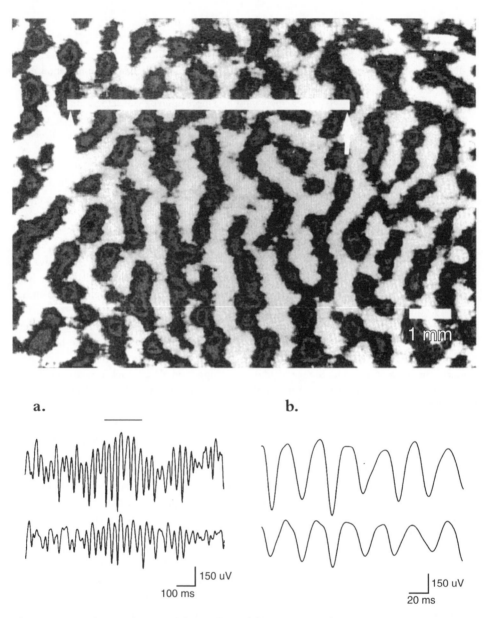

Fig. 1.18. Synchronized neuronal firing of two different groups of neurons in the visual cortex of a cat (area 17), shown in **a** and on a different time scale in **b**, during the observations of two vertically oriented light bars moving with the same speed and in the same directions, shown above on the surface of the cortex by two white arrows. (Bennett, 1997, fig. 3.5, after Gray and Singer, 1989.)

a.

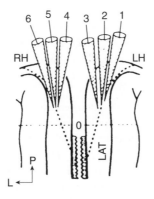

b.

Intrahemisphere

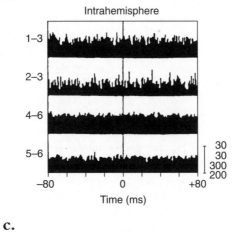

c.

Intrahemisphere

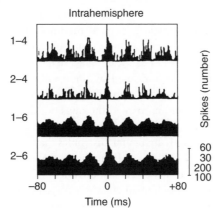

Fig. 1.19. Synchronized neuronal firing of three different groups of neurons in each hemisphere of the visual cortex of a cat. (Engel et al., 1991, fig. 3, p. 1178.)

neuronal groups in the visual cortex which are independently excited by the image on the retina of just one of the bars are now joined in a 'dynamic way' – that is, by a common frequency and phase of neuronal firing. This is an example of transient excitatory coupling of two neuronal groups within the same area of the neocortex, in this case the visual area.

Singer has also shown that there is interhemispheric synchronization of activity in the visual cortex when, he believes, a binding problem is being solved for a visual object. Suppose a single light bar is sufficient to stimulate three different neuronal groups, about 1 mm apart, in the visual cortex of one hemisphere. Electrodes are positioned in each of the groups, numbered 1–6 in area V1 of each hemisphere of the visual cortex of a cat, as shown in fig. 1.19a. The synchronization of the impulse firing and the phase of this firing, as measured by the different electrodes, can be shown by means of what is called a cross-correlogram. Fig. 1.19b depicts intrahemisphere cross-correlograms for the field recordings of pairs of neuronal group activity indicated by the electrode positions 1–3, 2–3, 4–6 and 5–6. If a periodic pattern is discernible in the cross-correlogram, then this indicates that the signals are correlated and gives information as to the common frequency and phase in the correlation. The cross-correlograms for the intrahemisphere recordings show a strong oscillatory modulation in the same frequency range of about 40 Hz, even though the electrodes may be separated by as much as 2 mm (fig. 1.19b). The cross-correlograms for interhemisphere recordings show surprisingly similar correlations, indicating that both hemispheres participate in the solution of the binding problem for the single white bar. This is not the case if the group of axons that join the two hemispheres (the corpus callosum) is cut. The cross-correlogram for recordings from the two hemispheres is now devoid of any periodic pattern and is flat, indicating that the firing of neuronal groups due to the light bar in each of the hemispheres is no longer correlated (fig. 1.19c). Singer takes it that the corpus callosum must mediate the synaptic connections between the two hemispheres that most likely participate in the solution of the binding problem.

Rodriguez and his colleagues (1999) have provided evidence for such long-distance synchronization of impulse activity in cortical modules of humans performing cognitive tasks. They recorded electrical brain activity from subjects who viewed ambiguous visual stimuli (perceived either as faces or as meaningless shapes). In this work they were able to show that face perception is accompanied by a long-distance pattern of synchronization, corresponding to the moment of perception itself and to the ensuing motor response. A period of strong desynchronization marked the transition between the moment of perception and the motor response. They suggest that this desynchronization reflects a process of active uncoupling of the underlying neural ensembles that is necessary to proceed from one cognitive state to another. Plate 1.8a and b shows the ambiguous visual stimuli used in their experiments, which are called 'Mooney' faces: namely, high-contrast pictures of a human face that are easily recognized as human faces when seen upright as in (a), but are difficult to recognize when inverted, as in (b). Subjects were asked to report as quickly as possible whether they had seen a face or not by pressing on one of two different keys. An electroencephalogram was recorded through 30 electrodes placed over the scalp of the subject and a precise time – frequency analysis carried out up to 100 Hz. Plate 1.8c and d show the spectral power following stimulation with the upright and the Mooney faces respectively.

Power peaks at about 230 ms after stimulus onset, and between 33 and 39 Hz. The perception condition elicits a significantly stronger response than the no-perception condition. The second peak lies at about 800 ms and 40 ± 5 Hz; it follows after the reaction time (645 $\pm$ 20 ms for perception; 766 $\pm$ 22 ms for no-perception), and no significant differences between conditions are found.

Thus humans as well as other animals show the synchronized oscillations of about 40 Hz over large areas of cortex during perception. This is perhaps more dramatically illustrated by means of Plate 1.9. This shows the average scalp distribution of about 40 Hz activity and phase synchrony. Colour coding indicates the power (averaged in a 34–40 Hz frequency range) over an electrode and during a 180 ms time window, from stimulation onset (0 ms) to motor response (720 ms). The frequency activity is spatially homogeneous and similar between conditions over time. In contrast, phase synchrony is markedly regional and differs between conditions. Synchrony between electrode pairs is indicated by lines. Black and yellow lines correspond to a significant increase or decrease in synchrony, respectively. Compared with the no-perception condition, which shows few synchronous patterns, the perception condition exhibits a sequence of localized spatial patterns that evolve over time. Synchrony first increases in the area between the left parieto-occipital and fronto-temporal regions. Desynchronization is then observed between the parietal and occipito-temporal area bilaterally. Rodriguez and colleagues propose that phase interactions between parietal and occipito-temporal regions are essential in the large-scale integration that is needed for the perception of upright Mooney faces. The second synchrony increase, which is probably linked to the motor response, is predominant between the right temporal and central regions. Phase synchrony, then, is directly involved in human cognition. Indeed, it has been suggested that the long-range character of the phase synchrony indicates that synchrony about 40 Hz and desynchrony may be viewed as a mechanism that subserves large-scale cognitive integration and not just visual-feature binding.

Both this work and that of Singer and his colleagues places emphasis on the solution of the binding problem itself as a necessary condition for us to be aware of something in the visual field – that is, to be conscious of that thing – without reference to an attentional mechanism. We will examine the nature of 'attention' and of 'awareness' further in chapter 2.

1.9.1 Misconceptions concerning the existence of a binding problem

The sense in which separate neural pathways carry information about colour, shape, movement, etc. is not semantic, but, at best, information-theoretic. In neither sense of 'information' can information be 'organized' into 'cohesive perceptions'. In the semantic sense, information is a set of true propositions, and true propositions cannot be organized into perceptions (i.e. into a person's perceiving something). In the engineering sense, 'information' is a measure of the freedom of choice in the transmission of a signal, and the amount of information is measured by the logarithm to the base 2 of the number of available choices – and this too is not something that can be 'organized' into perceptions. One cannot combine colour, form and dimensions into perceptions, just as one cannot put events into holes – this form of words makes no sense. And, correspondingly, when we see a square purple box, we do not 'combine' purple, squareness and boxhood – for this too is a nonsensical form of words. It is true that in order to see a coloured moving object with a given shape, separate groups of neurons must be active simultaneously. But it does not follow that, in the semantic sense of information, the brain must 'associate' various bits of information; nor could it follow, since brains cannot act on the basis of information or associate pieces of information. Whether the brain, in some sense that needs to be clarified, 'associates' information in the information-theoretic sense is a further question. But if it does, that is not because the features of the object perceived have to be 'combined in the brain', for that is a nonsense.

Above all, to see an object is neither to see nor to construct an image of an object. The reason why the several neuronal groups must fire simultaneously when a person sees a coloured three-dimensional object in motion is not because the brain has to build up a visual image or create an internal picture of objects in the visual field. When we see a tree, the brain does not have to (and could not) bind together the trunk, boughs and leaves, or the colour and the shape, or the shape and the movement of the tree. One may see the tree clearly and distinctly or unclearly and indistinctly, and one may be sensitive to its colour and movement, or one may suffer from one or another form of colour-blindness or visual agnosia for movement. Which neuronal groups must simultaneously be active in order to achieve optimal vision, what form that activity may take, and how it is connected with other parts of the brain that are causally implicated in cognition, recognition and action, as well as in co-ordination of sight and movement, are what needs to be investigated by neuroscientists. Since seeing a tree is not seeing an internal picture of a tree, the brain does not have to construct any such picture. It merely has to be functioning normally so that we are able to see clearly and distinctly. It does not have to take a picture apart, since neither the visual scene nor the light array falling upon the retinae are pictures. It does not have to put a picture back together again, since what it enables us to do is to see a tree (not a picture of a tree) in the garden (not in the brain).

1.9.2   On the appropriate interpretation of synchronicity of neuronal firing in visual cortex

Kandel and Wurtz are not correct in suggesting that the brain 'constructs a perceived world'; rather, it enables the animal to see a visible scene. Moreover, the brain does not create a three-dimensional perception which is different from the 'two-dimensional image' on the retina. It confers depth vision upon the animal, but the ability visually to discriminate depth is neither different from nor the same as an inverted reflection on the retina (which is incidental to vision anyway) – it is categorially distinct. The binding problem arises only if we consider that perceiving involves an internal picture or image of the external scene, so that the picture must be constructed, and the image 'built up'. And then one might indeed wonder how the brain produces such coherent pictures or images, correctly associating the shape, motion, depth and colour of the perceived object and not 'jumbling them up'.

To be sure, the cells that respond to motion, those that respond to shape, and those that respond to colour had better be active at (more or less) the same time; otherwise the person or animal will not see a coloured moving object of the relevant shape (or the asynchronicity will simply be reflected in a corresponding delay in the perception). And presumably the simultaneous activity of these cell groups had better be connected in some way to the centres that control recognition, movement and co-ordination. That much seems obvious. And indeed the first step towards clarifying the processes involved has been taken by the discoveries of Singer and his colleagues on the synchronous 40 Hz oscillations of neuronal firing in different neurons in the different parts of the brain that are involved in seeing.

1.10 Images and Imagining

The problem of identifying the different parts of the human brain associated with visual experience has been greatly illuminated by the introduction of non-invasive visual imaging techniques such as positron emission tomography (PET) and fMRI, especially in the 1990s. One of the pioneers of these techniques, Kosslyn, has made extensive observations concerning the identification of those cortical areas that are active during the period in which he claims his patients 'visualise things in their imagination'. For example, when one perceives an object – for example, the Sydney Opera House – then the image of the Opera House on the retina is said to be 'reconstructed' in area V1 of the cortex, involving the forward projection from the retina to the lateral geniculate nucleus and from there to V1 in the occipital cortex and beyond as shown by the forward projecting arrow in fig. 1.20. Kosslyn set out to determine if one closed one's eyes and imagined the structure of the Opera House, instead of actually perceiving it, whether area V1 is involved in reconstructing the image of the Opera House again on the basis of information reaching it from higher centres such as those in the temporal lobes. This would require a backward projection to V1 as indicated by the arrow in fig. 1.20. Such a problem would seem to be ideally suited to

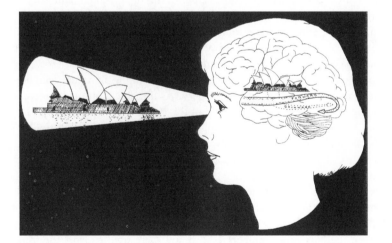

Fig. 1.20. Forward and backward projections to the primary visual cortex (area 17, V1) when viewing or imagining a scene. (From Bennett, 1997, fig. 5.3.)

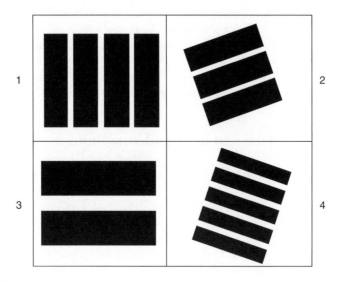

Fig. 1.21. Illustration of the stimuli used to determine the role of visual area 17 in visual imagery. (Kosslyn et al., 1999, fig. 1.)

study with PET or fMRI. However, although there has been general agreement using non-invasive imaging that both the temporal-occipital and parieto-occipital visual association areas of the cortex are involved in imagining a visual scene such as the Opera House, there has been little agreement as to whether area V1 is involved (see Kosslyn and Ochsner, 1994; Roland and Gulyas, 1994). The probable causes of this disagreement almost certainly reside in what are called the baseline conditions in setting up the PET or fMRI studies. They involve, in some experiments, determination of the areas of the brain that are active during the imagery test compared with the activation present when the subject is not performing a requested imagery task but simply lies motionless with eyes closed. However, this does not guarantee that the subject is not 'imagining something in visual consciousness', i.e. day-dreaming accompanied by mental imagery. As the detection of the increased activity in the imaging task requires the subtraction of this background activity, it is easy to see that activation of V1 during a day-dreaming episode could remove the indications of activity in this area of the brain during the imaging task.

However, Kosslyn and his colleagues devised approaches that seemed to avoid this problem and establish the role of area 17 (V1) in imagining. They used two convergent techniques, in one of which subjects closed their eyes during PET while they visualized and compared properties (e.g. relative length) of sets of stripes. Fig. 1.21 shows the stimuli used, which consisted of stripes that vary in length, width, orientation and the amount of space between the bars. The numbers 1, 2, 3 and 4 are used to label the four quadrants, each of which contains a set of stripes. After memorizing the display, the subjects closed their eyes, visualized the entire display, heard the names of two quadrants, and then heard the name of a comparison term (e.g. 'length'); the subject then decided whether the stripes in the first named quadrant had more of the named property than those in the second, and the response time was noted. The results showed that when people perform this task, area 17 (V1) is activated. The results of the PET scan, showing activation of area V1 (and areas 18/19) during imagery compared with baseline are shown in Plate 1.10, with the strength of the activation given by the colours, with blue, green, yellow and red representing increasingly higher activation.

In the other technique used by Kosslyn, repetitive transcranial magnetic stimulation was applied to the medial occipital cortex before presentation of the same task, thus transiently disrupting activity in this area of the cortex. This led to impaired performance after stimulation compared with sham control conditions, as it did when the subjects performed the task by actually looking at the stimuli. These results when stimulation was delivered before the imagery and perception conditions are given in fig. 1.22. In this figure 'Real' refers to when stimulation occurred with the magnetic field directed into area 17 (V1), whereas 'Sham' stimulation occurred when the field was diverted away from this site. The response times during Real stimulation were greater than those during Sham stimulation in both imagery and perception (1945 ms versus 1759 ms, and 1002 ms versus 827 ms, respectively). As shown, this response time increases in all five subjects in both modalities (digits next to each line indicate the subject number).

In other experiments, Kosslyn and his colleagues have shown that many different parts of the brain are involved when one visually imagines each of the letters of the alphabet in turn, compared with just naming the letters of the alphabet to oneself in one's imagination. Kosslyn takes this to provide evidence that the former is a much more complex task than the latter. He claims that the neural network modules involved in the visual imagination are the same as those involved in seeing, and that these modules are also involved in the processes of visual attention (Kosslyn, 1994).

1.10.1 Misconceptions concerning images and imagining

The claim of Kosslyn and his colleagues is that visualizing something (i.e. conjuring up visual images of it) involves the excitation of much the same neural systems as would the corresponding visual experience. Whether or not much the same neural systems are involved in the exercise of the faculty for producing eidetic imagery (which we shall call 'fantasia') as are involved in the corresponding perceptual experience is an empirical question which Kosslyn believes he has solved. Before accepting that this is the case, it is important to be clear about differences between seeing and its objects, on the one hand, and between visualizing and its objects, on the other.

Secondly, it is mistaken to suppose that recognition involves comparing a mental image with what one perceives. This is a confusion that we have already encountered in Marr's theory of vision, since he supposed that to generate a 3D model representation in the brain, a 2½ D sketch has to be compared with a stored catalogue of 3D model descriptions. This is indeed required for 'machine vision' − but then machine vision is no more a kind of vision than computers are kinds of mathematicians. It is a fiction that human recognition involves matching a perception with a mental image.

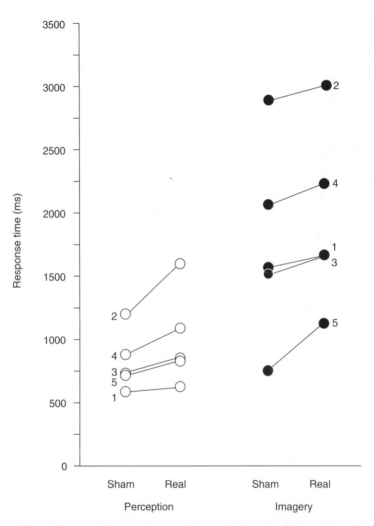

Fig. 1.22.   Effects of transcranial magnetic stimulation applied to visual cortex (area 17, V1) on the response time for perception and imagery tasks. (Kosslyn et al., 1999, fig. 3.)

Thirdly, to perceive something is not to have, construct, or reconstruct an image of it in the mind. To perceive is not to have or to form images, and what is perceived is not an image save in the cases in which one perceives pictures. To form a mental image of a scene is not to imagine an image of that scene. That is something a painter might do when he is trying to visualize the painting he intends to paint. But to form a mental image of a scene is visually to imagine *that scene* (not an image of it).

Finally, it is incoherent to suppose that one can discover things by reading off visual or spatial information from one's mnemonic image or 'visualized display' of an antecedently seen object. According to this conception, a mental image is a pictorial representation, akin to a private photograph, from which one can derive information about what it is an image of by observation. It is uncontentious that one might try to recollect the different lengths of stripes in experiments of the kind carried out by Kosslyn. What is problematic, however, is the idea that one might determine the length of the stripes in a particular quadrant in one's mental image by observation. One may visualize a set of stripes in one quadrant, and other sets of stripes in other quadrants. One may imagine the stripes in one quadrant to be longer that those in another. But one cannot *discover* that the stripes in one imagined quadrant are longer or shorter than the stripes in another (after all, one cannot *see* them). One may indeed come to *realize* that one has imagined the stripes in one quadrant to be longer than the stripes in another quadrant, but one cannot *find that out* by *looking* – since there is no such thing as looking at one's mental images. But one cannot make the comparison between the lengths of the stripes in the different quadrants that one is visualizing in order to find out their comparative length. (Similarly, one cannot measure, but only imagine measuring, the objects one visualizes.) Mental (visual) images are not like private pictures that only the subject can see.

2

Attention, Awareness and Cortical Function: Helmholtz to Raichle

2.1 The Concept of Attention

The concept of attention is closely connected with the concepts of awareness, concentration, consciousness and noticing. It is also linked with taking an interest in something, with enjoying and thinking about something. Lack of attention is correspondingly linked not only with unawareness of, failure to concentrate on, or to notice, something, but also with carelessness, inadvertence and absent-mindedness.[1]

The various forms of attention all require an object – one cannot attend without attending *to* something or other. Similarly, one cannot describe the paying of attention to something without referring to the object, since the characterization depends upon what one is attending to. The surgeon's attention to the operation is altogether unlike the student's attention to the lecture or the bird-watcher's to the birds. Being informed that someone is paying attention or is concentrating no more tells one what he is doing than being informed that he is rehearsing, repeating, working, practising or obeying. For, like the latter verbs, attention verbs are polymorphous – what counts as V-ing on one occasion or in one circumstance may not count as V-ing on another occasion or in another circumstance. A person attends, just as he rehearses, practises or works, by doing something *else*, such as looking, listening, writing, drawing, driving, etc. What he does in attending to what he is looking at may not differ at all from what he does in looking at the same thing without attention – although what he consequently may be able to do may differ greatly.

What a person attends to is what he pays attention to; what he is interested in is what he is prone to pay attention to. A person notices what captures his attention, and he is conscious of what holds his attention. He takes care when paying attention to the risks involved in his own activities, so *care* has a much more restrictive range than *attention*. Similarly, enjoyment typically involves attention, but is limited to what *affects oneself*. Attention concepts may qualify many different aspects of what a person or an animal does. For the qualifying description may signify attention or inattention to the doing, action or activity

---

[1] The following remarks are indebted to White, 1964, chs 1–4. His book should be studied by all neuroscientists doing empirical research on this topic.

itself (if, for example, done inadvertently), or to the manner of doing it (if done mechanically or inattentively), or to its effects (if done carelessly) or to its circumstances (if done regardless of them).

Attending, although not an activity, has affinities with activity concepts. It applies to what we do or are engaged in doing. Like activities, it takes time, can be intermittent or continuous, may be interrupted and later resumed. It has a manner (e.g. reluctant, eager, careful, conscientious). Unlike noticing, it is something that can be done willingly or unwillingly, and on purpose. One can order someone to pay attention, decide, promise, or refuse to pay attention. Because it can be voluntary, it can also be the object of praise or blame.

We pay attention in doing something else, such as looking or listening, walking or climbing, reading or writing. What makes what we do a case of attending in one or other of its various forms is that when we do it, something is made the centre, object or topic of whatever it is we are doing. So we attend to audibilia or their features by listening, to visibilia by looking (observing, watching, scrutinizing) and to intelligibilia by thinking (reasoning, calculating). Among possible objects of attention are one's own acts and activities. These one may attend to either *qua* observer – as when one 'watches oneself', as it were, while one is doing whatever one is doing – or *qua* agent – as when one does what one does attentively or carefully.

Noticing is a form of attention, and its objects are generally things to which attention may be paid. Unlike attention, however, noticing lacks affinity with activities. For one cannot be engaged in noticing something, or be interrupted in the middle of noticing it. One cannot notice something intermittently or continuously, and there are no methods or manners of noticing things. One does not notice things voluntarily, willingly or unwillingly, and one cannot decide, agree or refuse to notice something as one can decide, agree or refuse to attend to something. One cannot order another to notice, only to attend and to try to spot something.[2] Some things – for example, saliencies – we cannot help noticing, whereas others are easy to overlook.

Noticing has an affinity with achievements, like arriving, finding, discovering, discerning, detecting, winning, but 'to notice' is not an achievement verb.[3] Like 'to discover' and 'to detect', 'to notice' is factive and signifies not an activity but a result or upshot. Its factivity is patent in that, unlike believing, one cannot notice something that is not the case, and unlike looking for, one cannot notice something that does not exist. 'To notice', like 'to detect', signifies the acquisition of correct information. Unlike arriving, discovering or winning, but like realizing, becoming conscious or aware of something, noticing is a form of *cognitive receptivity*. Reception concepts, unlike achievement concepts, do not signify something brought about or brought off, gained or produced; they signify various forms of receiving, as opposed to achieving, knowledge and information. When we notice something, we are struck by it, it makes an impression on us, attracts our attention. One may be skilled at spotting or detecting something, but not at noticing something. There are methods for

---

[2] Nevertheless, 'to notice' does have an imperative from, as in 'Notice the fine brush work'. Here 'to notice' means 'to take note of'.

[3] The concept of an achievement verb was introduced by Gilbert Ryle (1949, pp. 149–54).

spotting or detecting things one wants to spot or detect, but there are no methods for noticing things. What is noticed is what is given or received, not what is attained or achieved.

Neuroscientists have concentrated upon visual and auditory attention, and have, on the whole, paid little attention to other forms of receptivity such as noticing, becoming conscious or being aware of something, concentrating on or being conscious of something.

2.2   The Psychophysics of Attention

Psychophysics, the psychological study of the relationship between physical stimuli and the effects they produce in humans, was first applied to the subject of attention by Hermann von Helmholtz in his great work *Handbuch der physiologischen Optik* of 1894. His research had a profound effect on ideas concerned with selective attention in vision. He comments as follows:

> I refer now to the experiments . . . with a momentary illumination of a previously completely darkened field on which was spread a page with large printed letters. Prior to the electric discharge the observer saw nothing but a slightly illuminated pinhole in the paper. He fixed his gaze rigidly upon it, and it served for an appropriate orientation of directions in the dark field. The electric discharge illuminated the printed page for an indivisible instant during which its image became visible and remained for a very short while as a positive after-image. Thus, the duration of the perceptibility of the picture was limited to the duration of the after-image. Eye movements of a measurable magnitude could not be executed within the duration of the spark, and movements during the brief duration of the after-image could no longer change its position on the retina. Regardless of this I found it possible to decide in advance which part of the dark field surrounding the continuously fixed pinhole of light I wanted to perceive, and then actually recognized upon the electric illumination single groups of letters in that region of the field, though usually with intervening gaps that remained empty. After strong flashes, as a rule, I read more letters than with weak ones. On the other hand, the letters of by far the largest part of the field were not perceived, not even in the vicinity of the fixation point. With a subsequent electric discharge I could direct my perception to another section of the field, while always fixating on the pinhole, and then read a group of letters there.
>
> These observations demonstrated, so it seems to me, that by a voluntary kind of intention, even without eye movements, and without changes of accommodation, one can concentrate attention on the sensation from a particular part of our peripheral nervous system and at the same time exclude attention from all other-parts. (Helmholtz, 1894b, pp. 258–9)

It is perhaps noteworthy that Helmholtz's conclusion confuses sensations with perceptions and having sensations with perceiving. What he had found was that he could concentrate on (intentionally direct his attention to) what was perceptible at the periphery of his visual field, not on 'a sensation from a particular part of his peripheral nervous system'.

To Helmholtz (1871, 1894b) these experiments indicated that there 'is a change in our nervous system, independent of the motions of the external movable parts of the body, whereby the excited state of certain fibres is preferentially transmitted to consciousness' (1894b, p. 263). This was a misdescription of the phenomena. It was not the 'excited state of neural fibres' that was 'transmitted to consciousness'. It was rather that as a result of the excited state of certain neural fibres, he *became* conscious of certain features at the periphery of his visual field. 'In this respect,' he continued, 'our attention is quite independent of the position and accommodation of the eyes, and of any known alteration in these organs; and free to direct itself by a conscious and voluntary effort upon a selected portion of a dark and undifferentiated field of view. This is one of the most important observations for a future theory of attention' (Helmholtz, 1890, 1894b, p. 263). Furthermore, he added:

> The natural tendency of attention when left to itself is to wander to ever new things; and so soon as the interest of its object is over, so soon as nothing new is to be noticed there, it passes, in spite of our will, to something else. If we wish to keep it upon one and the same object, we must seek constantly to find out something new about the latter, especially if other powerful impressions are attracting us away. . . . we can set ourselves new questions about the object, so that a new interest in it arises, and then the attention will remain riveted. The relation of attention to will is, then, less one of immediate than of mediate control. (See Van der Heijden, 1992, pp. 32–3)

The most interesting developments in investigations into processes involved in selective attention of the kind studied by von Helmholtz had to wait a further 60 years, until the research of Cherry (1953). Cherry studied selective auditory attention (rather than selective visual attention) in which one notices, for example, a word or sentence uttered amidst the hubbub of a cocktail party. In Cherry's experiments, competing recordings are played to the two ears through headphones and the subject is asked to attend to and immediately repeat the train of speech directed at one ear. Cherry discovered that whilst the subjects could remember the speech directed at the 'attending' ear, they could not remember that directed at the other. One of the most interesting results to emerge from Cherry's introduction of natural speech into the study of selective attention involved experiments in which a subject is presented with two mixed speeches recorded on a tape and is asked to repeat one of them word by word or phrase by phrase. The subject is allowed to play the tape as many times as he wishes and in any way. His task is simply to separate one of the speeches from the other, and to repeat the various identified portions, but without writing them down. Fig. 2.1 shows one example of two messages, with his reconstructions. The subject matters are markedly distinct in the case shown. The phrases recognized are underlined, and errors are indicated by the capitalized subscripts. It is remarkable that no transpositions of phrases between the speeches occurred in the example shown in fig. 2.1. In other examples, there were a few transpositions, but when these occurred, they were highly probable from the text. These observations (and others) suggested to Cherry (1953, p. 976) that 'The logical principles involved in the recognition of speech seem to require that the brain have a vast "store" of probabilities, or at least of probability rankings. Such a store enables prediction

Message 1 (a) "It may mean that our religious convictions, legal systems

and politics have been so successful in accomplishing their ends
~~ends~~ AIMS

during the past two thousand years, that there has been no need to

change our outlooks about them. Or it may mean that the outlook has not

changed for other reasons. I will leave the first hypothesis
~~will leave~~ BELIEVE IN

to those who are willing to defend it, and choose the second. As the
~~to~~ AND IN

reader may have guessed, I am interested in learning how obsolete

structure of languages preserves obsolete metaphysics."

Message 1 (b) "This very brief discussion will serve to give a slight

indication of the really complex nature of the causes and uses of birds'

colors, and may serve to suggest a few of the many possibilities that

may underlie them. There is a very great opportunity here for close and

careful observation of the habits of birds in a free state, with a view to

shedding light on these problems. But the observer, in interpreting what

he sees, must ever be on his guard lest he lose sight of alternative

explanation."

Fig. 2.1. An example of two speeches (Message 1(a) and Message 1(b)) reconstructed by a subject to whom they had been presented as mixed speeches by Cherry (1953, p. 976).

to be made, noise or disturbances to be combated, and maximum-likelihood estimates to be made.'

However, this conclusion is too hasty. It is not clear what could be *meant* by the claim that the brain 'has a store', let alone 'a vast store', of probabilities or probability rankings of word sequences. Even less clear is the suggestion that this cerebral store enables the human being whose brain it is to predict word sequences. Certainly the human ability to make such predictions does not involve *consulting* stores of probability sequences. To be sure, normal speakers of a language can predict probable sequences in common sentential contexts. Without a normally functioning brain they would not be able to do so. Is anything added to this platitude by the claim that the brain contains stores of sequences coupled with probability rankings?

In 1958, Broadbent proposed a means by which such selective auditory attention could be attained. His proposal is summarized by means of his 'information-flow diagram' shown in fig. 2.2. According to his theory, several sensory inputs to the brain (indicated by the arrows at the left of the diagram) fail to reach 'higher levels of analysis', as they are screened out by a 'limited capacity channel' found at an intermediate stage between the sensory input channels and the higher-order analysis, so that the limited capacity channel acts as a gate. He comments:

> A nervous system acts to some extent as a single communication channel, so that it is meaningful to regard it as having a limited capacity. A selective operation is performed upon the input to this channel, the operation taking the form of selecting information from all sensory events having some feature in common. Physical features identified as able to act as a basis for this selection include the intensity, pitch, and spatial localisation of sounds. The selection is not completely random, and the probability of a particular class of events being selected is increased by certain properties of the events and by certain states of the organism. Properties of the events which increase the probability of the information conveyed by them passing the limited capacity channel include the following: physical intensity, time since the last information from the class of events entered the limited capacity channel, high frequency of sounds as opposed to low (in man), sounds as opposed to visual stimuli or touch as opposed to heat (dogs). States of the organism which increase the probability of selection of classes of events are those normally described by animal psychologists as 'drives'. When an organism is in a drive state it is more likely to select those events which are usually described as primary reinforcements for that drive. Thus food has a high probability of being selected if the animal has been deprived of food for 24 hrs. (Broadbent, 1958, p. 297)

Broadbent's theory, with its gating mechanism, could explain Cherry's observations on the 'cocktail party effect' but not those of the phenomenon in which speech directed at the unattended ear was noticed if it contained words of high priority, such as the subject's name.

However, one might have deeper qualms about Broadbent's description. The phenomenon to be explained is the human ability to attend selectively to speech and the correlated disposition to notice (to have one's attention caught by) speech that mentions themes of interest and concern. The intensity, pitch and spatial localization of sounds are undoubtedly

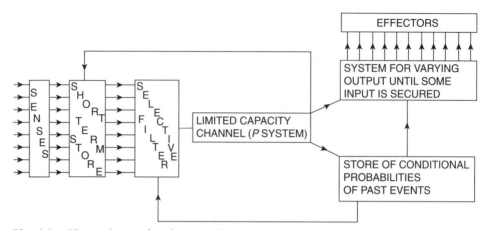

Fig. 2.2.   The mechanism for selective auditory attention proposed by Broadbent (1958, fig. 7).

among the factors relevant to the ability to focus one's attention as well as to the disposition to notice certain sounds rather than others. How much is added to the explanandum by the explanans that there is 'a limited capacity channel' in which something (?) operates on the input to the channel and selects 'information from all sensory events having some feature in common'? What, in this context, counts as 'input'? Is the input the words I hear, or the sound waves that hit my eardrum, or the consequent neural impulses? What count as 'sensory events'? Or as 'information'? Is the 'information' what I am trying to hear? – for example, what N.N. is saying, or his comments on topic X? Or is it the relative frequencies of neural signals along the auditory nerve? Certainly 'the probability of a particular class of events being selected is increased by certain properties of the events and by certain states of the organism' – namely, whether the 'organism' (the person) is interested in topic X and not in topic Y, and whether the audible utterances include talk of X. But this is part of the explanandum, not of the explanans. No doubt hungry animals are prone to attend to food (if there is no danger). Moreover, one might add, human animals are prone to attend to talk about what interests them. But these platitudes, which Broadbent dresses up in scientific jargon, add nothing to what we knew antecedent to theory.

In 1969, Treisman suggested that the model present in fig. 2.2 must be modified by removing the selectivity filter so that stimuli to which one is not attending are not excluded but simply 'attenuated'; that is, little attention is paid to them compared with the stimuli to which one is attending, thus still allowing the former to be 'available for analysis at higher centres' where their salience might lead to a change in attention. Her research led to the idea of parallel pathways of analysis, like those given for the detection of the letter 'G' in a display in which it is coloured red, as shown in fig. 2.3. As she explains it:

> An example of a complex visual search task may help to illustrate some different strategies or models for selective attention. We might ask S to decide whether a display of coloured letters in different sizes and orientations contains the letter 'G' or not. To do this he must first direct his attention to the display and not elsewhere in the room, that is, he must select the

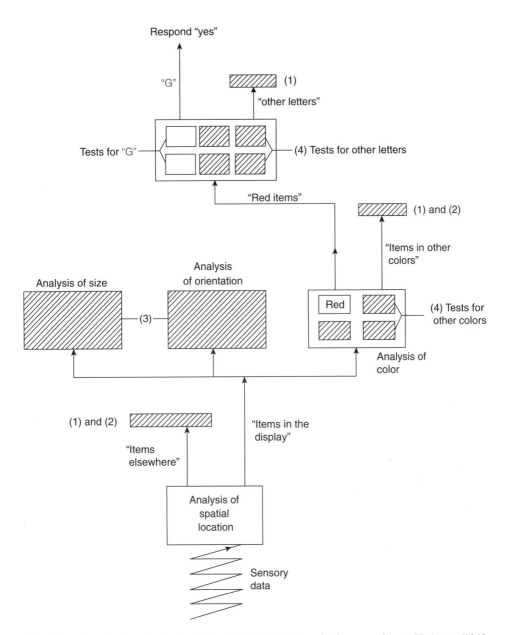

Fig. 2.3. A mechanism for the detection of the letter 'G' in a display, according to Treisman (1969, from fig. 1).

class of sensory data coming from one particular area as the input to the perceptual system. Second, he must attend to the shapes of the letters and not their colours, sizes or orientations, that is, he must select the analysers for shape and reject those for colour, etc. Next he must identify the target letter 'G' if it is present, and if possible ignore differences between the other letters. To do this he may be able to modify the function of the shape analysers so that they perform only the subset of tests for those critical features necessary to identify 'G'. He would therefore distinguish among the other letters only those which also differed by one or more of the critical features in 'G'. Finally, he must select the appropriate output of the shape analysers to control the response, 'G', giving a positive response and all other outputs a negative one.

In another form of the experiment S might be told that the target letter 'G' will be red if it is present at all. This might enable him further to restrict the inputs to the shape analysers of selecting only red items for analysis. To do this, of course, he would have to use the colour analyser at some earlier stage to distinguish red items from others, but he could still reject analysers for size and orientation, and perhaps also reject tests for colours other than red and so ignore the differences between green and black letters. (Treisman, 1969, p. 284)

She concludes from these studies that:

Four types of attention strategy are distinguished: the first restricts the number of inputs analysed; the second restricts the dimensions analysed; the third the items (defined by sets of critical features) for which S [the subject] looks or listens; and the fourth selects which results of perceptual analysis will control behaviour and be stored in memory. (Triesman, 1969, p. 282)

That someone who is asked to identify a plastic letter G among a group of vari-sized and vari-coloured letters has to look at the letters and attend to their shapes, while disregarding their sizes, orientations and colours is not an experimental result, but an explanation of the requirements of the task. But whether this means that he must 'select the class of sensory data coming from one particular area as the input to the perceptual system' is debatable. He must attend to the shapes and disregard differences of colour, size and orientation, but whether this means that 'he must select the analysers for shape and reject those for colour, etc.' is questionable. We have no idea of what, in this context, an 'analyser' is. Presumably it is whatever neural mechanism enables a human being to attend to shapes of visibilia, etc. But human beings do not *select* the neural mechanisms that enable them to do what they do. So all we are really being told is that in order to attend to the shapes of visibilia, we must possess such neural mechanisms that will enable us to attend to the shapes of visibilia. To suggest that a human being is able to 'modify the function of the shape analysers so that they perform only the subset of tests for those critical features necessary to identify "G"'' does not obviously amount to more than that a person, when picking out the letter 'G', must have such neural structures activated as will enable him to pick out specific shapes. 'Shape analyser', after all, means little more than 'a neural something, I know not what, that enables one to identify shapes'. Similarly, the supposition that a human being 'must select the appropriate output of the shape analysers to control the response "G", giving a positive response and all other outputs a negative one' is surely incoherent. Human beings cannot *select* outputs of neural 'shape analysers' (if there are any such things). But they can say 'G' when they see the letter and recognize it.

Triesman and her colleagues further developed this model of mechanisms for visual attention into a 'feature-integration' theory. In experiments designed to test this model, attention is directed serially to each stimulus in a display whenever conjunctions of more than one separable feature are needed to characterize or distinguish the possible objects presented. This is well illustrated by the following experiment. If the reaction or search time is measured for displays of different sizes, containing up to 30 letters, where targets are specified by a single feature (e.g. pink target amongst brown and purple colour distracters or 'O' amongst 'T' and 'N' shape distracters), then the function relating search times to display size is flat when a single feature is sufficient to define the target (fig. 2.4). On the other hand, for targets specified by a conjunction of features (e.g. a pink O amongst green Os and pink Ns), then the search time increases linearly with display size (fig. 2.4). Essentially the same results are obtained when a subject fixates on a certain spot in a display which possesses brown Ts and green Xs in equal numbers, and is asked to respond if there is a green T in the display (conjunction condition). Alternatively, in what is called the 'feature condition', the subject was asked to respond if a blue letter or an S was present in the display, with blue Ts and Xs matching half the distracters in shape, and the brown or green Ss matching half the distracters in colour.

When a single feature is sufficient to distinguish the target, it is immediately detected by the subject irrespective of the number of distracters present (fig. 2.4). On the other hand, when the target is defined by a conjunction of features severally shared with the distracters, the slopes of the curves relating reaction time to display size are positive, indicating that the items in the display are searched one at a time. Treisman took these results as evidence for the 'feature-integration' theory of attention. According to this theory, features, rather than objects, are detected first in perception,

> being registered early, automatically, and in parallel across the visual field, while objects are identified separately and only at a later stage, which requires focused attention. We assume that the visual sense is initially coded along a number of separable dimensions, such as colour, orientation, spatial frequency, brightness, direction of movement. In order to recombine these separate representations and to ensure the correct synthesis of features for each object in a complex display, stimulus locations are processed serially with focal attention. Any features which are present in the same central 'fixation' of attention are combined to form a single object. (Treisman and Gelade, 1980, p. 98)

Again, it is unclear whether this conclusion is warranted. It is not clear what is meant by 'the visual sense is coded along a number of separable dimensions', other than that the ability to see involves the power to detect a variety of features in the object seen. That is doubtless true (indeed, a conceptual, not an experimental, truth). But the claim that when we perceive something, we perceive its features *before* perceiving the thing itself, is questionable, even if it is true that the parts of the brain that respond to features react prior to those parts of the brain that respond to the objects whose features they are. The claim that

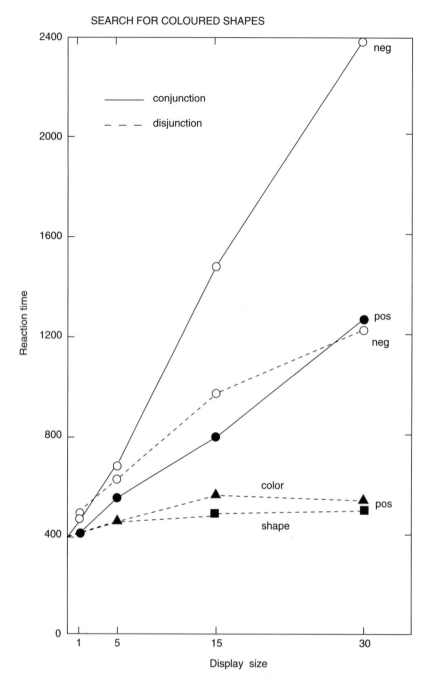

Fig. 2.4. The reaction time (or search time) of a subject measured for displays of different sizes, containing up to 30 letters, for targets specified by a single feature or a conjunction of features. (Treisman and Gelade, 1980, fig. 1.)

'representations' are involved presumably means that neural correlates of each of the detectable dimensions of visibilia can be found. This is an experimental claim, and has experimental warrant. But the further contention that these separate 'representations' must be 'recombined' is surely misconceived. It confuses two quite different senses of 'representation' – the causal correlate sense just mentioned and the symbolic or iconic sense (in which a picture is a representation of what it pictures). For the neural correlates, the various cells firing in the various locations of the 'visual' striate cortex, cannot be 'recombined', and do not need to be. The thought that the features a perceiver perceives must be correctly *synthesized* 'to form a separate object', the so-called 'binding problem', is confused. (For critical discussion see pp. 32–8.) To perceive is not to form an image of what is perceived, either in one's brain or in one's mind. What is perceived is the tree in the quad, not a representation of a tree in the quad. The brain does not have to synthesize a representation of the tree out of representations of its size, shape, colour and orientation – it has to enable the perceiver to see the tree and its features clearly.

2.3   Neuroscience of Attention

In order to attend, one must be awake rather than asleep, and alert and attentive rather than drowsy and inattentive. But if one is inattentive, one may have one's attention caught by changes in one's surroundings that are salient – e.g. sudden noises or movements. The neuroscience of attention was dominated in the 1940s by studies of the neural processes concerned with sleep versus arousal and wakefulness. Small voltage fluctuations accompany neuronal activity in the brains of animals during both sleep and arousal. Transitions from drowsiness to alertness and attention, or from sleep to wakefulness, are accompanied by breakup of the synchronous discharge of neuronal elements in the cerebral cortex in which high-voltage slow waves in the EEG (electroencephalogram) are replaced by low-voltage fast activity (Berger, 1930).

In 1949 Moruzzi and Magoun showed the existence of a system of neurons in the brainstem reticular formation, stimulation of which desynchronizes the EEG of the cortex, replacing high-voltage slow waves with low-voltage fast activity, as shown in fig. 2.5. This figure shows the effects of stimulation of the brain-stem reticular formation upon electrocortical activity in a cat. In this figure, the origins of the different channels is given at the left: L.SEN.MOT signifies left sensory-motor cortex; R.SEN.MOT, right sensory-motor cortex; L-R.CPU., left to right cruciate proteus; L-R.PRO, left to right gyrus proteus; L.VIS., left visual area. In A and B, stimulation of the left reticular formation in the brainstem at 300 Hz for the periods indicated by the horizontal bars leads to the replacement of high-voltage slow waves with low-voltage fast activity in both the left and right hemispheres of an 'encephale isole' cat – that is, one in which the spinal cord has been transacted at a high level (cervical 1). In C, the same stimulation of the left reticular formation almost completely blocks the high-voltage slow waves and outlasts the period of stimulation bilaterally in a deeply anaesthetized cat. In D, the frequency of stimulation of the reticular formation was reduced to 100 Hz, and under these conditions the reduction in high-voltage slow waves is restricted to the left cortex and does not outlast the period of stimulation.

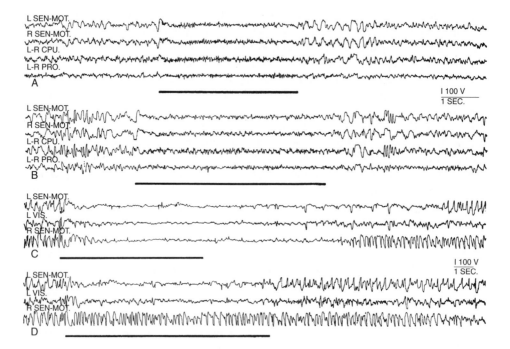

Fig. 2.5. Effect of stimulation of the brain-stem reticular formation upon electrocortical activity. (Moruzzi and Magoun, 1949, fig. 1.)

Moruzzi and Magoun (1949, p. 472) conclude from experiments such as these that 'a background of maintained activity within this ascending brain stem activating system may account for wakefulness, while reduction of its activity either naturally, by barbiturates, or by experimental injury and disease, may respectively precipitate normal sleep, contribute to anaesthesia or produce pathological somnolence'.

2.3.1   Attention and arousal

With the advent in the late 1960s of techniques for signal averaging of the EEG, such as the Computer of Average Transients (CAT), it was possible to isolate the components of the EEG measured in humans that directly relate to a stimulus in a particular sensory modality, such as vision. These averaged and very small potentials, referred to as 'event related potentials' (ERPs), were used by Eason, Harter and White in 1969 to show the effects of arousal on visually evoked ERPs in man. These results are shown in fig. 2.6, in which the ERPs measured over the occipital cortex (primary visual area V1) that are evoked by a flash of light in the right visual field are indicated for both 'high' and 'low' arousal states. These states were induced by the presence or absence of a shock threat when the flashes of light were presented. Attention was varied by having the subject react to flashes appearing in

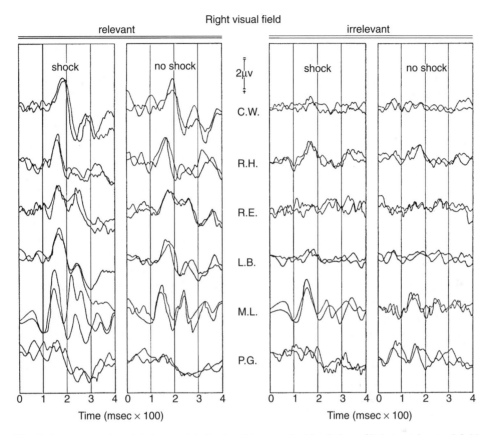

Fig. 2.6. Averaged occipital potentials for six subjects evoked by flashes of light in right visual field during 'high' and 'low' arousal states (shock *vs* no shock) when flashes were relevant (in correct visual field) or irrelevant (in ignored visual field). (Eason, Harter and White, 1969.)

either his right or left visual field while ignoring flashes appearing concomitantly but not simultaneously in the opposite field. The figure, with superimposed tracings representing replications, shows that ERPs evoked under 'high' arousal (threat of a shock) are greater than those obtained under 'low' arousal. Thus the potentials evoked by flashes receiving attention are much greater than those evoked by the flashes being ignored. These experiments show that the ERP magnitude is related to both the state of arousal and specific attention. Eason, Harter and White (1969, p. 288) suggest on the basis of this research and that of others that 'the presentation of a stimulus to an organism in a low state of arousal is followed by a strong orienting response due to the arousing effect of the stimulus, and conversely, that the presentation of a stimulus to the animal during high states of arousal elicit weak orienting responses due to the distracting effects of other environmental stimuli'.

2.3.2   Selective attention

The effects of selective attention on auditory evoked ERPs was determined for humans by Hillyard and colleagues (1973). They obtained ERPs related to the 'cocktail party' effect in which people are able to have their attention caught by, or to restrict their attention to, something they hear in a noisy environment, thus disregarding equally intense but irrelevant sounds or utterances. The auditory ERP possesses both a negative component (N1) which peaks at 80–110 ms after an abrupt sound and a subsequent positive component (P2) at 160–200 ms (see fig. 2.7a). The N1 but not the P2 component is larger when the sound presented is attended to compared with when it is not attended to. This is shown clearly by the results of fig. 2.7a, which indicate in the left column that N1 evoked by right-ear tones is considerably larger when these stimuli are attended to (solid tracings) than when the left-ear tones are receiving attention (dotted tracings); conversely, in the right column of fig. 2.7a, larger Ns are evoked by left-ear tones during the attend-left condition (dotted tracings) than during the attend-right runs (solid tracings). It will be noted that the amplitude of N1 evoked by right-ear tones (measured baseline to peak) is between 20 and 75 per cent smaller during the attend-left than the attend-right condition; conversely, the N1 evoked by the concurrent left-ear sequence is between 22 and 78 per cent smaller under attend-right conditions than under attend-left. Thus, when attention is switched from one ear to the other, the reciprocal effects of selective attention suppression of N1 evoked by tones in the ear one is not using to attend, and enhancement of N1 evoked in the ear one is using to attend, are approximately symmetrical.

The auditory evoked potentials (or ERPs) produced by occasional higher-pitched signals in the ear one is using to attend manifested a component which peaked at 250–400 ms, as shown by the shaded area in fig. 2.7b as an extended time base, and this is elicited only after the signal tones and not by the standard tones. These observations were interpreted by Hillyard and his colleagues in the following terms:

> Our results suggest that N1 and P3 are signs of fundamentally different selective attention processes, corresponding closely to the 'stimulus set' and 'response set' modes of attention, respectively, described by Broadbent (1970) and others. A stimulus set preferentially admits all sensory input to an attended channel (stimuli having in common a simple sensory attribute such as pitch, position in space, receptor surface, or the like) for further perceptual analysis, while blocking or attenuating inputs arriving over irrelevant channels (for example, the unattended ear) at an early stage of processing. Response set is a subsequent processing stage in which sensory information as compared against memorised 'templates' or 'models' for selected stimuli which are not distinguishable simply by virtue of belonging to a particular sensory input channel; a response set acts to facilitate the recognition of these specific task-relevant signals.
>
> These two hierarchical modes of attention generally operate together. At a cocktail party, for example, it is necessary to establish a stimulus set in favour of the location and pitch characteristics of a speaker's voice, and a succession of response sets to recognize the specific contents of his speech. In the present experiment we propose that the amplitude of N1 indexes the stimulus set which selectively excludes sensory input to the unattended ear from further

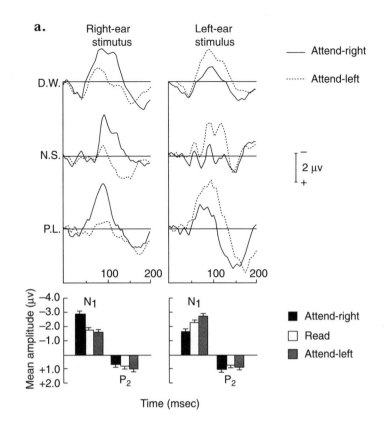

a.

Right-ear stimutus / Left-ear stimulus

Attend-right
Attend-left

D.W.

N.S.

P.L.

100   200   100   200

2 μv

Mean amplitude (μv)

N₁   N₁

Attend-right
Read
Attend-left

P₂   P₂

Time (msec)

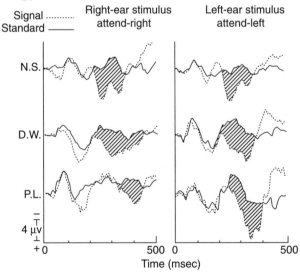

b.

Signal ·········
Standard ———

Right-ear stimulus attend-right   Left-ear stimulus attend-left

N.S.

D.W.

P.L.

4 μv

0   500   0   500

Time (msec)

Fig. 2.7. Auditory event-related potentials (ERPs) from three different subjects. **a:** tracings of the ERPs when stimuli were presented to each ear under attend-right (solid lines) and attend-left (dotted lines). Bar graphs give the baseline to peak amplitudes of N1 and P2 evoked via each ear (filled bars, attend-right; open bars, read; grey bars, attend-left). Read condition – 'Read a novel and disregard the tones'. **b:** the P3 component of the ERP (indicated by the shaded area) evoked by signal tone pips in attended ear. (Hillyard et al., 1973, figs 1 and 2.)

processing. The P3, on the other hand, reflects the selective recognition of the higher pitched tones in the attended channel by a response set mechanism which is coupled with an appropriate cognitive response (counting) (Broadbent, 1970). (Hillyard et al., 1973, p. 179)

This conclusion is problematic. It shares the unclarities we have already noted in Broadbent's account, unclarities concerning the appropriate mode of describing the 'sensory input', and concerning the very idea of neurons 'analysing' anything, let alone engaging in anything that can be called 'perceptual analysis'. The supposition that sensory information is compared with memorized 'templates' or 'models' for selected stimuli is of doubtful intelligibility. For the only 'information' involved here is information in the information-theoretic sense, and that is not *sensory* information. Moreover, it is wholly unclear what can be meant by neural 'templates' or 'models'. Before we can accept this speculative (mechanical) hypothesis, we need to be told much more about what would *count* as a neural template or model. When we have some conception of what such a thing would be, we can speculate on and investigate whether there are any in the brain. The supposition that *there must be* is no more than the dogmatic application of an engineering principle to neurobiology.

2.4   Attention Related to Brain Structures

2.4.1   Superior colliculus

In 1973, Poppel, Held and Frost examined in humans the effects of flashing a light briefly in different locations on a monitor screen in the visual field of subjects with visual defects caused by gunshot wounds that had damaged area V1 of the visual cortex. They asked their subjects to look in the direction of the flash, and to their surprise found that subjects could sometimes do so, even though, as the subjects themselves complained, they could not actually see the flash. Following on this work, Weiskrantz and colleagues (1974) made a comprehensive study of the capacity of a subject (DB), who had parts of V1 removed in an operation on one hemisphere. In these studies, DB was asked to guess whether a line was vertical or non-vertical, on the one hand, or whether a letter was an 'X' or an 'O' when presented on a screen projecting to the 'blind' part of his visual field (the 'scotoma') Figs 2.8a and b show that, under conditions in which either the size of the symbols was increased (fig. 2.8a) or the duration over which they were presented was increased (fig. 2.8b), DB was able to guess correctly well above the chance level of 15 (the maximum score possible was 30), provided the stimulus was greater than a certain size or exceeded a certain duration.

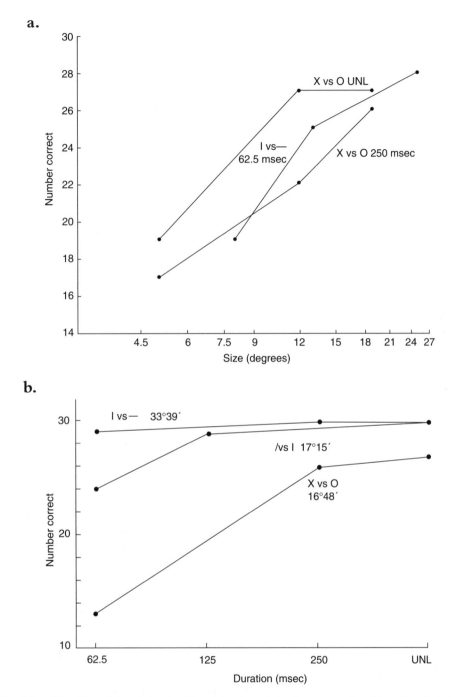

Fig. 2.8. The effect of size of stimulus (**a**) and duration of stimulus presentation (**b**) on forced-choice performance of a subject whose primary visual cortex (V1) was mostly removed by operation. UNL: unlimited duration; i.e. stimulus not extinguished until the subject responded. (Weiskrantz, 1986, figs 15 and 16.)

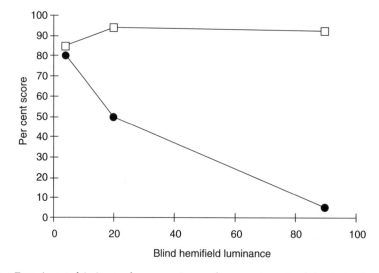

Fig. 2.9. Experiment claiming to show conscious and unconscious visual discrimination following lesions to primary visual cortex (V1). (Weiskrantz et al., 1995, fig. 2.)

This capacity of a subject with V1 missing was dubbed 'blindsight'. In all these experiments, DB had to make a choice (i.e. vertical or not, 'X' or 'O') even though he frequently commented that he saw nothing at all and was at a loss to describe any conscious perception. Thus object detection, it was argued, is in general not accompanied by any awareness. However, if the object was moving, DB sometimes reported that despite not seeing an object, he had a contentless kind of awareness of something happening and sensed a definite pinpoint of light. However, when questioned further, DB commented that what he sensed did not 'actually look like a light'.

Tests were made on DB in order to determine the extent to which the contrast between the light spot and its background on the monitor could be discriminated in the scotoma, with or without awareness. Fig. 2.9 depicts the results of such an experiment. Discrimination of horizontal or vertical motion of the light spot was made at different levels of contrast. The luminance of the light spot was held constant, and background luminance on the monitor was altered systematically, thus changing the contrast. DB had to indicate whether the spot was moving horizontally or vertically by pressing one of two keys. In addition, he had to indicate whether he was aware or not aware of the stimulus by pressing one of two other keys. The line of filled circles in fig. 2.9 indicates the percentage of trials in which DB signalled awareness. The line of open rectangles gives the percentage of trials when he signalled unawareness yet gave a correct response. The graph shows that there is a stable high level of performance independent of contrast, if only those occasions in which DB was unaware are counted. However, if only those occasions when DB was aware are considered, then there is a steep decline with a decrease in contrast of the object as a consequence of an increase in the background luminance level. This experiment shows that detection of the stimulus is excellent in the absence of acknowledged awareness but deteriorates rapidly for acknowledged awareness.

Weiskrantz (1986, p. 174) concludes his book on blindsight with the comment that 'the results, incomplete as they are, indicate unambiguously that the visual system damaged at the cortical level has a greater visual capacity for discrimination than is revealed by even quite searching clinical methods, or by the subject's own experience'. But this is not an illuminating characterization of the puzzling phenomenon. If 'the visual system' consists of those parts of the brain that enable a human being (or other animal) to see, then the *visual system* has no capacity for discrimination at all, since it is not the visual system that sees and discriminates, it is the human being, whose visual system endows him with the power of sight. But what one can say, and all one can say, is that human beings, with such-and-such damage to their visual system, display a greater sensitivity to visual phenomena in their scotoma than they are aware of.

The types of retinal ganglion cells that project to subcortical rather than cortical structures on the main visual pathway involving V1 structures, such as the superior colliculus that is involved in eye movement, have been identified. It is presumably the activity in these ganglion cells that mediates the capacity of DB to discriminate in the way indicated by fig. 2.8. Units in the superior colliculus of monkeys are selectively sensitive to flashed and moving stimuli. Indeed, while lesions to V1 block the capacity to identify visually presented objects, this does not interfere with detection and localization, which, as we know from animal studies, are dependent on the integrity of the superior colliculus. The residual function in DB's vision appears, then, to be related to the functioning superior colliculus.

In 1976, Wurtz and Mohler showed that neurons in the superior colliculus of primates are part of an eye movement system and are not involved in visual selective attention, so that the 'awareness' condition in blindsight patients is not likely to be associated with their intact superior colliculus, although their residual visual capacities, illustrated in figs 2.8 and 2.9 are. The original observations of Wurtz and Mohler (1976) involving training a monkey to fixate on a spot of light (the fixation point) for several seconds in order to detect a brief dimming of the spot, at which time the monkey released a bar and was rewarded by a drop of water (fig. 2.10a; Wurtz et al., 1982); if the monkey looked away from the fixation spot, he missed the dimming and so missed the reward. If the fixation spot went out and another came on, the monkey learnt to make a saccadic eye movement from the fixation point to the new point (fig. 2.10b). When the monkey fixated on the spot, the receptive fields of neurons in the superior colliculus were determined. On completion of this task, one point within the receptive field was chosen, and the response of the neuron to a spot of light at that point determined (see also fig. 2.11a). During these trials the monkey only had to look at the fixation point in order to obtain a reward, as the receptive field stimulus was not related to the reward. A new procedure was then introduced in which, when the spot in the receptive field came on, that at the fixation point went off. As the monkey knew from previous training sessions that the spot of light in the receptive field would eventually dim, providing an opportunity for a reward, the monkey made a saccade to the receptive field stimulus in order to detect the dimming more easily (fig. 2.10b and see also fig. 2.11b). This saccade was accompanied by vigorous firing of the neuron (fig. 2.10b and see also fig. 2.11b). Of considerable interest is the fact that the firing of the neuron was elevated before saccadic

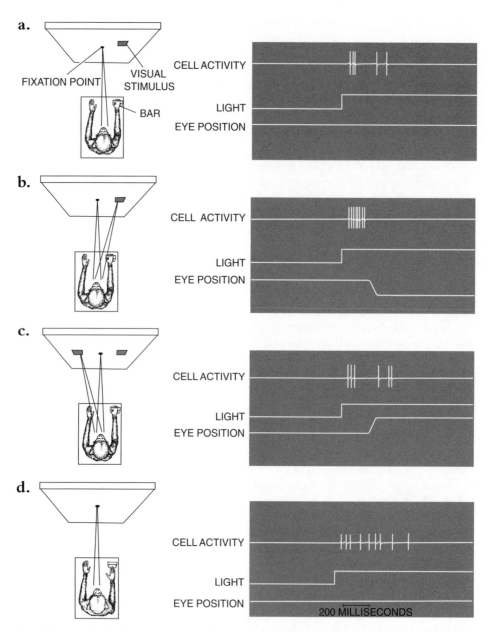

Fig. 2.10. Activity of neurons in a monkey's superior colliculus when a spot of light appears on a screen depends on how the monkey reacts to the spot. (Wurtz et al., 1982, p. 103A.)

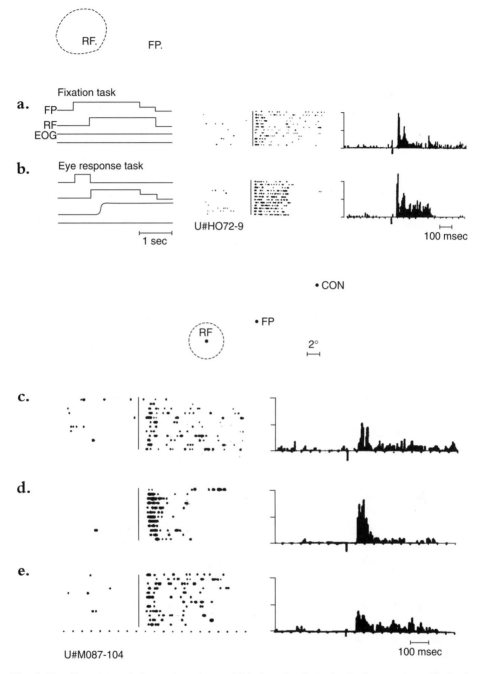

Fig. 2.11. Experimental observations that establish the role of neurons in the superior colliculus in eye movement regulation. (Wurtz et al., 1980, figs 3 and 5.)

eye movements were made (fig. 2.10b). The enhanced firing of the neuron is not due to the eye movements *per se*, as this firing does not occur before spontaneous eye movements made in the dark, and the enhanced firing begins in synchrony with the onset of the visual stimulus and not with that of the saccadic eye movement.

Fig. 2.11 illustrates the experimental observations that establish the role of neurons in the superior colliculus in eye movement regulation. The diagram on the upper left shows the location of the fixation point (FP), with the dashed circle outlining the extent of the excitatory central area of a visual receptive field (RF). The spot in the receptive field is the stimulus for experiment (a) and the saccade target for experiment (b). (a) (left) illustrates the time of onset of the fixation point, when the monkey fixates it, as indicated by the representative horizontal (top) and vertical (bottom) electro–oculogram traces (EOG). The receptive field stimulus comes on 0.5 seconds later. In the experiment for (b) (left) the fixation point comes on after the monkey presses the bar and then goes off when the light in the receptive field comes on. The monkey makes a saccadic eye movement to fixate the saccade target, as indicated by the deflection in the horizontal electro–oculogram trace. The data in (a) (right) show the consistent response of a superior colliculus cell to the spot of light in the receptive field while the monkey fixates. The data in (b) (right) show the enhanced response of this cell to the onset of the same stimulus when the monkey uses it as the target for a saccadic eye movement. Each dot represents an action potential, and each horizontal row of dots represents a single fixation trial for the monkey. The vertical line indicates the time of onset of the visual stimulus. Histograms sum the data in the adjacent dot pattern (raster) (Wurtz and Mohler, 1976).

That the enhanced firing described above is due to a selective increase of firing associated with eye movements to the receptive field is shown by the following experiment. When the fixation point goes off, two spots of light come on, so the monkey can saccade to either one of the stimuli (see fig. 2.10c and see also figs 2.11c–e). In this case, one spot of light was in the receptive field, and the other, the control stimulus, was outside the receptive field, as shown by lack of response of the neuron when the stimulus was presented alone. If the monkey made saccades to the receptive field spot, the usual increase in firing of the neuron was observed (fig. 2.10b and see fig. 2.11d), whereas when the saccades were made to the control spot, there was no large enhancement of firing (fig. 2.10c and see fig. 2.11e). Thus the increased firing of the neuron was spatially selective inasmuch as it was related to saccades made to the receptive field stimulus, but not to stimuli outside the receptive field. The increased firing was not related to general alerting or arousal effects involved in saccadic eye movements or to pupil dilation.

Fig. 2.11c–e shows the experimental observations which indicate that the increased firing of neurons during saccades to the receptive field spot was spatially selective. (c) shows the discharge of a collicular neuron to a spot of light in the receptive field (RF) and a control spot (CON) in the ipsilateral visual field while the monkey looks at the fixation point (FP). (d) shows the enhanced response on those trials when the monkey makes a saccadic eye movement to the receptive field stimulus, whereas (e) illustrates the lack of enhancement on the trials when the monkey saccades to the control stimulus. Since the stimulus conditions are the same in all three experiments, these data demonstrate that there is a selective increase in firing associated with eye movements to the receptive field (Wurtz and Mohler, 1976).

Wurtz and his colleagues concluded that neurons in the superior colliculus provide an eye movement system but do not contribute to a visual selective attention mechanism.

2.4.2   Parietal cortex

Clinical studies and experimental research have indicated for more than 100 years that the neurons in the posterior parietal cortex are involved in the mechanism underlying visual attention (Critchley, 1954). The attentional deficit in which humans neglect their contralateral visual field following damage to ipsilateral posterior parietal cortex is well established (see Heilman, 1979). In this case, presentation of a stimulus in the visual field of both hemispheres to a subject with damage to the right parietal cortex is followed by the subject's reporting that the stimulus is apparent only in the visual field contralateral to the normal hemisphere. On the other hand, if the stimulus is presented only in the visual field subserved by the damaged hemisphere and the subject told to attend to that field, he reports the presence of the stimulus. These observations indicate that the damaged parietal lobe has not led to sensory deficits, but rather that the subject is unable to select and attend to the stimulus in a complex environment. A dramatic example of this is provided by self-portraits made by the artist Anton Raederscheidt during his period of partial recovery from a stroke that affected his posterior parietal cortex in one hemisphere. Plate 2.1 shows four self-portraits carried out at successive times after the stroke, before he died, showing his failure to represent portions of his own body contralateral to the lesioned hemisphere. There is progressive recovery immediately after the stroke, although the final portrait (lower right-hand corner) still shows some deficits on the contralateral side.

In 1984 Posner and his colleagues investigated the extent to which humans can covertly attend to a target that is contralateral to a hemisphere with a parietal lobe lesion. In these experiments, subjects were required to keep their eyes fixed on the centre of a screen and to detect a bright square (the target) at one of two positions in the visual field ipsilateral and contralateral to their lesion. Prior to the target, cues were introduced (such as a pointing arrow) that directed the subject's attention either to the location of the target or to some other location. The reaction time to the target was measured as a function of the location of the cue and of the time between the appearance of the cue and of the target. On some occasions, the target occurred on one side of the cue, and in others, the target occurred equally often on both sides. The results of these experiments for patients with lesions in their right parietal lobe or left parietal lobe are shown in figs. 2.12a and b respectively. The continuous lines give the reaction times for different cue–target intervals for targets on the cued side, and broken lines give the reaction times for targets on the uncued side (triangles are contralateral targets and circles ipsilateral targets). It is evident that very long times occur when the target is contralateral to the hemisphere which is lesioned while the cue is ipsilateral, and that the longest reaction times are associated with right parietal lesions (fig. 2.12a). This effect of ipsilateral cues in slowing responses to contralateral targets recalls the notion of extinction as it is used in neurological testing of patients (Weinstein and Friedland, 1977). In this case, there is failure to perceive or respond to a stimulus contralateral to the lesion when presented with a simultaneous stimulus ipsilateral to the lesion. Such patients neglect stimuli contralateral to their lesioned hemisphere, as did the artist of Plate 2.1. However, they do not neglect such stimulus if instructed to attend to it, as is indicated by

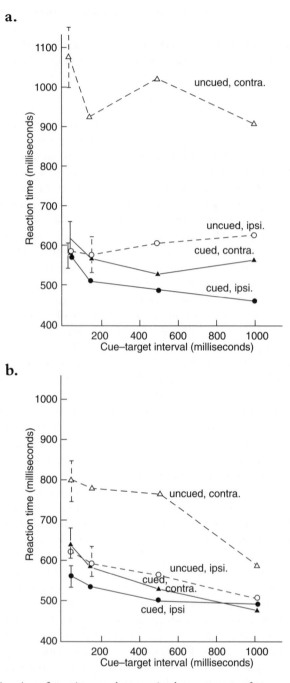

Fig. 2.12. Reaction times for patients to detect a visual target at one of two positions in the visual field ipsilateral and contralateral to their parietal cortex lesion. **a:** right parietal lesion. **b:** left parietal lesion. (Posner et al., 1984, figs 2 and 3.)

the cued contralateral experimental results of fig. 2.12. Nevertheless, without the cue or instruction, their relative neglect of stimuli in the contralateral visual field is reflected by the relatively very long reaction times indicated in fig. 2.12 for the case of uncued contra-lateral stimuli.

Neurons in the parietal cortex, as well as in the superior colliculus, also show enhanced firing when a spot is presented to monkeys in their receptive fields and a monkey makes a saccade to the spot. However, Bushnell, Goldberg and Robinson, following observations of Mountcastle (1976), discovered in 1981 that such neurons also showed considerably enhanced firing when the monkey correctly attended to the spot without a saccade from the fixation point. This is illustrated in fig. 2.13, which shows in (a) the response of a monkey's parietal neuron to the onset of a spot of light in its receptive field while the monkey fixated, with a much greater enhancement shown in (b) when the monkey was required to detect (attend to) the dimming of the spot while still fixating (the vertical lines denote when the stimulus was turned on, and the histograms sum the data in each horizontal scan). This figure also shows that another parietal neuron is slightly enhanced with the onset of a visual stimulus while the monkey fixates (fig. 2.13c), but shows a greatly increased firing when the spot was a target for a saccadic eye movement ('covert attention'; fig. 2.13d). A further increase occurs if there is a hand reach in the direction of the spot confirming the 'covert attention' (fig. 2.13e). Bushnell and colleagues (1981, p. 770) concluded their study with the comment that 'In studying neuronal discharge patterns, we can only propose that area 7 [parietal cortex] participates in a general mechanism for visual attention by providing an amplified signal corresponding to an important visual stimulus. The nature of the response that the animal will make to that stimulus is generated by other areas.'

Posner and his colleagues concluded from these experiments that

> The parietal lobe should be regarded as the neural system most responsible for the efficiency of processing that we associate with attention. . . . a covert attention shift provides an efficient routing of the stimulus to centres responsible for awareness (as measured by the ability to make an arbitrary response, such as a key press). . . . it appears that the attention–orienting system in the human may be asymmetric, in that right-side lesions have greater effects. While this result is consonant with much clinical observation, such hemispheric differences do not appear to be characteristic of the monkey. Moreover, we had thought it likely that the clinical observations arose because the right hemisphere was responsible for the spatial representation of the outside world rather than because the attention–orienting system was itself asymmetric. Thus, if our results had proven symmetric, we would have been inclined to the view that the act of orient-ing was controlled equivalently by the two hemispheres but that the spatial organization of the outside world was primarily a right-sided function. (Posner et al., 1984, p. 1873)

Note that by the phrase 'responsible for the spatial representation of the outside world' they must be presumed to mean 'responsible for the ability to see spatial relations'. Similarly, it is not the 'spatial organization of the outside world' that they might have supposed to be a 'right-sided function', but rather the *perception* of the spatial organization of visibilia.

Finally, Posner and his colleagues comment that 'It should be possible to determine whether the neural tissue involved in disengaging attention in these spatial tasks is also used

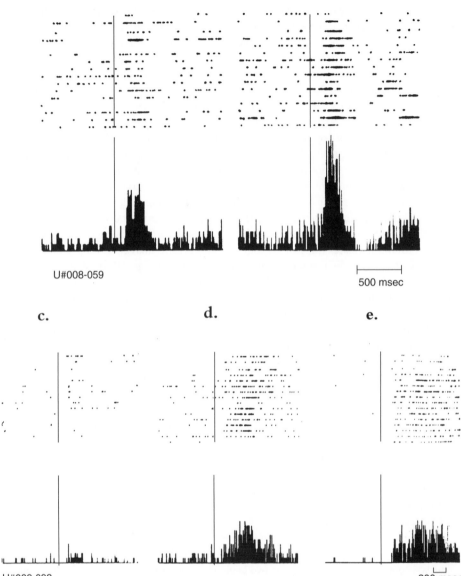

Fig. 2.13.   **a:** response of a parietal neuron to the onset of a spot of light in its receptive field while a monkey fixates. **b:** enhanced response to the onset of the same stimulus when the monkey was required to detect a dimming of the peripheral stimulus while fixating. **c–e:** enhancement in the same cell for eye and hand-reaching movements. **c:** the cell responds weakly to onset of a visual stimulus when the monkey fixates. The response to onset of the same stimulus is enhanced when the stimulus is a target for a saccadic eye movement (**d**) or a hand-reaching movement (**e**). (Bushnell et al., 1981, figs 5 and 9.)

for other nonspatial operations. Such findings would advance our understanding of the brain's control of cognition' (p. 1874).

2.4.3 Visual cortex

In chapter 1 we discussed evidence for the proposition that the visual cortex possesses two pathways, one concerned with feature analysis and object discrimination (the ventral 'what' pathway) and the other with the position of objects in space (the dorsal 'where' pathway). Moran and Desimone in 1985 investigated the question of whether spatial attention was associated with the gating of neuronal firing in the 'what' pathway (area V4). In their experiments, they first recorded the firing from a neuron in area V4, and determined its receptive field while the monkey fixated on a small target. Next they determined the most effective and ineffective stimuli, such as bars of various colours, orientations and sizes placed in the receptive field. Effective stimuli were then presented at one location in the receptive field concurrently with ineffective stimuli at a second location. The monkey was then trained on a task that required it to attend to the stimuli at one location but ignore the stimuli at the other. After a set of trials, the monkey was cued to switch its attention to the other location. Although the stimuli at the two locations remained the same, the animal's attention was repeatedly switched between the two locations. As the identical sensory conditions were maintained in the two types of blocks, any difference in the neuronal response could be attributed to the effects of attention. Fig. 2.14a shows the extent of firing of these neurons under the experimental conditions described above. The monkey attended to one location in the receptive field (RF) while fixating on a point and ignored the other. At the focus of attention, indicated by the circled 'searchlight of attention', two stimuli (sample and test) are presented sequentially. The monkey responded differently, depending on whether they were the same or different, as indicated by the density of dots under 'S' and 'T'. Irrelevant stimuli were presented simultaneously with the sample and test, but at a separate location in the receptive field. In the initial mapping of the receptive field, the cell responded well to horizontal and vertical red bars placed anywhere in the receptive field, but not at all to green bars of any orientation. Horizontal or vertical red bars (effective sensory stimuli) were then placed at one location in the field, and horizontal or vertical green bars (ineffective stimuli) at another. The responses shown are to horizontal red and vertical bars, but are representative of the responses to the other stimulus pairings. When the animal attended to the location of the effective stimulus at the time of presentation of either the sample (S) or the test (T), the cell gave a good response (left). But when the animal attended to the location of the ineffective stimulus, the cell gave almost no response (right), even though the effective stimulus was present in its receptive field. Thus the responses of the cell were determined by the object to which the animal was attending. Fig. 2.14b shows the same stimuli as in (a), but in this case the ineffective stimulus was placed outside the receptive field.

The neuron responded similarly to the effective sensory stimulus, regardless of the locus of attention. The neuron fires impulses when an object is presented within any part of a fairly large receptive field of the neuron. A red bar (hatched bar in fig. 2.14c presented anywhere within the area of this receptive field produced vigorous firing of the neuron, whereas a green bar (open bar in fig. 2.14c) failed to excite the neuron at all. The animal was then taught to attend to different locations within the receptive field, using an appropriate reward procedure. In the first experiment, the monkey attended to the location of the red bar (the attention being indicated in fig. 2.14c by a searchlight), while a green bar was also introduced into the receptive field; under these conditions the neuron fired vigorously, as shown in the lower part of fig. 2.14c. In the second experiment, the monkey was taught to attend to the location of the green bar (fig. 2.14d), even though the red bar was still within the receptive field of the neuron and might therefore be expected to cause vigorous firing of the neuron. It is clear that lack of attention to the red bar greatly decreases the rate of firing of the neuron. This experiment shows that neuronal mechanisms that are responsible for attention must be engaged in order for a neuron that is involved in visual phenomena of the kind described here to fire impulses at an optimal rate.

The conclusions reached from this study by Moran and Desimone are that:

> Our results indicate that attention gates visual processing by filtering out irrelevant fields of single extrastriate neurons. This role of attention is different from that demonstrated previously in the posterior parietal cortex, to our knowledge the only other cortical area in which spatially directed attention has been found to influence neural responses. In the posterior parietal cortex, some neurons show enhanced responses when an animal attends to a stimulus inside the neuron's receptive field compared to when the animal attends to a stimulus outside the field.
>
> Since parietal neurons have large receptive fields with little or no selectivity for stimulus quality, these cells may play a role in directing attention to a spatial location, but by themselves do not provide information about the qualities of attended stimuli. By contrast, in area V4 and the IT cortex selective attention may allow the animal to identify and remember the properties of a particular stimulus out of the many that may be acting on the retina at any given moment. If so, then the attenuation of response to irrelevant stimuli found in V4 and the IT cortex may underlie the attenuated processing of irrelevant stimuli shown psychophysically in humans. (Moran and Desimone, 1985, p. 784)

It is unclear what can be meant by the suggestion that *cells* may play a role in directing attention to a spatial location, as opposed to facilitating it. And it is surely confused to speak of cells *not providing information about the qualities of the stimuli*, since there is no such thing as a cell's *providing information* about anything. *Providing information* is not something a cell can intelligibly be said to fail to do (any more than a cell might fail to get married). What is evidently meant is that these cells play no role in enabling the subject to apprehend the qualities of some perceptual stimulus that has caught the subject's attention.

2.4.4 Auditory cortex

We noted in relation to fig. 2.7b that the P3 component of the auditory event related potential (ERP) was interpreted as due to sensory (auditory) information being 'compared with memorized "templates" or "models" for selected stimuli'. This P3 component of the ERP is generated when attention is drawn to infrequent novel stimuli. In 1989 Knight and his colleagues set out to determine the brain structures that produce the P3 component

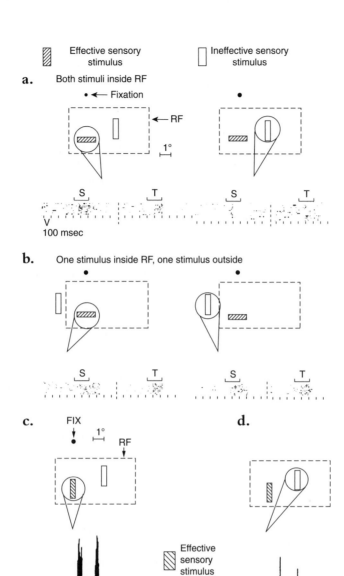

Fig. 2.14. The effect of selective attention on the responses of a neuron in monkey visual cortical area V4. (**a** and **b:** Moran and Desimone, 1985, fig. 1; **c** and **d:** Desimone et al., 1988, p. 172.)

of the auditory ERP in humans. Patients were studied with focal unilateral damage centred in the temporal-parietal junction. Fig. 2.15a shows the location of such a lesion, with the lines on the lateral reconstruction (upper left-hand corner) indicating the location of the axial sections used in CT scan transcription (1 to 7). The lesion was produced by an infarct of the parietal and temporal cortex caused by occlusion of the posterior trunk of the middle cerebral artery. In 1 to 7 the lesion of the patient is traced on to templates of horizontal brain sections through lower (top left, 1) and upper (lower right, 7) regions. In patients with lesions in this temporal-parietal junction the P3 component of the auditory ERP was eliminated, as shown in fig. 2.15b and c. In this figure, group-averaged ERPs were recorded to target and novel stimuli. The experiment consisted of patients listening to monaural tone bursts, presented at fixed 1.0 second intervals. Frequent standard tones occurred on 80 per cent of the trials. Infrequent target tones occurred randomly on 10 per cent of the trials. Novel sounds (unexpected complex tones and environmental noises) occurred randomly on 10 per cent of the trials. The solid lines in fig. 2.15b give the ERPs from control subjects (without lesions), the dotted lines from patients with temporal-parietal lesions, and the dashed lines from patients with just parietal lesions; scalp recordings are from sites both ipsilateral (subscript i) and contralateral (subscript c) to the lesioned hemisphere for patients or on the left and right for controls (F, C and P refer to an accepted international nomenclature for referring to the position of electrodes on the scalp for recording ERPs; the 'S' at the bottom of the figure refers to the time of onset of the stimulus). Note that lesions in the temporal-parietal junction (labelled in the figure 'temporal') abolished P3 (normally consisting of P3a and P3b components). The results show that the temporal-parietal junction in humans (containing the auditory association cortex) is required to be intact for auditory P3 generation. Knight et al. (1989, pp. 114–15) suggest that:

> The auditory P3 is generated by a neural system involved in orientation to and encoding of environmental events. . . . A Tpt (auditory association area)-mesial temporal network has been proposed to be critical for acoustic learning and memory in animals and humans and area cSTP (multimodal area) has been implicated in the control of global attention. The present results suggest that the auditory P3 is generated by engagement of these regions during encoding of significant environmental events in humans.

The use of the phrase 'during encoding' is singularly unhelpful. To notice something, or to focus one's attention upon something, is not to encode anything. One must presume that what is meant in this context is no more than 'during the apprehension of significant events'.

2.5   Conclusion

The introduction in the late 1980s of non-invasive imaging techniques to measure regional cerebral blood flow (rCBF) using positron emission tomography (PET) made it possible to determine which regions of the brain are active during attention to specific stimuli (Petersen

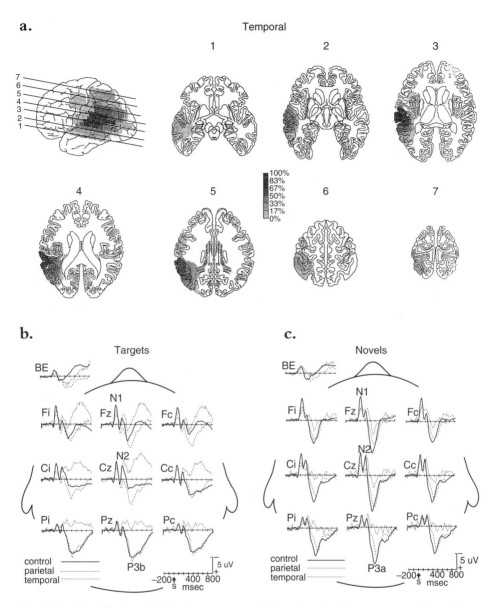

Fig. 2.15. Identification of the brain structures which produce the P3 component of the auditory evoked response potential (ERPs) in humans. The P3 component is generated when attention is drawn to infrequent novel stimuli. **a:** lesion extent in patients with focal unilateral damage centred in the temporal-parietal junction. **b** and **c:** group-averaged ERPs recorded in response to target and novel stimuli in a monoaural tone detection task. (Knight et al., 1989, figs 1 and 3.)

et al., 1988; Posner et al., 1988). In 1991 Corbetta and his colleagues showed that attention to visual features such as form, movement and colour activated different regions outside the primary visual cortex area V1. They comment that:

> It is a common experience that searching for a friend in a crowd is aided by the knowledge that he or she is wearing a red coat. The ability to select, or focus on, a small fraction of the incoming sensory information eases the computational load in analysing environmental scenes and planning responses coherent with behavioural goals. Understanding how the brain solves the problem of selecting relevant information is a major goal of both cognitive and neural sciences. (Corbetta et al., 1991, p. 2383)

It is noteworthy that here too, as in the older experimental approaches to the study of attention described above, the computational language of information technology is invoked without any obvious warrant, and indeed without any genuine explanatory role. What someone attends to when searching for a friend known to be wearing a red coat is the colour of the garments worn by people in his visual field, not 'a small fraction of the incoming sensory information'. What can be said to be 'incoming' is the light that hits the retinae, but since that is not what a person *sees*, it is not something that he could possibly attend to. Moreover, even if he could attend to the light hitting his retinae, it would be the wrong thing to attend to if he wanted to spot his red-coated friend. Similarly, what passes from the retinae to the visual cortex is not sensory information, but electrical impulses, and whatever the brain or its parts can be said to do to these, it surely cannot be described as 'analysing environmental scenes'. Finally, it is mistaken to suppose that *the brain* 'solves the problem of selecting information'. It makes no sense to speak of the brain's solving problems, understanding or misunderstanding problems. That is something that human beings, not brains, do. And for the same reason, it makes no sense to suppose that the brain could *select information* relevant to solving a problem. Rather, the normal function of the brain enables *the human being* to select information relevant to the problems the human being wishes to solve. As this chapter has emphasized, it is human beings that pay attention, not their brains or parts of their brains.

3

Memory and Cortical Function: Milner to Kandel

3.1 Memory

3.1.1 The hippocampus is required for memory, which decays at two different rates

Brenda Milner and her colleagues discovered in the 1950s that the medial structures of the temporal lobe in humans, including the hippocampus, are important for memory. Studies on the patient H.M., who had undergone a bilateral resection of these medial structures in an attempt to prevent severe epileptic seizures, were particularly informative. Although H.M. was able to converse about immediate events if not distracted, there was no retention of non-verbal stimuli for longer than a minute. Indeed, even the retention of verbal memory depended on his continual use of mnemonic schemes. Once his attention was diverted and these were lost, the memory was not retrieved. Thus, there was a loss of perceptual memory and of verbal memory so that what had been apprehended was forgotten within less than a minute (Milner and Taylor, 1972). These studies were confirmed in other patients who had undergone temporal lobe resection and who also had varying degrees of retrograde amnesia after the operation that extended from months to years (fig. 3.1a and b; Scoville and Milner, 1957; Penfield and Milner, 1958; Milner, 1965a, b). The components of the medial temporal lobe that are necessary for memory were subsequently established as the hippocampal formation together with the adjacent perirhinal and parahippocampal cortices (Squire and Zola-Morgan, 1991). The studies of H.M. by Milner and others led to the conclusion that there was a gradual decline in the ability of H.M. to retain new perceptual memories over a period of about a minute, indicating that there were two kinds of processes in the brain that underpin memory, one with a rapid decay and the other of much longer duration which in normal people allows them to remember over long periods of months or years (fig. 3.1c; Milner, 1972).

3.1.2 Memory is of two kinds: declarative and non-declarative

Further studies of H.M. by Milner and others, in which H.M. was challenged, for instance, to learn new visual and motor skills such as those required in drawing objects observed in a mirror, showed that he could learn and retain these skills in a normal way even though

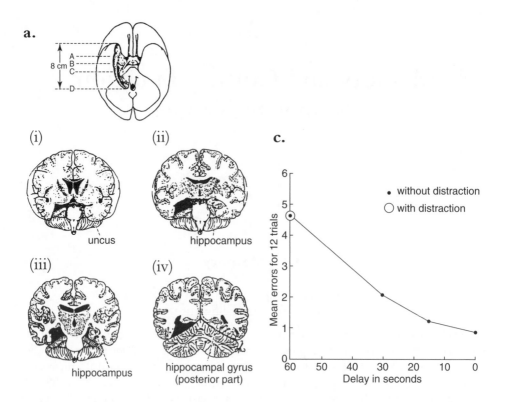

a.

8 cm — A, B, C, D

(i) uncus

(ii) hippocampus

(iii) hippocampus

(iv) hippocampal gyrus (posterior part)

c.

Mean errors for 12 trials (y-axis, 0–6)
Delay in seconds (x-axis: 60, 50, 40, 30, 20, 10, 0)

• without distraction
○ with distraction

b.

Classification of cases

Cases	Age at time of follow-up (yr.)	Sex	Diagnosis	Operation	Bi- or uni-lateral	Approximate extent of removal along medial temporal lobes (cm)	Time between operation and testing (months)	Wechsler scale Intelligence Quotient	Wechsler scale Memory Quotient
Group I: Severe memory defect									
Case 1, H. M.	29	M	Epilepsy	Medial temporal	B	8	20	112	67
Case 2, D. C.	47	M	Paranoid schizophrenia	Medial temporal and orbital undercutting	B	5.5	21	122	70
Case 3, M. B.	55	F	Manic-depressive psychosis	Medial temporal	B	8	28	78	60
Group II: Moderate memory defect									
Case 4, A. Z.	35	F	Paranoid schizophrenia	Medial temporal	B	5	40	96	84
Case 5, M. R.	40	F	Paranoid schizophrenia	Medial temporal and orbital undercutting	B	5	39	123	81
Case 6, A. R.	38	F	Hebephrenic schizophrenia	Medial temporal and orbital undercutting	B	4.5	47	Incomplete	
Case 7, C. G.	44	F	Schizophrenia	Medial temporal	B	5.5	41	Incomplete	
Case 8, A. L.	31	M	Schizophrenia	Medial temporal	B	6	38	Incomplete	
Group III: No memory defect									
Case 9, I. S.	54	F	Paranoid schizophrenia	Uncectomy	B	4	53	122	125
Case 10, E. G.	55	F	Incisural herniation	Inferior temporal lobectomy	U-Rt.	9	16	93	90

he could not remember ever having been trained in these skills on previous occasions (Milner, 1962; Milner et al., 1968). This work initiated research on the possibility that there is more than one kind of memory that is manifest in behaviour. Subsequent research in neuroscience has endorsed this view and so come to distinguish between two main forms of memory: declarative memory (that is explicit) and non-declarative memory (that is implicit). Declarative memory is held to be 'what is ordinarily meant by the term memory'; it is 'propositional'; it can be true or false; and it is involved 'in modelling the external world and storing representations about facts and episodes' (Milner et al., 1998, p. 450). It is roughly equivalent to what can be expressed by the phrase 'remembers that such-and-such'. Non-declarative memory, which is roughly equivalent to 'remembering how (to do something)', is concerned with the retention of motor skills (as are involved in driving a motor car). It is held to be manifest in the procedure called 'priming' whereby one is better able to identify or carry out procedures as a consequence of previous encounters or training, a process that depends on the integrity of the neocortex. Non-declarative memory has also been taken to be involved in classical conditioning (as in the eye-blink response, see below) and sensitization (in which there is a strengthening of a reflex response to a previously neutral stimulus, following the presentation of a noxious stimulus), each of which can be found early in phylogenesis (fig. 3.2; Carew et al., 1983; Carew and Sahley, 1986). We argue below in §3.2.1 that conditioning and sensitization are not forms of cognition at all, and that since memory is essentially the retention of knowledge acquired, the term 'non-declarative memory' should not be applied to these cases.

Furthermore, each of these forms of non-declarative memory are taken to possess both short (minutes) and long (days) time courses (Carew and Sahley, 1986). One example of non-declarative memory is indicated in the rabbit eye-blink response, involving a classical conditioning paradigm, for which the neuronal pathway has been determined. The conditioning stimulus used is a tone and the unconditioned stimulus an air-puff with the conditioned response being an eye-blink from the rabbit. This work showed that a neural network involving the cerebellum is required in this form of what is alleged to be non-declarative memory (Thompson and Krupa, 1994).

Another form of putative non-declarative memory involves emotional responses. Memories which have their behavioural manifestation in fear are dependent on the integrity of the amygdala. Joseph LeDoux's work indicates that rats show such behaviour towards a

---

Fig. 3.1 (opposite)   The hippocampus is required for memory in humans. a: diagrammatic cross-sections of human brain illustrating extent of attempted bilateral medial temporal lobe resection in the radical operation (for diagrammatic purposes the resection has been shown on one side only. (Scoville and Milner, 1957, fig. 2.) **b:** table shows the histories and individual test results for 10 cases following hippocampal lesions. These cases have been divided into three groups representing different degrees of memory impairment. (Scoville and Milner, 1957, table 1.) **c:** effect of bilateral medial temporal lobe resection on the ability to compare stimuli that are separated by a short time interval. The graph shows the mean error scores of patient H.M., for five tasks, as a function of the intratrial interval. Six errors would be chance performance. (Prisko, 1963, p. 126, and Milner, 1972, fig. 25.2.)

harmless stimulus such as a tone if this is coupled with a mild electric shock in a fear conditioning task (LeDoux, 1995a, b). Later work supports the idea that LeDoux's identification of the amygdala in rats as required for the consolidation of what have come to be called emotional memories also holds for humans (Damasio, 1994). Electrical stimulation of the amygdala produces feelings of apprehension and environmental stimuli that engender fear in humans and involves an increase in neuronal activity in the amygdala (LeDoux, 1995a, b). The fact that the amygdala is involved in the non-declarative experience of fear is emphasized by LeDoux in his comment that it is 'possible for your brain to know that something is good or bad before it knows exactly what it is' (LeDoux, 1998, p. 69). Knowing what it is, involves the declarative memory systems of the brain, whereas the experience of good or bad involves the non-declarative systems such as the amygdala.

3.1.3   Cellular and molecular studies of non-declarative memory in invertebrates

The existence of so-called non-declarative forms of memory in the invertebrates, such as the gill withdrawal reflex in *Aplysia*, feeding in *Limax*, and phototaxis in *Hermissenda* provided relatively simple preparations, compared with those in the vertebrates, to study the neuronal changes accompanying various forms of putative non-declarative memory. Kandel and his colleagues have searched for the molecular changes in neurons and their synapses that occur during the different temporal phases of supposed non-declarative memory that are manifest in sensitization of the gill withdrawal reflex in the sea slug *Aplysia* (fig. 3.2). They have shown that both the short- and long-term changes in this reflex can be traced to short and long-term changes in the increases in efficacy of synapses between the sensory neuron and the motoneuron that is responsible for the movement of muscles in the reflex (Carew et al., 1983; Byrne and Kandel, 1996).

The short-term enhancement over minutes following a single trial is due to the release of serotonin (5-hydroxytryptamine) from interneurones that are activated by the sensitizing stimulus. The serotonin activates cAMP-dependent protein kinase A (PKA) and protein kinase C (PKC) which in turn produce covalent modifications in proteins that directly modify transmitter release from the sensory terminal on to the motoneuron. In sensitization of the gill withdrawal reflex, the PKA closes potassium channels in the sensory terminal that results in an increase in the duration of the action potential initiated in the terminal and so increases the calcium influx and transmitter release, as well as directly acts on the machinery responsible for the exocytosis of transmitter from the sensory terminals (Castellucci et al., 1978). The long-term enhancement over at least days, following repeated trials, is due to the translocation of PKA and a mitogen recruited by PKA — namely, mitogen-activated protein kinase (MAPK) — to the nucleus of the sensory neurons. Here, the kinases activate CREB1 (a cAMP response element-binding protein), which in turn activates immediate response genes whose products are responsible for the increase in efficacy of transmission from the sensory neuron to the motoneuron, which is at least in part due to the formation of new transmitter release sites (Bartsch et al., 1995). This work has led to a model of non-declarative memory at the molecular level in which short-term memory is dependent on covalent modifications of pre-existing proteins leading to an increase in the

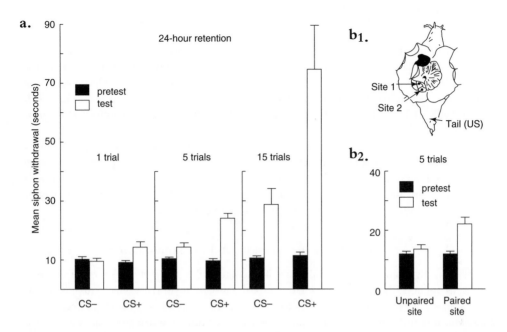

Fig. 3.2. Differential classical conditions of a defensive withdrawal reflex in *Aplysia californica*. The defensive siphon and gill withdrawal reflex of *Aplysia* is a simple reflex mediated by a well-defined neural circuit. This reflex exhibits classical conditioning when a weak tactile stimulus to the siphon is used as a conditioned stimulus and a strong shock to the tail is used as an unconditioned stimulus. The siphon withdrawal component of this reflex can be differentially conditioned when stimuli applied to two different sites on the mantle skin (the mantle shelf and the siphon) are used as discriminative stimuli. The differential conditioning can be acquired in a single trial, is retained for more than 24 hours, and increases in strength with increased trials.

a: the effect of the number of training trials on differential conditioning. Different groups of animals were given 1, 5, and 15 trials and tested twice, once within 1 hour after training (not shown) and again 24 hours later. A significant differential effect was present after one trial, and the differential effect increased progressively with more trials. Sensitization (comparing pretest and test conditioned stimulus scores) was not evident after one trial, but did appear after 5 trials and was larger after 15 trials.

b: differential conditioning of two sites on the siphon skin. **b₁:** dorsal view, illustrating the approximate location of the two implanted conditioned stimulus electrodes in the siphon and the unconditioned stimulus electrodes in the tail. **b₂:** pooled test scores from paired and unpaired sites compared to their respective pretest scores. Significant differential conditioning was exhibited 15–30 minutes after 5 training trials. (Carew et al., 1983, fig. 2.)

efficacy of transmission at the synapses in which this occurs. Long-term memory arises as a consequence of CREB-mediated activation of gene expression giving rise to the formation of new transmitter release sites. Genetic studies using *Drosophila*, which in part parallel those on *Aplysia*, have emphasized the role of the cAMP pathway and of CREB in the generation of both short- and long-term non-declarative forms of memory (Yin et al., 1995).

These experiments, and those on the other invertebrate preparations mentioned above, have been taken to point to the fact that there are no specialized neuronal networks committed to these simple forms of 'non-declarative memory'. Rather, it is modification of the efficacy of synapses working in the pathways that produce the reflexes under investigation, which, it is argued, is responsible for 'non-declarative memory'.

3.1.4   Declarative memory and the hippocampus

The claim by Milner and her colleagues in the late 1950s and early 1960s that the hippocampus might be the main site in the brain for the processing of recent declarative memories was followed by the discovery of O'Keefe and Dostrovsky (1971) that a particular set of pyramidal neurons in the rodent hippocampus fire optimally when the rodent is in a particular place (fig. 3.3). This initiated a period of intense study of the properties of these neurons as 'place cells' and of the hippocampus as essential for the declarative memory involved in identifying a particular place. Although rodents cannot 'declare' anything, the study of place cells in these animals has proceeded on the assumption that such cells also occur in humans. Research and speculation on this topic in the 1970s is summarized in the fascinating book *The Hippocampus as a Cognitive Map* (O'Keefe and Nadel, 1978). Subsequent work has supported the idea that a unique set of pyramidal neurons is active when an animal is in a particular area, identified as the neurons' 'place field'. New place fields are formed over periods of minutes when a rodent enters a new environment; but once they are formed, they remain for long periods of the order of months. Each pyramidal neuron in the hippocampus, which participates in the formation of a place field, can also participate in the formation of other such fields.

How are these place field cells in the hippocampus of rodents detected? A mouse, for instance, will have its head fitted with a device connected to electrodes that are placed in the hippocampus so as to record action potentials from one or several pyramidal (place) cells. In addition, a light source is attached to the head so as to be able to record the location of the mouse with an overhead TV camera as it moves. Next, the mouse is placed in a round chamber and a cable connected to the device so that recordings of the firing of the cells can be made as the mouse moves around the chamber, its location being ascertained by the light source and TV camera. In this way, the firing rate of the neurons can be correlated with the position of the mouse as it explores the environment of the round chamber. It is found that as the mouse explores the chamber, having previously been introduced to the chamber before the recording session, each place cell fires action potentials only when the mouse is in a particular location in the chamber. If the mouse is returned to the chamber at some later time, the place cells retain their specificity and fire action potentials only when the animal occupies the same location that it did on the

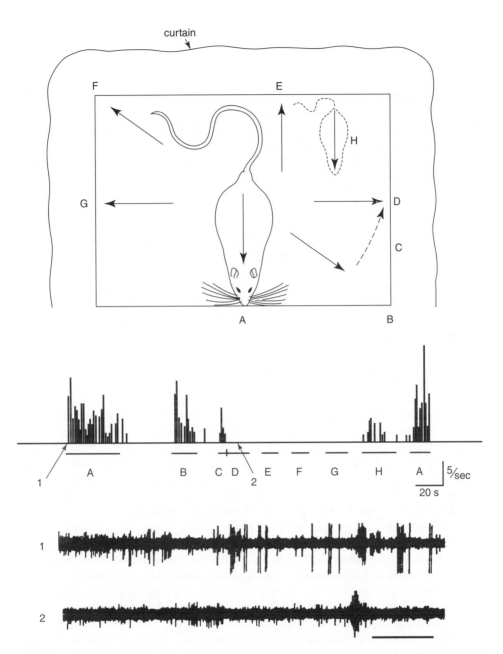

Fig. 3.3. The discovery of neurons in the hippocampus that fire optimally when the animal is in a particular place. Responses of a hippocampal (CA1) neuron to a restraining tactile stimulus as a function of the rat's spatial orientation. The arrows and associated letters mark the positions at which the animal was restrained as it was pushed or coaxed in a counter-clockwise direction around the test platform. The firing rate of the neuron during this procedure is illustrated by the continuous frequency histogram in the middle of the figure. The letters correspond to the positions, and the lines indicate the periods when the rat was restrained. In between these periods, the rat sat immobile in the same position for a few seconds and then was moved on to the next position. The bottom two lines show the raw data taken at the onset of the neuron response at A (1) and during the absence of a response at D (2). Time calibration for these data is 400 msec. (O'Keefe and Dostrovsky, 1971, fig. 1.)

previous occasions when these place cells fired. This procedure defined the meaning of 'place cells'.

This important work of Milner and her colleagues has been accepted as showing that the hippocampus is central to the 'laying down' of declarative memories. The contribution of O'Keefe and his colleagues has been taken as identifying the participation of particular hippocampal neurons in a particular form of declarative memory. Both these contributions initiated a tremendous amount of interest in this structure in the last decades of the twentieth century. The reason for this interest arises from the premiss that conscious declarative memory probably 'provides the possibility of recreating in memory a specific episode from the past' (Squire and Kandel, 1999, p. 212), with this memory being 'laid down' in the hippocampus. The fact that there is a convergence of synaptic inputs from a great deal of the neocortex to the medial temporal lobe, and from there to the hippocampus, led naturally to the suggestion that the different neocortical regions that are engaged when one is perceiving something 'send information' concerning this perception to the hippocampus. There, 'the resulting memories are stored as changes in strength at many synapses within a large ensemble of interconnected neurons' (Squire and Kandel, 1999, p. 212). These stored memories in the brain then enable one to 'recreate in memory' a past episode. We shall consider further, in §3.2.2, the coherence of these claims.

3.1.5   Long-term potentiation (LTP) of synaptic transmission in the hippocampus

The first intracellular recordings of synaptic transmission to the pyramidal cells in the hippocampus by Kandel et al. (1991) as well as by Andersen et al. (1963) were made at the time of Milner's pathfinding investigations implicating this structure in declarative memory. However, these early investigations on transmission did not consider the possibility that long-term changes might be sought in the efficacy of transmission at these synapses, and that these might subserve the neuronal mechanisms involved in establishing a declarative memory. This was left to Lomo (1966), who showed that stimulation of the entorhinal input to the granule cells of the hippocampus could give rise to an increase in efficacy of transmission at the synapses formed on the granule cells which lasted for hours, an observation later verified by Bliss and Lomo (1970). Subsequent work showed that these increases in synaptic transmission, referred to as long-term potentiation (LTP), could last for periods of months following the initial period of stimulus conditioning (figs. 3.4d and e). Bliss and his colleagues were well aware of the potential that this discovery of LTP might have in providing a mechanistic explanation for the observations of Milner: 'Our experiments show that there exists at least one group of synapses in the hippocampus whose efficiency is influenced by activity which may have occurred several hours previously – a time scale long enough to be potentially useful for information storage' (Bliss and Lomo, 1973, see fig. 3.4).

The problem posed by this prescient comment concerning whether LTP is involved in a memory process in the hippocampus is still not resolved. However, much has been revealed concerning how LTP is induced and maintained as a consequence of intense study of the phenomenon over the past decade or so. McNaughton et al. (1978) showed that the induction of LTP at synapses following high-frequency stimulation is a cooperative process requiring coactivity of a large number of axons. Their research led to the conclusion that 'the results of these two sets of studies separately and jointly indicate that enhancement (LTP) is a cooperative phenomenon'. They saw this work as contributing to the 'minimal logical requirement for a physical theory of associative memory': namely, that 'there be some change in the potential for interaction between input and output elements of a system, resulting from use. This change must be such that a previous output may be reactivated by some subset of the corresponding previous input' (p. 14).

At the end of 1983, three facts had been established concerning the induction of associative LTP. They were: (i) that a threshold depolarization is necessary; (ii) that NMDA (*N*-methyl-D-aspartate) receptors must be occupied by the transmitter glutamate (fig. 3.5a–c; Collingridge et al., 1983); and (iii) that an increase in calcium in the postsynaptic cell is necessary (Lynch et al., 1983). The work of Nowak et al. (1984; and fig. 3.5d) provided a complete explanation for both the voltage-dependent properties of the NMDA receptor and the criteria that had to be met for the induction of associative LTP. Their work indicated that in magnesium-free solutions, glutamate opens voltage-independent cation channels, but that in the presence of physiological levels of magnesium, the single-channel currents measured at the resting potential are chopped into bursts, and the probability of the channels opening is greatly reduced. The voltage dependence of the NMDA receptor-linked conductance increase to cations is, therefore, attributed to the voltage dependence of the magnesium block. In the case of the induction of LTP, the fact that a threshold number of axons that form synapses on NMDA receptors must be stimulated follows from the requirement that in order for these receptors to allow cations to pass in any quantities, it is first necessary to remove the magnesium block of the channels by depolarization (Wigstrom and Gustafsson, 1985a, b). As these cations include calcium ions, the open NMDA channel provides a major pathway for increasing the calcium concentration in the postsynaptic cell, thus fulfilling the intracellular calcium requirement for the induction of LTP.

Elaboration of this scheme also provides an explanation for how the NMDA receptor mediated LTP is associative. Consistent with the above observations, Wigstrom and his colleagues (Wigstrom et al., 1986b) as well as Malinow and Miller (1986) showed that LTP could be induced by pairing single afferent volleys with intracellularly injected depolarizing current pulses in the postsynaptic cell, and that LTP could be blocked by intracellular injection of hyperpolarizing currents in the cell during conditioning high-frequency volleys (fig. 3.6). These results explain why a strong conditioning input coincident with a weak input leads to potentiation of the response of the weak input: postsynaptic depolarization induced by the strong input is electrotonically propagated to the site of the weak input so that the summed depolarization at the weak input is sufficient to remove magnesium ions from the NMDA receptors that have been activated by glutamate there, thus allowing an influx of calcium ions to occur at the weak input, leading to an induction of LTP at the previously weak synapses.

The question next arises as to why this associative LTP should be confined to just the excited synapses if a rise in intracellular calcium in the postsynaptic cell is to be taken as the necessary and sufficient condition for induction. Why do not all the terminals on the cell, once calcium increases, have LTP induced? One possible explanation for this is that only synapses on the spinous processes of pyramidal cells possess NMDA receptors. In this

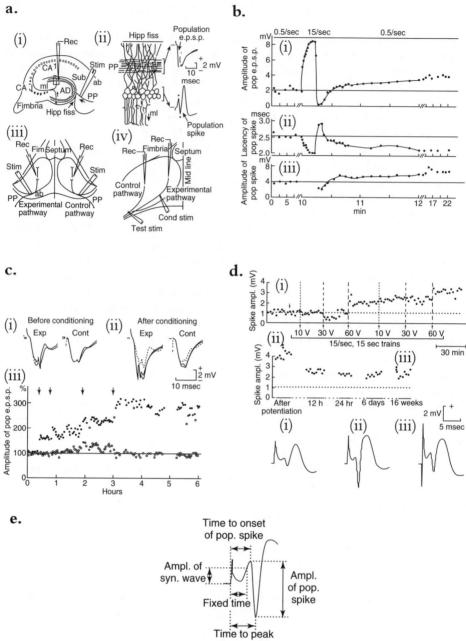

Fig. 3.4. The discovery of long-term potentiation (LTP). a(i): diagrammatic parasagittal section through the hippocampal formation, showing a stimulating electrode placed beneath the angular bundle to activate perforant path fibres (pp), and a recording microelectrode in the molecular layer of the dentate area. (ii): the region enclosed in the rectangle in (i), enlarged to show the apical dendritic field of the granule cells, with the perforant path fibres confined to the central one-third of the field. The population responses evoked by a strong perforant path volley in the synaptic layer (upper trace) and in the cell body layer (lower trace) are displayed on the right. The spots (lower trace) mark the peaks between which the amplitude of the population spike was measured. (iii): arrangement of electrodes for experiments in which the control pathway was situated in the contralateral hippocampus. (iv): electrode arrangement for experiments in which both test and control pathways were on the same side. Abbreviations: ab, angular bundle; AD, dentate area; CA$_1$, CA$_3$, pyramidal fields CA$_1$ and CA$_3$; Fim, fimbria; Hipp fiss, hippocampal fissure; inf, mossy fibres; pp, perforant path. (Bliss and Lomo, 1973, fig. 2). **b:** frequency potentiation and the immediate after-effects of a conditioning train. The graphs show the changes produced in three parameters of the evoked response by increasing the rate at which the perforant path was stimulated from 0.5 sec to 15 sec for 15 sec. The points obtained during the conditioning train and the following 1 min 45 sec are shown on an expanded time scale. Note immediately after the train the brief period of spike potentiation followed by depression, and the subsequent maintained potentiation. The value of the population excitatory postsynaptic potential (EPSP) during the train could not be accurately measured from the film record and is not plotted. (Bliss and Lomo, 1973, fig. 2). **c:** an experiment in which all three standard parameters of the evoked response were potentiated. Three superimposed responses obtained in the synaptic layer for both the experimental and the control pathways are shown in (i) (before conditioning) and in (ii) (2–5 hours after the fourth conditioning train). (iii): Graph showing the amplitude of the population EPSP for the experimental pathway (•) and the ipsilateral control pathway (○) as a function of time. Each point was obtained from the computed average of 30 responses by measuring the amplitude of the negative wave 1 msec after its onset. The values are plotted as percentages of the mean preconditioning value. Conditioning trains (15/1 sec for 10 sec) were given through a medially placed conditioning electrode at the times indicated by the arrows. (Bliss and Lomo, 1973, fig. 4). **d:** measurements of spike amplitude (from averages of 16 responses to 30 V stimuli) plotted as several trains of stimuli (15-1 sec, 15 sec) were given at the indicated strengths, and at various indicated times afterwards. The approximate mean spike amplitude before the conditioning trains is shown by the dotted lines. Average responses at the times marked i, ii, and iii are shown beneath. (Bliss and Gardner-Medwin, 1973, fig. 7). **e:** a typical average response recorded using a computer, with the derived parameters labelled on it. Average of 16 responses. (Bliss and Gardner-Medwin, 1973, fig. 1).

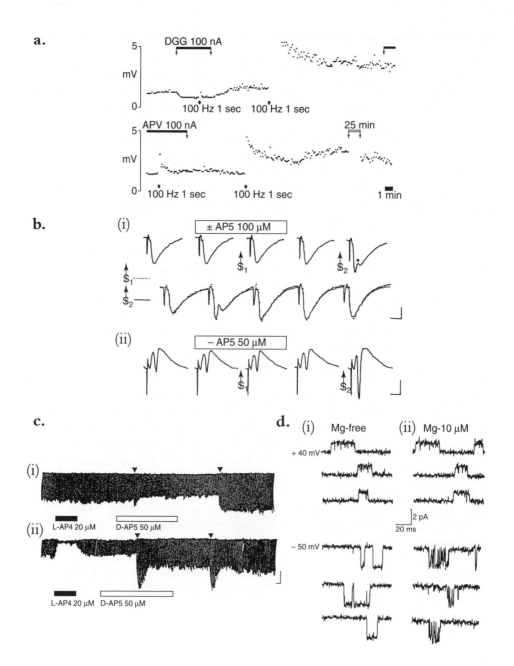

a.

DGG 100 nA

5

mV

0

100 Hz 1 sec   100 Hz 1 sec

APV 100 nA

5

mV

0

25 min

100 Hz 1 sec   100 Hz 1 sec   1 min

b. (i)

± AP5 100 μM

$_1

$_2

(ii)

− AP5 50 μM

$_1 $_2

c.

(i)

(ii)

L-AP4 20 μM   D-AP5 50 μM

L-AP4 20 μM   D-AP5 50 μM

d. (i) Mg-free   (ii) Mg-10 μM

+ 40 mV

2 pA

20 ms

− 50 mV

Fig. 3.5. **N-methyl-D-aspartate (NMDA) receptors implicated in associative long-term potentiation (LTP). a:** effects on the population spike and on the generation of LTP of NMDA receptor antagonists. The amplitude of the population spike was recorded in stratum pyramidal in response to 0.1 Hz stimulation of the Schaffer collateral-commissural projection, and antagonists were administered ionophoretically in stratum radiatum for the durations indicated by the bars. The pathway was stimulated at 100 Hz at the times shown by the arrows below the trace. Gamma-D-glutamyl glycine (DGG) reduced the amplitude of the population spike and prevented LTP in response to high-frequency stimulation. Following recovery from the effects of DGG, LTP was produced using a period of identical high-frequency stimulation. After 17 min, the NMDA antagonist DL-2-amino-5-phosphononalerate (APV) was applied and had no effect on the population spike; 2 min later the stimulus intensity was reduced (lower record), and 3 min later the effects of high-frequency stimulation were again tested. Although some short-lasting post-tetanic potentiation resulted, LTP was prevented. After the APV injection had been terminated for 8 min, 100 Hz stimulation for 1 sec was again able to produce LTP, which did not recover completely over the time that responses were measured (45 min). (Collingridge et al., 1983, fig. 5.) **b:** effects of NMDA receptor antagonist ±AP5 on Schaffer collateral response LTP. Constant current biphasic pulses were delivered to a bipolar electrode placed on the Schaffer collateral fibers in stratum radiatum of CA1 at one every 20 sec. A series of three high-frequency trains (50 or 100 Hz for 1 sec, one every 20 sec) was delivered at the times indicated by S_1 and S_2. Antagonist was present in the medium bathing the slice during the time indicated by the bar. (i): upper trace: responses recorded by an electrode placed in stratum radiatum. Representative responses from the following conditions: before and during drug application; ten minutes after the first high-frequency stimulation (S_1) following drug washout; and 10 min after the second high-frequency stimulation (S_2). Following the high-frequency stimulation in the absence of drug (S_2), the synaptic response is increased in amplitude, and a population spike appears (fifth trace, asterisk). Lower trace: frequency potentiation during the high-frequency stimulation. The first five responses recorded during high-frequency stimulation in the presence of ±AP5 (S_1) and after washout (S_2) are superimposed (dotted and solid traces respectively). (ii): extracellular evoked responses recorded by an electrode placed near the CA1 pyramidal cell layer. Experiment as in part i, except that the (—) isomer of AP5 (final concentration 50 μM) was applied before the first high-frequency stimulation (S_1). Calibration bars, 1 mV, 5 msec. (Harris et al., 1984, fig. 2) **c:** comparison of L- and D- isomers of AP4 and AP5 on the induction of LTP. L-AP4 and D-AP5 were present during the intervals indicated by the bars. High-frequency stimulation as delivered at the times indicated by arrowheads. The commissural/associational response (i) is insensitive to L-AP4, but the induction of commissural/associational LTP is completely blocked by D-AP5. In contrast, mossy fibre responses (ii) are profoundly reduced by L-AP4, and although there is a slight effect of D-AP5 on mossy fibre responses, induction of LTP is not blocked by D-AP5. (Calibration: top, 2 min, 0.5 mV; bottom, 2 min, 0.3 mV. (Harris and Cotman, 1986, fig. 2.) **d:** magnesium gates NMDA receptor channels. Glutamate-currents appear as simple events on both sites of the reversal potential (c. −5 mV in this experiment). After addition of Mg^{2+} (10 μM) (ii) the currents recorded at +40 mV are unchanged, whereas the currents recorded at −60 mV appear as bursts. The size of the single-channel current is not altered by the addition of 10 μM Mg^{2+}. In this experiment, $MgCl_2$ (2 mM) had been added to the internal solution. Note that the single-channel conductance is 51 pS at −60 mV, and only 33 pS at +40 mV. This discrepancy was observed in all experiments where Mg^{2+} (2 mM) was present in the internal solution, but was not seen when Mg^{2+} was absent. Thus, when Mg^{2+} was absent from both the internal and the external solutions, the I–V relationship of the glutamate-induced current was linear (between −60 and +60 mV) at the single-channel level as well as at the whole-cell level. (Nowak et al., 1984, fig. 2.)

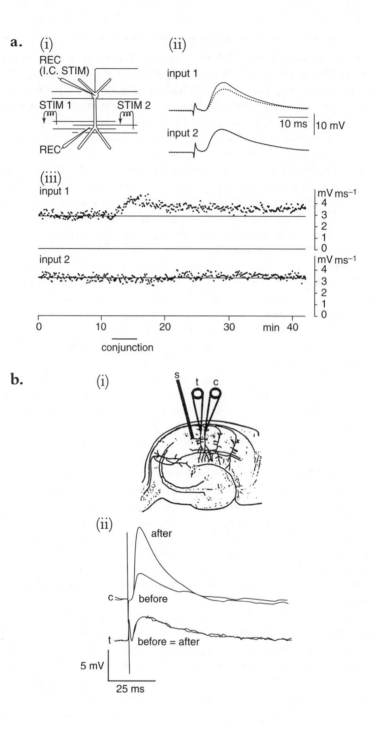

a.

(i)

REC
(I.C. STIM)

STIM 1   STIM 2

REC

(ii)

input 1

input 2

10 ms | 10 mV

(iii)

input 1

mV ms⁻¹
4
3
2
1
0

input 2

mV ms⁻¹
4
3
2
1
0

0   10   20   30   min 40

conjunction

b.

(i)

s   t   c

(ii)

after

c   before

t   before = after

5 mV

25 ms

case, the appropriate rise in calcium ion concentration necessary for induction of LTP, which is contingent on the opening of NMDA receptors, could be confined to the spines on which the active terminals form synapses. Evidence that spines are involved in LTP was provided as early as 1977 by Fifkova and Van Harreveld, who showed that stimulation of the perforant path could induce an increase in the area of the dendritic spines of granule cells in the distal third of the dentate molecular layer. Within a period of 1 hour after a tetanus, the area of these spines had increased by 38 per cent, whereas the density of vesicles in the nerve terminals on the spines had decreased by 19 per cent. There were no changes in the spines or terminals on them for those granule cells in the proximal third of the dentate molecular layer, which do not receive synaptic input from the pyriform pathway. These observations pointed to the possibility that the calcium increase does not occur throughout the granule cell on stimulation of the perforant path but is restricted to just those spines that receive input from the terminals of the perforant axons. This offered an explanation for why associative LTP is confined to just excited synapses whilst being dependent on an increase in the calcium concentration of the postsynaptic cell at the same time.

Bliss and Gardner-Medwin (1973) showed that LTP lasted for at least several days in the dentate gyrus following suitable stimulation of the pyriform pathway input. It was clear that such long periods of maintenance of LTP must involve new protein synthesis initiated by the stimulation protocol used to induce the LTP. However, it was not until 1981 that this was shown to be the case. At that time, Duffy et al. (1981) showed that LTP of the hippo-

---

Fig. 3.6. **The effects of polarization of neurons during stimulation on the generation of long-term potentiation (LTP). a:** effects of depolarizing currents. (i): diagram showing the arrangement of stimulating (STIM) and recording (REC) electrodes. (ii): Averaged records ($n = 10$) of intracellulary recorded postsynaptic potentials following single volleys. Potentials obtained before conjunction are shown as dotted lines, those obtained 5 min after the end of conjunction as solid lines. iii: Measurements of the initial slopes of the intracellularly recorded excitatory postsynaptic potentials (EPSPs) resulting from activation of STIM 1 (input 1) and STIM 2 (input 2) are shown for a series of test responses. During the whole recording period shown (except that indicated by a heavy bar) a 6 nA, 100 msec current pulse was given through the intracellular electrode 400 msec after the stimulus to input 1. (Malinow and Miller, 1986, fig. 1.)

b: effects of hyperpolarizing currents. (i): diagram of a hippocampal slice showing the location of the bipolar extracellular stimulating electrode (s), the intracellular electrode in the control cell (c), and the intracellular electrode in the test cell (t). (Adapted from Ramon y Cajal, 1904). (ii): the upper traces show an intracellular recording from a control cell (c), which did not receive any current passage during the conditioning high-frequency stimulation (HFS). Each trace is the average of five successive responses 4 sec apart recorded immediately before and 10 minutes after the conditioning HFS. The lower traces show a simultaneous intracellular recording from a nearby test cell (t) which received passage of a 3-nA hyperpolarizing current during the HFS. Averaged responses were recorded immediately before and 10 min after the HFS. The control cell's response was potentiated by the HFS whereas the EPSP of the test cell was not. (Wigstrom et al., 1986a, b, fig. 1.)

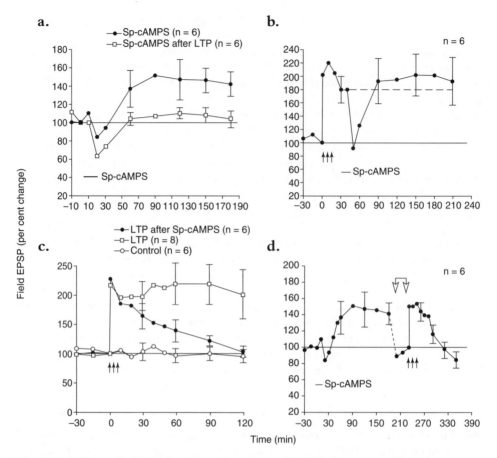

Fig. 3.7. Effects of cAMP simulate a late stage of LTP in hippocampal CA1 neurons.
Hippocampal long-term potentiation (LTP) is thought to serve as an elementary mechanism for the establishment of certain forms of explicit memory in the mammalian brain. As is the case with behavioural memory, LTP in the CA1 region has stages: a short-term early potentiation lasting 1–3 hours, which is independent of protein synthesis, precedes a later, longer-lasting stage (L-LTP), which requires protein synthesis. Inhibitors of cyclic adenosine monophosphate (cAMP)-dependent protein kinase (PKA) blocked L-LTP, and analogs of cAMP induced a potentiation that blocked naturally induced L-LTP.

The action of the cAMP analog was blocked by inhibitors of protein synthesis. Thus, activation of PKA may be a component of the mechanism that generates L-LTP. Long-term synaptic potentiation induced by tetanization and by a membrane-permeable analog of cyclic AMP, Sp-cyclic adenosine, 3′,5′-monophosphorothioate (Sp-cAMPS) occlude one another. **a** and **b:** pre-exposure to L-LTP induced by tetanization occluded the persistent facilitation produced by Sp-cAMPS. **a:** Sp-cAMPS (100 μM for 15 min) produced a persistent facilitation after an initial transient inhibition (solid circles). **b:** tetanization, with three high-frequency trains (arrows), produced L-LTP. Thirty minutes after the induction of L-LTP, Sp-cAMPS was applied and produced a depression that was larger than that campal slice in either the dentate gyrus following perforant path stimulation or area CA1 of the hippocampus following Schaffer collateral stimulation resulted in an increase in the incorporation of labelled valine into proteins destined for secretion into the extracellular medium from just those regions that had been stimulated. The expected link between LTP in a particular region and metabolic processes that lead to protein synthesis in that region was then established.

More recently, LTP that lasts for long periods of time, and therefore requires the synthesis of new mRNA and protein, has been shown to involve the same signalling pathway of cAMP, PKA, MAPK and CREB as identified in the mechanisms responsible for non-declarative memory in invertebrates, described above (fig. 3.7; Frey et al., 1993; Abel et al., 1997). Furthermore, the increase in the area of spines concomitant with long-lasting LTP, also mentioned above, indicates that new protein synthesis responsible for long-lasting LTP is likely to contribute to the formation of new synapses, a possibility that has been substantiated (Greenough and Bailey, 1988; Geinisman et al., 1991; Bolshakov et al., 1997). The similarity between the molecular mechanisms proposed for non-declarative memory formation in the invertebrates and that for LTP is striking. It has held out the promise that the storage of declarative memories in the hippocampus could soon be understood at the molecular level. However, the caveat remains as to what is meant by 'non-declarative' and 'declarative' memories, as well as of the concept of 'storage' in the brain, problems we shall return to in §3.2.

3.1.6   Cellular and molecular mechanisms of declarative memory in the hippocampus

The intense amount of research carried out in the closing decades of the last century on the mechanisms that generate hippocampal LTP was predicated on the assumption that LTP is involved in memory. The declarative memory for place, taken to be laid down in

←——

Fig. 3.7.   (*Continued*)

produced when Sp-cAMPS was given alone (**a**), but the synaptic facilitation that followed the depression was significantly reduced compared with a control without the preceding tentanus–induced L-LTP. The residual facilitation remaining after the occlusion by L-LTP is regraphed in (a, open squares) to compare it with the facilitation produced by Sp-cAMPS alone (solid circles).

c and **d:** pre-exposure to Sp–cAMPS occluded L-LTP induced by tetanization. **c:** 3 hours after Sp-cAMPS was applied (100 μM for 15 min), three high-frequency trains of stimuli were given. These trains produced an early facilitation that decayed in about 90 min. The residual potentiation present at 90 and 120 min was significantly reduced compared with L-LTP in the absence of Sp-cAMPS. **d:** 3 hours after Sp-cAMPS potentiation was induced (143 ± 13 per cent), the stimulus intensity was reduced (open arrows) so as to achieve an EPSP slope value comparable to control (0.4 ± 0.03 mV/ms), and a new baseline was taken. Three high-frequency stimuli (solid arrows) induced a transient facilitation (comparable to E-LTP) that decayed to baseline in about 90 min. This residual facilitation, measured 90 and 120 min after tetanization, was significantly reduced compared with L-LTP produced in the absence of Sp-cAMPS. (Frey et al., 1993, fig. 2.)

the hippocampus, has been thought to involve pyramidal neurons in area CA1 becoming place cells as a consequence of the induction of LTP at synapses on these cells. However, it has been found that pharmacological experiments involving the reduction of LTP with NMDA antagonists block the ability of rats to form spatial memories in some learning procedures (Morris et al., 1986) but not in others (Bannerman et al., 1995). Experiments involving gene-targeted mice have been designed to see if this issue can be resolved. These have been reported, and appear to arrive at contrary conclusions as to whether LTP is part of the mechanism for generating declarative memories concerning place. For example, knocking out the R1 subunit of the NMDA receptor on pyramidal cells (place cells) in the CA1 region of the mouse hippocampus does not affect normal synaptic transmission but blocks LTP at the synapses formed on these cells. Tests of spatial memory in these mice show that deficits in this form of declarative memory then occur, apparently showing a dependence of spatial memory on LTP (Tsien et al., 1996a, b). Another experiment implicating LTP in the formation of declarative memory involves regulation off and on of the expression of a transgene for a persistently active form of calcium/calmodulin-dependent protein kinase II. This technique provides a means of turning off and then on again the LTP induced by stimulation of the synapses to pyramidal neurons in the CA1 region of the hippocampus. When this mutated gene product is turned on, LTP is blocked, and there is a concomitant deficiency in spatial learning and memory; when the gene is turned off, the capacity for spatial memory and learning is restored (Mayford et al., 1996). More recently, however, gene-targeted mice lacking the L-alpha-amino-3-hydroxy-5-methylisoxazole-4-propionate (AMPA) receptor subunit CluR-A have been used to test the idea that spatial memory is conditional on the mechanisms for generation of LTP. This work has shown that the loss of the AMPA receptor subunit blocks LTP but does not produce any detectable changes in a wide variety of properties of CA3 neuronal terminals on CA1 pyramidal neurons or of the dendritic spines on which these terminals form synapses. The learning of spatial memories is completely unaffected in these gene-targeted mice, indicating that it is unlikely that LTP is required for this form of declarative memory formation (fig. 3.8; Zamanillo et al., 1999). It would seem, then, that the cellular and molecular mechanisms responsible for the formation of declarative memories in the hippocampus have yet to be clearly elucidated. However, increased clarity is also called for in relation to the meaning of the terms used to describe what are claimed to be different forms of memory. We attempt to provide this in §3.2.

3.1.7   Summary

We have traced some of the most important discoveries about memory made by neuroscientists in the last half of the twentieth century. In the next sections, we shall examine some of the claims made by leading neuroscientists in their attempts to give an overview of the bearing of their discoveries on the understanding of psychological capacities (such as memory) and their exercise. Our contention is that many of these claims are enmeshed in conceptual confusions. Our aim is to weed out the conceptual confusions in order to clarify what can be justified in such claims. This requires a conceptual analysis of a kind unfamiliar to most neuroscientists. We hope to demonstrate that careful application of these

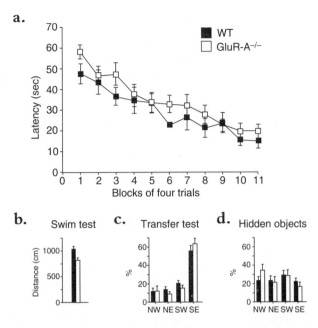

Fig. 3.8. AMPA receptors not required for long-term potentiation. Gene-targeted mice lacking the L-alpha-amino-3-hydroxy-5-methylisoxazole-4-propionate (AMPA) receptor subunit GluR-A exhibited normal development, life expectancy and fine structure of neuronal dendrites and synapses. In hippocampal CA1 pyramidal neurons, GluR-A$^{-/-}$ mice showed a reduction in functional AMPA receptors, with the remaining receptors preferentially targeted to synapses. Thus, the CA1 soma-patch currents were strongly reduced, but glutamatergic synaptic currents were unaltered; and evoked dendritic and spinous Ca^{2+} transients and Ca^{2+}-dependent gene activation; and hippocampal field potentials were as in the wild type. In adult GluR-A$^{-/-}$ mice, associative long-term potentiation (LTP) was absent in CA3 to CA1 synapses, but spatial learning in the water maze was not impaired. The results suggest that CA1 hippocampal LTP is controlled by the number or subunit composition of AMPA receptors and shows a dichotomy between LTP in CA1 and acquisition of spatial memory.

Spatial learning. **a:** in a Morris water maze the mean latency (±SEM) to escape from the pool to the submerged platform (eight trials per day in blocks of four) is presented as a function of trial block for male wild-type (filled squares) and GluR-A$^{-/-}$ (open squares) mice. **b:** swim test gives the mean distance covered by the two genotypes in 50 sec in the pool without a platform before training. **c:** in a transfer test after trial block 10, the platform was removed, and wild-type and GluR-A$^{-/-}$ mice were allowed to search for 60 sec. Both groups searched selectively in the target quadrant (SE). Ordinate, per cent time spent in each quadrant. **d:** quadrant preference was not observed when distal visual cues were invisible in the transfer test. (Zamanillo et al., 1999, fig. 7.)

kinds of analytic techniques is highly relevant to the correct understanding by neuroscientists of their achievements and for the eradication of misunderstandings. There is a pervasive problem that occurs in the neurosciences concerning the subject of psychological attributes. Such attributes are commonly ascribed by neuroscientists to the brain (and, occasionally, to the mind), and neuroscientists' explanations of the exercise of capacities such as sight or memory by an animal involve ascribing psychological attributes to the brain of the animal. This is conceptually incoherent in a multitude of ways. In §3.2 we outline what we take to be the correct account of the conceptual framework which neuroscientists need to employ in their reflections on the neural foundations of memory.

3.2 Memory and Knowledge

Perception is a primary source of knowledge, and, as noted, to perceive *that* something is so is to acquire knowledge of how things are in respect of objects in one's field of perception. To know that something is thus-and-so is trivially to be in possession of information. To possess information, however, is not to be in any kind of mental state. To acquire information is not to change from a mental 'state of ignorance' to a mental 'state of knowing'. The criteria for a person's knowing something are not criteria for his being in a certain state. We find out whether a person knows something by seeing *what he can do*, not by establishing what state he is in. To know something to be thus-and-so is ability-like, hence more akin to a power or potentiality than to a state or actuality. To learn that something is so is to come to be able to do a wide range of things (to inform others, to answer certain questions, to correct others, to find, locate, identify, explain things, and so forth). To forget that something is so is not to cease to be in some state, but to cease to be able to do certain things. We ask *why* someone is in a given state, but *how* someone knows. Mental states can be interrupted and later resumed (as when one's intense concentration is interrupted by a telephone conversation and later resumed), and such mental states as intense anxiety or excitement are broken off by sleep. But one cannot interrupt someone in knowing, and one does not cease to know when one falls asleep. To ask someone 'How long have you known such-and-such?' is not like asking 'How long have you been concentrating (agitated, feeling nervous)?', but more like 'Since when have you been in a position to . . . ?' and akin to 'Since when have you been able to . . . ?' If we know that things are thus-and-so, it is possible for us to act on the basis of that information. The information that things are so may provide us with reasons, in the context of our projects, not only for acting, but also for thinking or feeling something or other (e.g. feeling pleased or angry). What one knows is what can occur as a premiss in one's reasoning from truths to the conclusions one may draw. For language-using creatures such as ourselves, to know where, when, who, what, whether or how is, among other things, to be able to answer these questions. Of course, other animals, no less than human beings, know things, although their cognitive powers are less than ours: they can act for reasons, at best, only in an attenuated sense; and they cannot answer questions, but exhibit their knowledge only in their non-linguistic behaviour. A dog can be said to know how to get home if it is able to find its way home – an ability exhibited in its regularly doing so without getting lost; it knows where it buried its bone if it is able to go and dig it up – an ability exhibited in its going to the right place without hesitation and doing so; it knows its master if it is able to recognize its master; and so on.

Although knowledge can be said to be ability-like, being able to do something is not necessarily to know anything. Indeed, it is not necessarily even knowing how to do anything. (These distinctions, as we shall see, have an important bearing on neuroscientists' attempts to distinguish between declarative and non-declarative memory.) To justify these claims, we must clarify the relationship between being able to do something and knowing how to do something. Then we must shed some light on the relationship between knowing how to do something and knowing that something is so.

We may distinguish between innate abilities, such as the ability to breathe, to perceive or to move one's limbs, and acquired abilities, such as the ability to walk or talk. A further distinction we shall need is between one-way abilities (or powers) and two-way abilities (or powers). All inanimate abilities are one-way powers, and may be active or passive. The ability of an acid to dissolve a metal is a one-way active power: if the conditions are appropriate, the sulphuric acid will dissolve the zinc – the acid is the active agent, but it has, as it were, no choice in the matter. The liability or susceptibility of zinc to dissolve in acid is a one-way passive power. Some of the abilities of animate creatures are one-way abilities, e.g. the ability to see, hear or feel pain. Others are two-way abilities, which the animal can exercise at will or refrain from exercising if it so chooses, e.g. the ability to walk or talk. Abilities that are acquired may be acquired simply through natural maturation (e.g. the ability of animals to engage in sexual intercourse) or through learning (which may or may not include training or teaching). Not all successful learning results in the possession of knowledge – it may result in the possession of an ability or skill that does not involve knowing how to do anything. So, a child must learn, and indeed is taught, to be patient, or to be silent; but these do not involve acquisition of knowledge. The successful upshot of such learning is being able to do the relevant things, but not knowing, and hence remembering, the way to do them. What then distinguishes knowing how to V from merely being able to V? For us to speak of an animal's knowing how to V, its ability must be a two-way ability, which the animal can exercise or refrain from exercising as it pleases. That is not sufficient, since the ability to walk, for example, is an acquired two-way ability; but although we have to learn to walk, the upshot of learning to walk is being able to walk, not knowing how to walk. One may lose the ability to walk through paralysis, but one cannot forget (i.e. there is no such thing as forgetting) how to walk, and one cannot later be reminded or remember how to do it. To know how to do something differs from being able to do something inasmuch as knowing how to do something is knowing the way to do it (just as knowing when or where to do something is knowing the time and place to do it). To know the way to do something includes knowing the manner, means and method (where these are appropriate). Exercise of knowledge of the way to do something is plastic, adaptive and circumstance-sensitive. To know the way to do something typically involves knowing that it is done thus, and the 'thus' may, in the case of human beings, be stated or demonstrated.

One can learn how to do something by experience, by trial and error, by being trained or taught, by being shown how to do it, and, with human beings, by being told how to do it. What one knows how to do is something of which it makes sense to say that one has forgotten how to do it, that one remembers, recollects or can be reminded how to do it.

Of something of which it makes sense to say that one knows how to do it, it also makes sense to say that one made a mistake in trying to do it, that one realized that one was doing it wrongly, and that one tried to correct oneself. For to know how to do something is to know the way to do it, and knowing the way to do it implies an ability to distinguish between doing it correctly and doing it incorrectly. Of course, non-human animals cannot state how to do something whereas humans often can. But an animal's knowledge of the way to do something – e.g. a dog's knowing how to get home from a given point – is exhibited in the plasticity of the skill in response to circumstances, the recognition of error when it occurs, and its rectification in performance.

So, one may be able to do something, but not know how to do it, and conversely, one may know how to do something but be unable to do it. (i) Being able to do something does not imply knowing how to do it in those cases in which the concept of knowledge (and hence too of remembering and forgetting) is simply inapplicable. It may be inapplicable because knowledge is irrelevant to the kind of ability in question (e.g. to feel the heat of the fire from three feet away – a one-way passive ability, to walk – a two-way ability which involves no knowledge of a way of doing anything). It may be inapplicable because knowledge is irrelevant (because categorially inappropriate) to the type of possessor of the ability (e.g. a plant's ability to grow in the shade). (ii) Knowing how to do something does not imply being able to do it. For one may know how to do things for the doing of which one has lost the physical power or lacks the strength of will. The aged tennis coach may no longer be able to play tennis, but he surely knows how to; and one may know perfectly well how to lose weight, but be unable to.

We must distinguish not only between being able to do something and knowing how to do something, but also between knowing how to do something and knowing that something is so. But it is mistaken to suppose, as Gilbert Ryle (1949), who introduced and made much of the latter distinction did, that knowing how is always and essentially different from knowing that. Knowing how and knowing that are not so much two different forms which knowledge may take, as knowledge of two different kinds of thing. To know how to do something, as we have suggested, is to know the way to do it, and to know the way to do something is often (but not always) to know, and to be able to say or show, that it is done thus-and-so. Knowledge may be acquired, for example, by active or passive perception, or by reasoning. But it may be given one in the form of the authoritative judgement or testimony of others. Indeed, it should always be borne in mind (but is often forgotten by epistemologists and by psychologists) that much of what a human being knows is not perceptual knowledge but transmitted knowledge, learnt from the written or spoken word of others. Of course, to acquire knowledge thus, one must be able to perceive, i.e. to see (in order to read) hear (in order to listen to what is said) – but what is learnt is not what is perceived (one sees the words one reads, but what one learns is the information they convey). Knowledge is not only *given*, in the form of passive perception or of information imparted by others, it may also be *attained* by endeavour – by reasoning, or by discovery or detection, which may be the upshot of seeking, searching for, experimenting or trying to find out how things are. Further, it may also be *received*, without endeavour and independently of being given by others, by recognizing or noticing, becoming aware or conscious of something, or by realization, on the basis of information already possessed, that things are so.

Again, it must be emphasized, it is the human being, not his brain, that knows that things are thus-and-so, knows how to do things, and possesses the abilities constitutive of knowing something. It is not correct, we suggest, to say, as LeDoux does, that it is 'possible for your brain to know that something is good or bad before it knows exactly what it is' (LeDoux, 1998, p. 69), or for Crick (1994) to speak, as we have seen he does, of the brain's learning things about the outside world. It is a confusion to speak, as J. Z. Young does, of the brain's asking and answering questions (Young, 1978, pp. 119 and 126). It is misleading of Colin Blakemore to write that 'Somehow the brain knows about the properties of the retina and fills in the missing information' (Blakemore, 1973, p. 38). A person who knows what time the next train is, where the railway station is, whether the train is likely to be on time, who else might be on it, etc. can answer the corresponding questions. But there is no such thing as the brain's knowing when . . . , where . . . , whether . . . , etc., and there is no such thing as the brain's answering such questions. It is not the brain, but the person whose brain it is, that acquires knowledge by perception, reasoning or testimony. A concept-exercising creature that can know things may be knowledgeable or ignorant, learned or untutored, an expert or a charlatan who pretends to know. But brains cannot be said to be knowledgeable, ignorant, learned, untutored, experts or charlatans – only human beings can be such things.

It is also incorrect to speak, as Young does, of the brain's containing knowledge and information, which is encoded in the brain 'just as knowledge can be recorded in books or computers' (Young, 1978, p. 192). We may say of a book that it contains all the knowledge of a lifetime's work of a scholar, or of a filing cabinet that it contains all the available knowledge, duly card-indexed, about Julius Caesar. This means that the pages of the book or the cards in the filing cabinet have written on them *expressions* of a large number of known truths. In this sense, the brain *contains* no knowledge whatsoever. There are no symbols in the brain that by their array express a single proposition, let alone a proposition that is known to be true. Of course, in this sense a human being *contains* no knowledge either. To possess knowledge is not to contain knowledge. A person may possess, for example, a smattering of knowledge about seventeenth-century woodcuts, but he contains none. Hind's history of early woodcuts contains a great deal of such knowledge, but has none. The brain neither possesses nor contains any knowledge.

A great deal of information is contained in the *Encyclopaedia Britannica*. In that sense, there is none in the brain. Much information can be *derived* from a slice through a tree trunk or from a geological specimen – and so too from PET and fMRI scans of the brain's activities. But this is *not* information which the brain *has*. Nor is it *written in* the brain, let alone in the 'language of the brain', any more than dendrochronological information about the severity of winters in the 1930s is written in the tree trunk in arboreal patois.

3.2.1 Memory

The faculty of memory is a cognitive power of human beings. Again, it is at best misleading, to speak, as Milner, Squire and Kandel (1998, p. 446) do of the progress that has been achieved in our understanding of 'how the nervous system learns and remembers'. For it is not the nervous system that learns or remembers anything at all, but the animal. And the achievements that can be hoped for are of understanding the neural processes that make it possible for animals to remember whatever they can remember.

Memory is exercised in the *retention* of knowledge already acquired. It is logically possible to remember only what one previously *came to know, was aware of, noticed* or *otherwise appre-hended*. But *what* one remembers need have nothing to do with the past. For, apart from facts about the past that one remembers, one also learns and remembers facts concerning the present (e.g. where one's keys are), concerning the future (e.g. when the next train leaves), as well as general facts (e.g. laws of nature) that hold at all times, and truths of mathematics or logic that are atemporal. One must distinguish between the following three forms which memory may take. *Factual memory* is linguistically expressed by sentences in which the verb 'remember' takes as its grammatical object a that–clause or sentential-clause: e.g. 'I remember (that) the Battle of Hastings was fought in 1066'. *Experiential memory* is expressed by sentences in which the verb 'remember' is followed by a gerund which speci-fies a previous experience of the person: e.g. 'I remember seeing . . .' (or 'hearing', 'feeling', etc.), as well as 'I remember V-ing . . .' and 'I remember being V'd' (where 'V' is any verb signifying something an agent might do or undergo). Clearly, I may remember *that* I per-ceived something, did or underwent something, without remembering, perceiving, doing or undergoing it, although I cannot remember perceiving, doing or undergoing something unless I remember that I did or underwent it. So experiential memory implies factual memory, but not vice versa. *Objectual memory* is sometimes expressed by sentences in which the verb 'remember' is followed by a direct object signifying a perceptible thing or quality: e.g. 'I remember her smile (the house) well', 'I remember the scent of jasmine (taste of raspberries)', where a contrast with mere factual memory is intended (I may remember *that* she had a sweet smile, but not be able to remember *it*; I may remember much *about* the house, but not be able to *visualize it*). *Sometimes* we use such sentences to indicate our ability to conjure up images (visual or auditory) of something previously perceived. Imagist memory, in this sense, although it may be common, is not logically necessary for either factual memory or experiential memory. Moreover, having a mental image of something previously perceived is no more sufficient for remembering the object antecedently per-ceived than is having a photograph of it, since one must also remember what one's mental image (or photograph) is an image of. Memory of objects or qualities may involve any or all of the above forms.

Parallel to the previously discussed distinction between *knowing how* and *knowing that*, we must distinguish between remembering how to do something and remembering that something is so. And just as *knowing how* is not always essentially distinct from *knowing that*, so too, remembering how to do something is not always essentially distinct from remem-bering that something is so. For to remember how to do something is to retain one's previ-ous acquired knowledge of the way to do it. Not to have forgotten the way to V is to remember that one V's *thus* rather than *thus*. In many kinds of case, this is no different from remembering that V-ing is done thus-and-so (as is obviously the case in remembering how to open the combination lock, how to integrate, how to address the Pope, or how to spell 'Edinburgh'). This bears on a distinction widely invoked by neuroscientists investigating the neural underpinnings of memory. Cohen and Squire (1980), it is claimed (Milner et al., 1998, p. 450), 'suggested a fundamental distinction in the way all of us process and store information about the world': namely, between *declarative* and *non-declarative memory*. As we have seen, declarative memory is held to be 'what is ordinarily meant by the term memory'; it is 'propositional'; it can be true or false; and it is involved 'in modelling the external world and storing representations about facts and episodes' (ibid.). Non-declarative memory is held to underlie 'changes in skilled behaviour and the ability to respond appropriately to stimuli through practice, as the result of conditioning or habit learning'. It is held to be involved in priming, in so-called habit memory ('acquired dispositions or tendencies that are specific to a set of stimuli and that guide behaviour'), in Pavlovian conditioning (both emotional conditioning and eye-blink reaction conditioning). All these different phenomena are deemed to be kinds of memory, because 'performance changes as the result of experi-ence, which justifies the term memory'. Many forms of non-declarative memory, such as habituation, sensitization, classical conditioning, are already, it is held, well developed in invertebrates. Accordingly, the gill withdrawal reflex in *Aplysia* was found to be modifiable by habituation, dishabituation, sensitization, classical and operant conditioning. Similar investigations were carried out on the tail flick in crayfish, feeding in *Limax*, phototaxis in *Hermissenda*. These were held to show that 'non-declarative memory storage does not depend on specialized memory neurons or systems of neurons whose only function is to *store* rather than process information' (Milner et al., 1998, p. 454). Similar research on *Drosophila* was held to show that they 'can remember to avoid an odour that has been paired with an electric shock', but that accumulation of cAMP 'interferes with their ability to acquire and store new information' (Milner et al., 1998, p. 457).

Much of this pioneering research, we suggest, is not research on memory in any sense of the word, and the extent to which it bears on actual memory has to be demonstrated. We shall comment below on the misconception that we *store* information about the world in our brains. We shall not comment on the misconception that factual memory is involved in 'modelling the external world and storing representations about facts and episodes', save to remind neuroscientists that ordinary people do not go in for 'modelling the external world', unless they are sculptors, and they 'store representations about facts and episodes' primarily when they stick photographs into the family album. It should be noted, however, that it is not really correct to say that declarative memory 'is what is ordinarily meant by "memory"'. It would be more accurate to say that declarative memory is *included* in what is ordinarily meant by 'memory', for in the ordinary use of the term 'remember' we include both *remembering that* and *remembering how*, as well as *remembering V-ing* and *remembering M* (i.e. experiential and objectual memory). It is claimed that what is called 'conscious recol-lection' (Milner et al., 1998, p. 451) is central to declarative memory, but inapplicable to non-declarative memory, and that declarative and non-declarative memory 'use a different logic', viz. 'conscious versus unconscious recall' (Milner et al., 1998, p. 463). But it is unclear what is meant by 'conscious recollection'. It is possible that the phrase is being used to suggest that whenever one declaratively remembers something, one is aware of the past event in which one acquired the knowledge in question; or it may mean that whenever one remembers, one is aware that one is remembering. But it is not correct to say that whenever one remembers a piece of information previously learnt, e.g. that the Battle of Hastings was in 1066 or that $F = ma$, that one remembers the event of learning it. And it is also not true that whenever one remembers some fact, one is aware of remembering it, as when one remembers to turn off the light, or when, having spoken to Jack earlier and arranged a meeting for the next day, one remarks to one's wife that one is going to meet Jack tomorrow. It would be equally confused to suppose that when one exercises one's non-declarative memory, no conscious recollection is ever involved. For *if* non-declarative memory includes remembering how to do something, then one very often remembers how to do something by calling to mind the episode in which one was taught to do it, and one may well, in exercising one's memory of how to do something, be aware of the fact that one is. Of course, neither is necessary. But then they are not necessary for declarative factual memory either. These confusions are easily rectified. The confusions about non-declarative memory, however, are deeper. For the habituation, sensitization, desensitization, classical conditioning, etc. of invertebrates, as well as the conditioned eye-blink responses and fear reactions of mammals, are not forms of memory at all. The animal may indeed have learnt to respond in certain ways to certain kinds of stimuli, and its responses may change – for example, accelerate – as a result of continued exposure to a stimulus. So one might say that the animal, as a result of experience, has learnt to react more rapidly or has acquired the ability to react more rapidly. But that does *not* warrant characterizing the animal as remembering anything. For nothing *cognitive* is involved here. The animal learnt neither that something is so nor the way to do anything. An accelerated reflex or a conditioned reaction are not forms of *knowledge*. But memory is the *retention of knowledge acquired*, and remembering to V is *the use of knowledge retained*. One can indeed condition insects and molluscs to avoid a certain stimulus, but that, by itself, does not show that any knowledge was either acquired or retained. The primitive animals in question cannot be said to have come to know that things are thus-and-so; nor can they be said to have learnt the way to do anything. It is surely misconceived to hold that *Drosophila* 'can remember to avoid an odor that has been paired with an electric shock' (Milner et al., 1998, p. 457), for all that has been shown is that *Drosophila*s can, by conditioning, acquire the disposition to avoid an odour that has been paired with an electric shock. They can be said to have acquired *a primitive one-way ability*, but that is not sufficient to demonstrate any form of memory whatsoever. Indeed, even in the case of a mouse that is conditioned to fear an electric shock on hearing a tone, there is no reason to take the mouse to have acquired any knowledge. All that has been shown is that conditioning produces a regular, conditioned fear reaction.

It is possible that the neural phenomena that have been discovered to accompany such forms of conditioned reaction also characterize cases of genuine memory, but that is something that must be shown. What is clear is that these studies are not actually studies of memory. It is argued that the findings in question 'illustrate that non-declarative memory storage does not depend on specialized neurons or systems of neurons whose only function is to *store* rather than process information' (Milner et al., 1998, p. 454; our emphasis). But this, we suggest, is mistaken. For, first, no form of *memory* is involved in these investigations. And secondly, there is, as we shall argue below, no form of *storage of information* in the brain.

Failure to clarify the concept of memory is responsible for further difficulties in neuro-scientific reflection on this crucial capacity. So it is, for example, incorrect to suggest, as does LeDoux, that 'to remember is to be conscious of some past experience' (LeDoux, 1998, p. 181). For, first, what one remembers need not be anything past – it can be present, future or timeless, although, of course, one must have learnt such facts in the past. Secondly, what one remembers *need not* be an experience at all, and *is not* when what is remembered is, for example, the date of the Battle of Hastings. Thirdly, to remember the date of Hastings, who Caesar's wife was, or the way home is not to be conscious of 1066, of Calpurnia or of the way home. Moreover, even when remembering does take the form of experiential memory, to remember V-ing, i.e. a past experience, is not to be conscious of that past experience – to remember feeling ill last month is not to be conscious of feeling ill last month. It is merely to know now that one was ill then, and to know it *because* one then felt ill (and not because, having forgotten the episode, one was subsequently told that one previously felt ill).

Just as one can perceive, fail to perceive, misperceive or suffer from hallucinations, so too one can remember, fail to remember, misremember or suffer from mnemonic delusions. If one comes to know that things are so, and does not forget what one learnt, then one can be said to remember that things are so. One may be altogether unable to recollect something one previously knew, and such failure of memory may be a temporary lapse or it may be permanent. If one errs correctly in one's belief concerning something one previously knew, one misremembers. But one may also labour under a mnemonic delusion regarding one's own past experiences (as the Prince Regent did in thinking that he remembered fighting at Waterloo) – in which case what one believes is *so* out of line that it amounts no longer to a correctable *error*, but to a form of derangement.

3.2.2 Memory and storage

Memory, as we have emphasized, is knowledge *retained* (including the knowledge that one perceived, did or underwent this or that in the past, which may take the form of factual memory or of experiential memory, and may or may not involve mnemonic imagery). But it is incorrect to suppose, as do Squire and Kandel (1999, pp. 211–14), that memory is knowledge *stored*, let alone *stored in the brain*. It is, we suggest, confused to claim, as Milner, Squire and Kandel (1998, p. 463) do, that declarative and non-declarative memories 'are stored in different brain areas', for there is no such thing as storing memories in the brain. Rather, the capacity to remember various kinds of things is *causally dependent* on different brain areas and on synaptic modifications in these areas.

The notion of storage and the associated idea of memory traces long antedates neuroscience. It began life as a metaphor (of wax tablets) in Plato, and as a rudimentary speculative theory in Aristotle, who conceived of memory as the storage of an impression of a percept in the heart, functionally dependent upon the humidity of the tissues. The idea of memory as a 'storehouse of ideas' runs through the empiricist tradition of the seventeenth, eighteenth and nineteenth centuries. Indeed, this conception continues to cause confusion – the metaphor being taken to be what it is merely a metaphor for. So, for example, LeDoux recently listed an array of things one might be said to have learnt and not forgotten, and asks, 'What do all of these have in common?', to which he replies, 'They are things I've learned and stored in my brain' (LeDoux, 1999, p. 179). But one may surely be sceptical about the intelligibility of storing the things he cites, such as the smell of banana pudding, the meaning of the words 'halcyon days', and the rules of dominoes, *in the brain*. One can store smells in bottles, write down the meanings of words in dictionaries, and codify the rules of games in documents, which can then be stored – but one cannot *store* smells, meanings of words or rules *in a brain*! Of course, what LeDoux means is that these are things that he can remember – and that is right; where he errs, we suggest, is in the supposition that in order to be able to remember them, he must have stored them in his brain (or anywhere else). It is deeply tempting to insist that while what is stored is obviously not what is remembered (e.g. smells, meanings of words or rules of games), it is a *representation* of what is remembered. One is inclined to think that the knowledge antecedently acquired *must* be stored in one's mind or brain, either in the form of an image or in the form of an encoded description representing what is remembered. If it were not, it seems, one would not be able to remember what one remembers – the knowledge would not be *available* to one. The classical empiricists tended to think that what is stored is stored in the mind, and the manner in which it is stored, is as a mental image or picture that represents or is a copy of the original experience. Neuroscientists think that what is stored is stored in the brain, and the manner in which it is stored is given by a pattern of synaptic connections with efficacies that lead to the excitation of certain neurons under certain conditions, which excitation represents or encodes the original experience. We shall examine this pervasive idea in a moment.

Unsurprisingly, with the development of neurophysiology, the obscure idea of storing mental images *in the mind*, and the idea that these images are *unconscious* until recalled, fell from favour. In its place, the conception of brain-traces became popular. At the end of the nineteenth century, James wrote:

> The *retention* of n [the previously experienced event which is now remembered], it will be observed, is no mysterious storing up of an 'idea' in an unconscious state. It is not a fact of the mental order at all. It is a purely physical phenomenon, a morphological feature, the presence of these 'paths', namely, in the finest recesses of the brain's tissue. The recall or recollection, on the other hand, is a *psycho-physical* phenomenon, with both a bodily and a mental side. The bodily side is the functional excitement of the tracts and paths in question; the mental side is the conscious vision of the past occurrence, and the belief that we experienced it before. (James, 1890, p. 655)

It should be noted that according to James (in this passage), the memory trace ('tracts' or 'paths') is not *a condition* of retaining the knowledge acquired, i.e. a condition of being able to do something; it *is* the storage of that knowledge ('The *retention* . . . is a purely physical phenomenon, a morphological feature . . .'). This, as we shall see, fails to distinguish the retention of the abilities of which knowing something consists from the neural conditions for possession of those abilities, and from the storage of information in inscribed or otherwise recorded form. The background presupposition of James's reasoning is that remembering is repeating a past experience in attenuated form 'in memory' – 'the conscious vision of the past occurrence', as he puts it. This is part of the empiricist legacy, according to which to remember is to revive in one's mind a faint copy (an 'idea') of a previous experience (an 'impression'). The possibility of reproducing a facsimile of a past experience thus can be explained, James conjectures, if the original experience left a 'path' or 'tract', i.e. a brain-trace, which, if excited again, causes the recurrence of a faint copy of the antecedent experience together with a belief that one had 'experienced it before'.

The idea was repeated, with modifications, by such distinguished Gestalt psychologists as Koffka and Köhler, and became a commonplace among neuroscientists. The basic picture, which, as we shall see in a moment, informs neuroscientific reflection to this day, was nicely elaborated by Köhler:

> What does recognition mean? It means that a present fact, usually a perceptual one, makes contact with a corresponding one in memory, a trace, a contact which gives the present perception the character of being known or familiar. But memory contains a tremendous number of traces, all of them representations of previous experiences which must have been established by the processes accompanying such earlier experiences. Now, why does the present perceptual experience make contact with the *right* earlier experience? This is an astonishing achievement. Nobody seems to doubt that the *selection* is brought about by the similarity of the present experience and the experience of the corresponding earlier fact. But since this earlier experience is not present at the time, we have to assume that the trace of the earlier experience resembles the present experience, and that it is the similarity of our present experience (or the corresponding cortical process) and that trace which makes the selection possible. (Köhler, 1969, p. 122)

> All sound theories of memory, of habit, and so forth, must contain hypotheses about memory-traces as physiological facts. Such theories must also assume that the characteristics of traces are more or less akin to those of the processes by which they have been established. Otherwise, how could the accuracy of recall be explained, which in a great many cases is quite high. (Köhler, 1947, p. 252).

This conception is committed to the thought that an original experience created a brain-trace, which *represents* that experience. Recognition is a feeling of familiarity in response to an object perceived, caused by the excitation of a trace, which is itself caused by the neural stimulus which resembles the original cortical process. Recollection is a matter of *being reminded* of the antecedent experience by a current experience, which resembles it in producing a brain-trace that corresponds (at least in part) to the trace already laid down. Recalling something is a causal consequence of the excitation, by a partly corresponding neural stimulus, of the very same trace as was laid down by the original experience. This thought, as we shall see, continues to inform neuroscientific research on memory.

Squire and Kandel elaborate the Jamesian conception with the sophistication of late twentieth-century neuroscience. Conscious declarative memory, they claim, 'provides the possibility of re-creating in memory a specific episode from the past'. The 'starting point' is the set of cortical sites that were engaged when one perceived whatever one perceived. The consequent memory 'uniquely depends on the convergence of input from each of these distributed cortical sites into the medial temporal lobe and ultimately into the hippocampus'. This convergence, they claim, 'establishes a flexible representation' so that one can remember the object perceived and the episode of perceiving it. 'The resulting memories are stored as changes in strength at many synapses within a large ensemble of interconnected neurons.' Furthermore, 'the stored information in its specifics is determined by the *location* of the synaptic changes', although, they admit, 'we still know relatively little about how and where memory storage occurs'. Nevertheless, they have no doubts that what they call 'declarative information' is stored in the brain (Squire and Kandel, 1999, pp. 212f). This stored information enables one to 're-create in memory' a past episode.

Ian Glynn has recently articulated part of the present picture thus:

> Since the episodes that give rise to memories involve a variety of perceptions, it seems likely that the laying down of such memories involves nerve cells in the association areas and in secondary or higher order cortical areas concerned with the different senses. . . . It is also likely that recalling memories involves recreating something like the original pattern of activity in those same sets of cells, or at least some of them. . . . Initially then, both the hippocampal zone and the neocortical zone must act together. Eventually, when consolidation is complete, the memories are stored in such a fashion that they are available without the involvement of the hippocampal zone, implying that storage is then wholly in the neocortical zone. (Glynn, 1999, p. 329).

It should be noted that the thought that recollecting involves re-creating a part of the original pattern of neural activity follows both James and Köhler. And presumably the motivation for this hypothesis is that it seems to offer the hope of an explanation of the possibility of accurate recollection, on the assumption that recollection is a phenomenon of 're-creating in memory a specific episode from the past' (as Squire and Kandel put it). For the activation of the 'trace', like the movement of a stylus along the grooves of a gramophone record, is conceived to 're-create' the original experience 'in memory' (ideas of memory being thought to be, as the empiricists held, faint copies of the original impressions of which they are ideas). Building on the idea that recalling memories re-creates something like the original pattern of neural excitation, Bennett, Gibson and Robinson constructed a model of the mechanism of the putative associative memory network in the hippocampus. The fundamental idea is as follows: associative memory is construed as the disposition of a set of neurons (which previously fired according to a given pattern in response to a given input) to repeat the firing pattern when just part of the pattern is fed into them. If there are x neurons in the circuit, then these can be joined with connections that have properties such that a very large number of different patterns of inputs can use different overlapping sets of these x neurons, with each of these sets being made to fire when only a subset of the original input to the circuit is presented. This might be called 'a memorizing circuit'. This model is invoked to explain the neural basis for human memory. So, it is claimed,

> Memories are stored at the recurrent collateral synapses using a two-valued Hebbian. . . . The recall of a memory begins with the firing of a set of CA3 pyramidal neurons that overlap with the memory to be recalled as well as the firing of a set of pyramidal neurons not in the memory to be recalled . . . The CA3 recurrent potential network is shown to retrieve memories under specific conditions of the setting of the membrane potential of the pyramidal neurons by inhibitory interneurons. . . . The number of memories which can be stored and retrieved

without degradation is primarily a function of the number of active neurons when a memory
is recalled and the degree of connectivity in the network. (Bennett et al., 1994, pp. 167f)

The account provides a formal model of the brain-traces envisaged by James and
others.

However, a number of questionable ideas are involved in the received conception. First,
it is supposed that when we perceive something and remember what we thereby learnt,
then something is *stored*. Secondly, what is stored is a memory, which *represents* the original
perceptual experience. Thirdly, the memory is *laid down* in such-and-such parts of the brain,
in the form of changes in strength at synapses. So the neurons contain a *representation* of the
original experience. Fourthly, recollection involves re-creating the original pattern of activity in the relevant neurons. In particular, being reminded of something (associative memory)
involves having an experience, which bears some similarity to the antecedent experience
in which one acquired the information of which one is reminded by the associative experience. For recollecting results from stimulating the original memory trace by a neural input
of a part of the original pattern of neural excitation.

These four claims are debatable, and we shall raise some doubts and questions about
them.

(1) The thought that to remember is to store something confuses retention with storage.
To remember is to retain. But although storage implies retention, retention does not imply
storage. Memory, being the retention of knowledge acquired, is the retention of an ability
to just the extent that knowledge itself is an ability – but it is not the storage of an ability.
One may acquire and retain an ability, but that does not imply storage. For there is no such
thing as *storing* an ability, even though there is such a thing as retaining the neural structures
that are causal conditions for the possession of an ability.

The supposition that if one remembers, then one *must* have stored a representation rests
on the idea that unless there were a stored representation, the knowledge in question would
not be available to one. How could one remember unless it is 'written down' in encoded
form? But that is a confusion. Writing things down is indeed a way of storing information
(as long as one remembers how to read). Pictures do remind one of what one has seen (as
long as one remembers what the pictures are pictures of). But the idea that in order to
remember, there must be a *neural* record stored in the brain is incoherent. For even if there
were such a 'record', it would not be *available* to a person in the sense in which his diary
or photograph album is available to him – after all, a person cannot see into his own brain,
and cannot read neuralese. Moreover, the idea that there must be a stored memory, which
is available to a person and is a necessary condition of his being able to remember *presupposes* memory (in two different ways), and cannot explain it. For were such a record available
to one, one would have to *remember* how to read it, just as one can make use of one's diary
only if one remembers how to read. Similarly, one can use one's photograph album as an
aide-mémoire only if one remembers what the photographs are photographs of. The idea of
a store of knowledge makes sense only if the store is indeed available to one and one can
read or recognize the 'representation' – which is obviously not the case when it is supposed
that the relevant information is 'stored' in the brain. The idea of neural storage of *representations* (in the semantic or iconic sense) is incoherent.

If one perceives or learns that things are thus-and-so, one has come to know how things are. One may remember *what* one has thus learnt, retain the information one acquired, i.e. continue to possess the diffuse abilities constitutive of knowing things to be thus. To retain here simply means that one once knew, and has not ceased to know, that one acquired the ability, for example, to answer the question whether . . . or where . . . or when . . . and has not lost it, that it became possible for one to act on the information that things are so, and that it is still possible for one to do so, since one has not forgotten that things are so. Nothing is implied about *storage* of information. To remember that *p* is to *possess* the information that *p*, but it is not to *store* or *contain* the information that *p*. One stores the information that *p* if, for example, one writes it down, and stores the inscription in a filing cabinet or computer, which then contains it (but does not possess it). One cannot store information in one's head, and one's head, unlike one's diary, contains no information. Similarly, if one perceives an object, place or person M, and one does not forget M, then one will recognize M if one encounters it or him again. One's remembering M may therefore include, apart from facts about M, also a recognitional ability. But to remember M well, to be able to recognize M (or a picture of M), does not imply that one has stored anything. It implies the acquisition and retention of a recognitional ability. What the neural prerequisites of this are, merits investigation.

(2) When neuroscientists invoke the notion of storage, their thought is apparently that (a) what is stored when one remembers something is a memory; (b) this stored item is a representation; and (c) what it represents is the original perceptual episode. This is anything but clear.

First, we speak of 'a memory' and of having 'many happy (or sad) memories' of something or other. Thus used, the expression 'a memory' typically signifies *what is remembered* when one remembers *that such-and-such* or *having such-and-such an experience*. We say such things as 'My memory is that (things are so)', which means much the same as 'As I remember . . . (things are so)' or 'As far as I can remember . . .'. We say 'I have a dim memory of (Euclidean geometry, Toledo, my grandfather)', which means much the same as 'I remember . . . but dimly'. So *a memory* is an item of information (or putative information) that such-and-such or concerning this or that (or that one had such-and-such an experience), previously acquired and not forgotten. In so far as this is what is meant by 'a memory', it is evident that a memory is not a *representation* of what is remembered, any more than a belief is a representation of what is believed. But one might say that the *verbal expression* of what is remembered is such a representation (in the semantic sense of the word). Secondly, a memory, i.e. what is remembered – namely, *that such-and-such* or *having such-and-such an experience* – is not even a candidate for storage. For there is no such thing as storing *that such-and-such*, let alone storing *having an experience* – at most one might store an inscription which expresses what is remembered or a picture which represents what was experienced. But it would be absurd to suppose that what is allegedly stored in the brain is an English (or any other) *sentence or inscription* or an array of *pictures* (like a photograph album). Thirdly, the idea that what is remembered when one remembers something is necessarily an original perceptual episode is mistaken. As we have noted, what we remember need not be anything past. We have all long since forgotten how we acquired most of the knowledge we possess. In order to be able to remember the myriad facts we know, we need not, and typically do not, recollect the episode on the occasion of which we acquired the information in question.

When we learn by reading or by being told, for example, what we typically remember is *what* we read or were told, not the reading or the telling of it. But neuroscientists seem to suppose that *the original episode of knowledge acquisition* must be 'registered' in the brain in the form of a representation. For the excitation of this representation allegedly explains three things. First, it seemingly explains the aetiology of remembering when one is reminded of something previously learnt. The current stimulus, which causes one to remember (i.e. reminds one of what one then remembers), produces a neural correlate which is the same as part of the neural pattern which was laid down by the original episode. That is why it reminds one of the antecedent experience. Secondly, it explains the phenomenon of remembering. For the stimulus excites the very same neural structure, which has 'stored the memory', and that excitation causes the person to have a memory experience. Thirdly, it allegedly explains why repetition strengthens or reinforces memory. For changes in strength at synapses increase with repetition. We shall investigate these suppositions in a moment.

(3) Given that what is allegedly 'stored' or 'laid down' in the brain is not (and could not be) a verbal report or pictorial representation of an antecedent experience, it seems that the perceptions that 'give rise to memories' must be *encoded* in the nerve cells and synapses, and that this *neural representation* is what is stored. But this idea too is questionable.

First, perceiving something does indeed lead to neural changes, but it is altogether obscure what might be meant by the suggestion that *a perception* is *encoded*. One can *describe*, in words, what one perceives and one's perceiving of it – and then *encode the descriptions*, assuming that one knows the transformation rules. But there is no such thing as encoding a perception. Nor is there any such thing as *encoding* something in the brain (at any rate, not in the ordinary sense of 'encode') – for there is no such thing as a neural *code*. For a code is a method of encrypting a linguistic expression (or any other form of representation) according to conventional rules.

Secondly, it is unclear what is meant by the claim that a neural configuration may *represent* a memory. Suppose the relevant memory is that one was told that the Battle of Hastings was fought in 1066. What would count as a neural representation of this remembered fact? It is unclear whether, in the requisite sense of 'representation', *anything* could count as a representation, short of *an array of symbols belonging to a language*. Nothing that one might find in the brain could possibly be a representation of the fact that one was told that Hastings was fought in 1066 in the sense in which the English sentence 'I was told that Hastings was fought in 1066' can be said to be such a representation. But, of course, it may well be the case that but for certain neural configurations or strengths of synaptic connections, one would not be able to remember the date of the Battle of Hastings and would not recollect being told it. But it does not follow from that idea that what one remembers must be, as it were, written down in the brain, or that there must be some neural configuration in the brain from which one could in principle read off what is remembered. Nor can it be said that this neural configuration *is* a memory.

It might be supposed, however, that the original perceptual episode must have caused a set of neurons to fire in the brain, and the excitation of this pattern is precisely what causes one *to have the experience of remembering* whatever one remembers about the original episode. But even this relatively modest idea is problematic.

(4) The idea that when one remembers something on a given occasion, the brain must reactivate the pattern of neural excitation that was stimulated by the antecedent perceptual experience in which one came to know what one is now recollecting, rests upon a number of questionable assumptions.

1. Currently remembering something is a (mnemonic) experience variously described as 're-creating in memory' a past episode or 'the conscious vision of a past occurrence'. (In eighteenth-century jargon, it is having a current idea corresponding to an antecedent impression.)
2. What is remembered is a past experience or some feature of a past experience.
3. Currently remembering is triggered by a reminding experience. The reminding experience in certain respects resembles the past experience that is remembered.

Correlative to these assumptions, current neuroscientific speculation adds a series of neuroscientific assumptions:

1. Currently recollecting something is the re-excitation of a neural firing pattern. It is this which causally explains the person's having the mnemonic experience.
2. The original experience now remembered laid down a neural trace (a neural structure which, when excited, will repeat the pattern of firing generated by the original experience). The reactivation of the memory trace causes a mnemonic experience (the 'conscious memory event'), which 'reproduces in memory' the original perceptual experience or some part thereof. (It is an idea or faint copy of the original impression.)
3. The current reminder triggers the brain-trace, and hence the mnemonic experience, by a pattern of neural input, which is part of the original pattern generated by the past perceptual experience. The similarity between the current memory experience and the original experience of which it is the memory is explained by its being caused by the reactivation of the brain-trace or pattern of neural firing, which was laid down by the original perceptual experience.

This reasoning, though tempting, is flawed. We have already noted that what is remembered need not be anything past. The information acquired in the past need not be about the past, and one typically does not remember the occasion of its acquisition. All that is logically required for remembering in such cases is that one came to know something and that one still knows it (i.e. one has not forgotten the knowledge one acquired).

Now a further two points need to be stressed. First, currently remembering something need involve no reproductive 'representation'. To remember that *p* (e.g. that Hastings was fought in 1066, that one did such-and-such last week), to remember perceiving, doing or undergoing something, or to remember M (a person, place, object or event), or to remember how to do something need not involve reproducing a 'representation', either in the form of a mental image or in the form of a sentence spoken aloud or in the imagination. So, for example, to remember the way home need involve no mental imagery, but only the exercise of the ability to go home without losing one's way. To remember how to drive need involve nothing more than exercising the ability to drive. To remember what someone said need involve nothing more than acting or reacting on the grounds of the information conveyed by the utterance. To remember perceiving, doing or undergoing something is not essentially an ability to 're-create' the experience in the imagination. It is, of course, exhibited in recounting the experience; but this is not necessary for currently remembering it. It is, as is evident from the above examples, sufficient that one act (or react) *for the reason* that one previously perceived, was told, did or underwent such-and-such. (And here, the reason is not a *cause* but a *justification*, which one might adduce in answer to the question of why one did what one did.)

Secondly, remembering what we remember on a given occasion is no more *an experience* than is knowing what we know on a given occasion. This should not be surprising, since to remember that something is thus-and-so is to know something previously learnt and not forgotten. Of course, I may suddenly remember something, and this may be accompanied by various experiences (e.g. a feeling of relief, or having a mental image).

But remembering something on an occasion (like knowing something) is not essentially a *phenomenon*; i.e. it is not akin to a feeling about which one may ask 'What did it feel like?'. Rather, there may be various *manifestations* of the fact that I remember something, none of which *is* the remembering. If you cancel this evening's meeting, there are indefinitely many things that I, remembering that the meeting is cancelled, may consequently do. I may go home, or go to the cinema, or phone any number of friends and arrange to dine together, or stay on at the office until late, or go to the bookshop to buy a book to read in the evening, and so forth. All these cases involve my remembering that the meeting is cancelled. But in none need I 're-create in memory' your cancelling this evening's meeting, or even say to myself that you have done so. All that is necessary is that part of my reason for doing what I do is that you have cancelled the meeting – and that is not an experience. If remembering something need not involve remembering the past episode in which the relevant information was acquired, it clearly need not involve exciting a hypothesized brain-trace or pattern of neural firing *in order to re-create* a reproduction 'in memory' of the original episode. And if memory need involve no reproductive mnemonic experience, it is not necessary that the hypothesized brain-trace be reactivated in order to produce the relevant experience. Of course, it is tempting to think that if one learnt that p (e.g. that Hastings was fought in 1066, or that $E = mc^2$) and one remembers these facts, then they must be 'laid down' or 'encoded' in the brain. Otherwise, how could one possibly recollect these facts? But, as we have seen, no sense has been given to the idea of encoding or representing factual information in the neurons and synapses of the brain. It is false that whenever one remembers something (e.g. the day of the week, the way home, one's last birthday, the opening bars of Beethoven's Fifth), one's remembering is triggered by a current experience that causes a neural excitation similar to part of the neural excitation that was caused originally by the perceptual event in which one learnt whatever one now remembers. It is not true that whenever one's reason for doing something is a fact one previously learnt, one must have been reminded of that fact by some current experience, let alone by an experience that bears some resemblance to the past experience from which one learnt what one now recollects. Consequently, the demand that the putative brain-trace be reactivated by a current experience that generates a part of the original pattern of neural excitation is altogether redundant. It was produced to meet the demands of a *picture* – a picture of what remembering consists in. But that picture is altogether misconceived.

Neuroscientists have discovered that damage to the hippocampus deprives one of the ability to recollect anything subsequently learnt or experienced for longer than about 30 sec. This certainly suggests that retention of certain neural firing patterns and synaptic connections is essential for the possibility of recollection. But it does not follow that 'memories are stored at recurrent collateral synapses', *if* the terms 'memory' and 'store' are being used in the normal sense. For, to repeat, there is no such thing as 'storing' what one remembers, e.g. *that Hastings was fought in* 1066, or *visiting Florence for the first time*, unless it is inscribed in symbolic form and the inscription is stored. It may be that retention of certain synaptic connections and creation of certain recurrent firing patterns are a necessary condition for one to be able to recall something – but that is all. The relevant synaptic connections and firing patterns cannot be said to *represent* 'a memory' or what is remembered. Remembering something is not a matter of retrieving something stored in the hippocampus. Nor is it having a special kind of experience – a mnemonic experience that re-creates 'in memory' some past experience. Memory is the retention of knowledge previously acquired. It is a capacity that may be exercised in indefinitely many forms, e.g. in *saying* what one remembers, affirming *that* one remembers it when asked, not *saying* anything but *thinking* about what is remembered, neither saying nor thinking anything, but acting on what one remembers in any of indefinitely many ways, recognizing something or someone, and so forth. It is very tempting to think that the diverse forms in which remembering something may be manifest are all due to the fact that what is remembered is *recorded* and *stored* in the brain. But that is a nonsense. *What is remembered* when it is remembered that such-and-such is not anything laid down in the brain (about which we know virtually nothing), but rather something previously learnt or experienced. What neuroscientists must try to discover is what are the neural conditions of remembering and the neural concomitants of recollecting something. For the time being, that is ambition enough.

In short, neuroscientists investigating memory must distinguish between the experience of information acquisition and the information acquired, and hence between remembering the information acquired and remembering the acquiring of it. They must be careful not to slip into the error of thinking that all remembering is remembering a past experience. When they are concerned with remembering a past experience, they must not suppose that remembering need be a form of imaginative reproducing, as opposed to recounting or otherwise acting, and they must not suppose that recounting involves reading off information from a mental image. And they should avoid thinking that remembering something is a kind of experience. So too, they must distinguish the memory, i.e. what is remembered, from the expression of the memory in words, symbols or images, and also between the verbal expression of a memory and the multiple forms in which the overt remembering may be manifest. The expression of a memory must be distinguished from the neural configurations, whatever they may be, which are conditions for a person's recollecting whatever he recollects. But these configurations are not the memory; nor are they representations, depictions or expressions of what is remembered.

3.3   The Contribution of Neuroscience to Understanding Memory

Few neuroscientists now subscribe to the Cartesian doctrine that there is a mind, conceived of as an immaterial substance, which in some mysterious and inexplicable way interacts with the neural networks of the brain and incorporates within itself a private 'world of consciousness'. Rather, many neuroscientists believe that it is the brain itself (or one or other hemisphere of the brain) that, for example, perceives and remembers. And they, as well as others who are not guilty of this error, are prone to explain how it is that we human beings perceive and remember by reference to the brain's exercising its alleged psychological abilities, such as its ability to construct hypotheses, to conjecture, to reason and to think. It is only because the brain can do such things (the very kinds of things that the dualists ascribed to the mind) that we ourselves enjoy the 'conscious experiences' of remembering what we experience and what we learn in the course of our experience. Or so it is customarily argued by contemporary neuroscientists. What is most striking about their overall conception is just how Cartesian it is, differing from the Cartesian view primarily in repudiating the conception of the mind as an immaterial substance, and substituting the brain for the Cartesian mind. But the *logical structures* of the dualist conception remain to a very large extent intact, being simply transferred from mind to brain. The causal relation between the Cartesian mind and the body is replaced, in current reflections, by the causal relations between the brain and the body, and the overall conception of the relation of the 'inner' to the 'outer' that was enshrined in classical dualist thought soldiers on more or less intact, the brain being conceived to fulfil much the same role as the Cartesian mind.

In §3.1 we briefly reviewed the triumphs of twentieth-century neuroscientific investigations of memory and endeavoured to give an overview of how neuroscientific work led to the emergence of the above conception of the relationship between neural processes and mental attributes. In §3.2 we have presented an analysis of the conceptual framework deployed by many neuroscientists today. In so doing, we offer a very different conception of the relationship between the functioning of neural networks in the brain and human experience.

The foundation upon which our study rests is the logico-linguistic analysis of the psychological concepts deployed by neuroscientists. These concepts are invoked in neuroscientists' descriptions of the relationships between neural processes and the concomitant psychological attributes for which these processes are causally necessary conditions. The logical structures of the conceptual framework thus deployed determine what does and does not make sense. The bounds of sense do not exclude any empirical possibilities, but only *logical impossibilities*. Logical impossibilities, however, are not possibilities that are impossible, but forms of words that lack any sense. They are, therefore, not constraints upon any intelligible investigations. Rather, they fence one in only from the void of nonsense. A fundamental point which informs our investigation is an aspect of the logic of psychological concepts. One cannot correctly and literally ascribe to parts of an animal (including human beings) properties which are logically ascribable only to the whole animal. We refer to this as the 'mereological principle' (mereology being the logic of part/whole relationships). It is a crucial feature of psychological concepts (with a qualified exception in the case of verbs of sensation, such as 'itching' and 'throbbing') that they apply to the animal as a whole, and not to its parts. It makes no sense to ascribe to parts of a creature, including the brain, such psychological attributes as being conscious or unconscious, thinking or being thoughtless, believing or disbelieving, perceiving or misperceiving, hypothesizing or inferring, knowing or remembering.

This is not a trivial convention that might simply be overridden by conceptual innovation. Rather, it has multiple ramifications, for the mereological principle is bound up with the kinds of grounds that constitute logically good evidence for the ascription of psychological attributes to a person and the complex relationships between the grounds for ascribing them to others and the possibility of ascribing them groundlessly to oneself. The received view among neuroscientists is that each person ascribes psychological predicates to himself on the basis of introspection, conceived as a form of inner perception. On this view, introspection is the means by which each of us gains privileged access to the 'inner world of consciousness'. This conception of a private inner world, to which each of us alone has access is, in our view, a far-reaching misconception, which infects much of the thought and reasoning of neuroscientists. In §3.2 we considered the extent to which neuroscientists' investigations of memory are flawed as a result of conceptual confusions, including the failure to comply with the logical requirements of the mereological principle. We endeavoured to survey the concepts of memory which neuroscientists employ in their investigations of the neural foundations of such human (and animal) capacities. We outlined the conceptual framework for the description of the phenomena of memory that are of concern to neuroscientists: i.e. the manifold connections, compatibilities and incompatibilities that obtain among members of this large network of concepts. And, from case to case, we demonstrated that many neuroscientists, including one of the authors, in commenting on their own work and in the explanations they offer for the phenomena they investigate, have failed to conform to the logical requirements determined by the very concepts they invoke. To this extent, they misinterpret the results and implications of their own research. And the price of failing to abide by the logical requirements of the concepts invoked (and failure to stipulate coherent novel rules for different uses of the expressions) is that what is said lacks sense. Many confusions came to the surface. Contrary to widespread views, it is a muddle to conflate retention of knowledge with storage of knowledge, and a worse muddle to suppose that knowledge can be *stored* in the brain. And so on. The moral of our tale is that neuroscientists need to devote as much care to ensure conceptual coherence and lucidity as they do to the experiments they undertake.

The most important point we wish to press is that the neuroscientific task, in respect of memory, is to inquire into the physical concomitants and causal conditions for the possession and exercise of such powers as are involved in remembering. These powers are the attributes of human beings, not of their brains, and explaining the conditions of the possibility of their possession and exercise cannot, on pain of transgressing the bounds of sense, involve the ascription of any psychological attributes to the brain.

4

Language and Cortical Function: Wernicke to Levelt

4.1 Introduction: Psycholinguistics and the Neuroanatomy of Language

In the middle of the nineteenth century Broca (1861), and later Wernicke (1874), identified a number of asphasic syndromes in speech production and auditory comprehension that became associated with their names: in particular, Wernicke's aphasia, which involves a major disturbance in auditory comprehension of speech, and Broca's aphasia, which involves a major disturbance in speech. Lesions of the brain which appeared to be localized were associated with these different syndromes. With reference to the Brodmann Area (BA) determination of different architectonic parts of the brain, observed in lateral view in Plate 4.1, Broca's aphasia is associated with lesions in the inferior frontal cortex (pars opercularis (BA44) and pars triangularis (BA45)), whereas Wernicke's aphasia is associated with lesions in the superior temporal cortex (namely, the planum temporale (BA42), the superior temporal gyrus (BA22) and the superior part of the middle temporal gyrus (BA21)). A third area, related to disturbances in the production of single words and their comprehension (anomic aphasia), is associated with lesions in the parieto-temporal cortex (the angular gyrus AG (in BA39)) and the supramarginal gyrus (SMG in (BA40)), and is called AG/SMG.

In 1885 Lichtheim speculated that 'language is localized in structures interconnected anatomically in order to produce a language system' (fig. 4.1a). The language system proposed for this connected set of localized cortical regions by Lichtheim (1885), and later elaborated by Geschwind (1965) and Caplan (1994), is shown in fig. 4.1b. These authors suggested that Wernicke's area is, in Caplan's words, 'an auditory centre for word processing in which word sounds are stored so forming a kind of phonological lexicon'. Broca's area is identified as a 'motor centre for speech planning and programming taken as a problem in syntax' (Caplan, 1994). Finally, the AG/SMG area is required for 'the storage of conceptual information and is therefore concerned with syntax'. Fig. 4.1a shows this 'language system' – that is, a neural system necessary for mastery of a language, in which A is located in Wernicke's area and is associated with word sounds now called a phonological lexicon; M is located in Broca's area, associated with movements involved in executing speech intentions; B is a centre allegedly associated with possession of concepts. Lichtheim's (1885) isolation of a centre that is required for 'auditory word representations' from a centre for

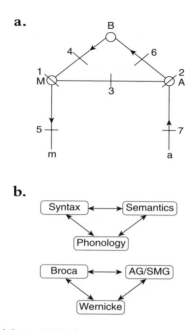

Fig. 4.1. **a:** the classical Lichtheim (1885) 'language system' (Caplan, 1994, fig. 3). **b:** (*upper*): sug-gested interaction between 'language modules'; (*lower*): suggested areas of cortex for language and their interactions. (Sakai et al., 2001, figs 2 and 3.)

'motor representations' – that is, Wernicke's area from Broca's area – follows the experimental discoveries of Wernicke (1874). The 'a priori' argument for a connection between the two centres rests on the claim that as children learn to speak by imitation, allegedly before con-cepts are acquired, a centre on which the acquisition of concepts is dependent (AG/SMG) must be located elsewhere than in Wernicke's or Broca's areas. The classical clinical aphasic syndromes given in the top half of table 4.1 are then predicted to be consequences of the lesions shown in table 4.2 (see bottom half of table 4.1):

The Wernicke/Lichtheim theory is concerned with what is now called 'psycholinguis-tics': namely, 'the empirical and theoretical study of the mental faculty [*sic*] that underpins our consummate linguistic ability' (Altmann, 2002). The theory is concerned with deter-mining the functional neuroanatomy of the brain on which this faculty depends. However, the above sketch of the Wernicke/Lichtheim theory contains unanalysed terms which are now part of the vocabulary of that discipline, such as 'language system', 'storing word sounds', 'word processing', 'speech planning and programming', 'conceptual information', 'auditory word representation'. The account of language abilities developed by Wernicke and Lichtheim has had a profound effect on modern students of the subject. For instance, Sakai et al. (2001) comment that 'Human language is a unique faculty of the mind'. The grammaticality of a sentence, they assert, needs to be made explicit by the adoption of an appropriate 'theoretical framework' for linguistic structures. Grammatical rules arise from the human brain, so language must be considered to be a 'subsystem of the mind', with

Table 4.1. The classic aphasic syndromes

Sydrome	Clinical manifestations	Hypothetical deficit	Classical lesion location
	A. Syndromes attributed to disturbances of cortical centres		
Broca's aphasia	Major disturbance in speech production with sparse, halting speech, often misarticulated, frequently missing function words and bound morphemes	Disturbances in the speech planning and production mechanisms	Primarily posterior aspects of the third frontal convolution and adjacent inferior aspects of the precentral gyrus
Wernicke's aphasia	Major disturbance in auditory comprehension; fluent speech with disturbances of the sounds and structures of words (phonemic, morphological, and semantic paraphasias)	Disturbances of the permanent representations of the sound structures of words	Posterior half of the first temporal gyrus and possibly adjacent cortex
Anomic aphasia	Disturbance in the production of single words, most marked for common nouns with variable comprehension problems	Disturbances of the concepts and/or the sound patterns of words	Inferior parietal lobe or connections between parietal lobe and temporal lobe
Global aphasia	Major disturbance in all language functions	Disruption of all language-processing components	Large portion of the perisylvian association cortex

(*Continued*)

Table 4.1. *Continued*

Sydrome	Clinical manifestations	Hypothetical deficit	Classical lesion location
	B. Syndromes attributed to disruptions of connections between centres		
Conduction aphasia	Disturbance of repetition and spontaneous speech (phonemic paraphasias)	Disconnection between the sound patterns of words and the speech production mechanism	Lesion in the arcuate fasciculus and/or corticocortical connections between temporal and frontal lobes
Transcortical aphasia	Disturbance of spontaneous speech similar to Broca's aphasia with relatively preserved repetition	Disconnection between conceptual representations of words and sentences and the motor speech production system	White matter tracts deep to Broca's area
Transcortical sensory aphasia	Disturbance in single word comprehension with relatively intact repetition	Disturbance in activation of word meanings despite normal recognition of auditorily presented words	White matter tracts connecting parietal lobe to temporal lobe or in portions of inferior parietal lobe
Isolation of the language zone	Disturbance of both spontaneous speech (similar to Broca's aphasia) and comprehension, with some preservation of repetition	Disconnection between concepts and both representations of word sounds and the speech production mechanism	Cortex just outside the perisylvian association cortex

Table 4.2. Lesions

Injury to Broca's area (M)	Lesion 1	Broca's aphasia with disturbances in speech production and auditory comprehension
Injury to Wernicke's area (A)	Lesion 2	Wernicke's aphasia with disturbances in auditory comprehension and choice of word sounds
Injury to the input to Wernicke's area (A)	Lesion 7	Spontaneous speech normal but comprehension and repetition disturbed
Injury to output of Broca's area (M)	Lesion 5	Misarticulation of repetition and spontaneous speech with comprehension preserved
Injury between AG/SMG (B, concept centre) and Broca's area (M)	Lesion 4	Reduction in spontaneous speech but repetition left intact
Injury between Wernicke's area (A) and AG/SMG (B, concept centre)	Lesion 6	Disturbance of comprehension with normal repetition ability retained
Injury between Broca's area (M) and Wernicke's area (A)	Lesion 3	Altered spontaneous speech and repetition without affecting auditory comprehension

the language system a 'distinct module', which in turn possesses its own modularity or subsystems 'such as phonology, semantics, and syntax, which interact systematically with each other through the "information flow" between them' (fig. 4.1b). However, this rudimentary account of language is incoherent, and the vocabulary is systematically misleading or worse.

Language is not a faculty of anything, let alone of the mind, although the ability to speak a language may be a unique human ability. Furthermore, there is no need of a 'theoretical framework' for a speaker of a language to understand the language he speaks. The most that can be claimed is that the neuroscientist or psycholinguist needs a framework for the description of the speech phenomena with which he is concerned, and for the description of their neural correlates. Arguably, the less theoretical baggage this vocabulary carries, the fewer the hostages to fortune.

A competent speaker of a language can, for the most part, judge whether a sentence of his language is grammatical. But there is nothing 'implicit' about such a judgement. Not judging a sentence to be ungrammatical must not be conflated with judging a sentence to be grammatical. Rendering explicit *general criteria* for a sentence's being grammatical in a given language is a task for grammarians, not for psycholinguists.

Language is not a 'subsystem' of the human mind, although the ability to learn a language is innate, and it is above all the mastery of a language that endows human beings with those abilities that are characteristic of creatures that can be said to have a mind. To have a mind is to have a certain array of abilities. But a mind is not a system of anything, and it is altogether unclear what is meant, if anything, by the claim that the mind has subsystems. Of course, the character of human languages can be presumed to reflect the biological and other properties of the human brain, in various, as yet unknown ways.

It is unclear what Sakai and his colleagues mean by the claim that 'language' consists of modules. It is even less clear what they mean by the claim that the modules of language *interact*, and totally obscure what they mean by the assertion that they interact 'through information flow'. Information flow can occur between people or institutions. Can it occur between language modules? Can well-formedness interact with truth valuation? Can it occur between language modules in *the brain*? Can the phonological module inform the semantic module what it is up to? This surely makes no sense. Can talk of a language module in the brain mean anything more than that certain parts of the cortex are causally associated with certain kinds of linguistic abilities? Although parts of the cortex may interact, it does not follow that the several abilities interact. We shall explore these doubts as our survey progresses.

We provide below an analysis first of the Wernicke/Lichtheim theory (§4.2), and then of more recent developments (§4.3) that have led to a renaissance in modular theories of language comprehension (§4.4) and speech (§4.5). This is followed (§§4.6 and 4.7) by consideration of the extent to which modern functional neuroanatomical studies have illuminated how linguistic abilities depend on brain structure. Finally (§4.8) consideration is given to the recent claims concerning models of speech and its comprehension with respect to their neuroanatomical dependence.

4.2   The Theory of Wernicke/Lichtheim

4.2.1   Introduction: Wernicke

Wernicke (1874) is credited with beginning the process of developing models, given in diagram form, of how aphasia arises. These models were thought to provide a succinct way of summarizing the bewildering array of syndromes reported at the time by clinicians. Thus he comments that 'The theory of aphasia presented here is capable of subsuming under itself the exceedingly varied clinical picture of aphasia. The very multiplicity of these pictures, which until now has provided every new observer with new riddles to solve, will no longer be so striking' (p. 93). Aphasic patients gave Wernicke the opportunity to probe the relationships between different linguistic abilities and the anatomy of the cortex. Most of what he says is couched in anatomical terms intermingled with cognitive ones. The anatomical terms were often inaccurate, and Lichtheim (1885) stripped out the anatomical descriptions, leaving the cognitive ones and their supposed relationships, as indicated by diagrams (fig. 4.1a). It is of some importance to examine the application of these cognitive terms by Wernicke and Lichtheim, as they were used uncritically in the twentieth century by those developing a modular description of language acquisition and use.

Wernicke introduces first the idea of 'memory images of sensations' (§4.2.1.1) and then that of 'images of movement' (§4.2.1.2). The essential properties of voluntary movement as compared with reflex movement are next considered (§4.2.1.3), with the former alleged to consist of movements caused by mental images of kinaesthetic sensations. This was the standard late nineteenth-century ideo-motor conception (or misconception) of voluntary movement advanced by such eminent scientists as von Helmholtz, Wundt, Mach and, later, James. Wernicke then introduces his famous flow diagrams, superimposed on diagrams of the cortex, to illustrate how voluntary movement is related to cortical function. All of this is preparatory to an understanding of the supposed causal role of movement images in the cortex in the production of phonemes and to an explanation of how aphasia might arise (§4.2.1.4). Finally, Wernicke attempts to give an account of how patients might retain their mastery of a concept but be unable to recollect the word associated with it (§4.2.1.5).

4.2.1.1 *Images of sensations*

Wernicke suggests that the surface of the brain exhibits a mosaic of simple elements which are characterized by their relatively direct anatomical connections with the periphery of the body, as is the case with the visual cortex and the projection of the optic nerve or the olfactory cortex and the projection of the olfactory nerve. The 'elementary psychic functions' can be assigned to these elementary areas, as in visual or olfactory perception. Everything beyond these elementary functions, such as the linking of different sense impressions to form a concept, thought and consciousness, is a function of the fibre tracts that connect different cortical regions with each other – i.e. a function of the association systems, to use Meynert's term. Sense impressions, Wernicke argues, can be projected: 'The sense impressions projected onto the cerebral cortex from the outside world last longer than the external stimulus affecting the sense organ; they can reappear in the form of memory images (*Erinnerungsbilder*) independently of the stimulus that produced them, although in less vivid form' (p. 35). He suggests that the first convolution of the temporal lobe at the Sylvian fissure (now called the superior temporal gyrus) is the site for the 'deposition of acoustic images of words' where the central terminations of the acoustic nerve occurs, that is at the auditory cortex. Wernicke then envisages that, as the number of neurons in the cortex is in excess of 10^{10}, there is 'a sufficient number of storage areas in which the countless sense impressions delivered by the outside world can be stored in succession'.

These comments, at the beginning of his seminal work, introduce the venerable empiricist confusion that ideas or concepts, indeed thoughts, are 'formed by the linking of different sense impressions'. In this tradition, sense impressions are taken as psychological entities that a perceiver apprehends – indeed perceives – when his nerve endings are stimulated by objects in the external world. Many confusions are embedded in this classical empiricist (Lockean) conception. First of all, what we perceive when we perceive our environment are not sense impressions, but the indefinitely varied array of perceptibilia that humans are able to perceive: material objects, properties of material objects (sizes, shapes, textures, etc.), sounds and smells, distances between things, gaps and holes, events and processes that are occurring, states of affairs that obtain, and so on. The fact that light waves have to impact upon our retinae or sound waves upon our eardrums in order for us to see what is before our eyes or hear the sounds being made in our vicinity does not imply that what we perceive are not public visibilia and audibilia. The fact that complex neural events have to occur within the cortex in order for us to be able to perceive whatever we perceive does not imply that what is perceived is within the cortex. What one sees when one sees a tree is the tree, not a sense impression of a tree. It may appear to one to be other than it is, but it does not follow that what one sees is something other than a tree – only that it looks to one like something else.

Secondly, it is mistaken to suppose that *sense impressions* are 'projected onto the cerebral cortex from the outside world'. Rather, nerve impulses are conducted from sense-organs to the brain. It is a further confusion to think that something called 'a sense impression' might 'last longer than the external stimulus affecting the same organs'. It is true that we can have an after-image that persists after the object perceived has ceased to exist (e.g. a flash of light), but an after-image is not a sense impression – having an after-image is not perceiving something (after-images are *had*, not perceived), nor is it how something one perceives strikes one as being. It is even more confused to suppose that sense impressions 'reappear' in the form of memory images, as if memory images were what sense impressions become when they are first stored in the memory (that 'warehouse of ideas' as Locke called it), and then pulled out of cold storage. But there is no such thing as *storing* something called 'a sense impression', and the brain is no storehouse.

Thirdly, neither sense impressions nor combinations of sense impressions are concepts. In so far as sense impressions are supposed to be akin to mental images, then possession of a sense impression of X is neither necessary nor sufficient for possession of the concept of an X. We shall discuss this matter below.

4.2.1.2 Movement images

Wernicke next extends the concept of memory images of perceptions to what he called 'movement images' (i.e. memories of kinaesthetic sensations). He suggested that bodily movements and changes in the state of the musculature give rise to sensation, memory images of which also remain in the cerebral cortex. Such 'movement images' are allegedly deposited in the cortical area anterior to the fissure of Rolando. The content of consciousness supposedly consists of 'memory images of sensations [perceptions] on the one hand, of the forms of movement of one's own body [memories of kinaesthetic sensations] on the other hand', both of which are 'elements acquired from the outside world'.

Wernicke's conception of movement images is confused. There is no reason to suppose, and every reason not to suppose, that whenever one moves a limb, one has a characteristic kinaesthetic sensation. *Sometimes* one may have kinaesthetic sensations. Commonly, if one attends carefully to a movement one is engaged in, one apprehends a kinaesthetic sensation. But even if one has a kinaesthetic sensation there is no reason to suppose that there is a *distinctive* sensation for every muscle or group of muscles that one can contract when making a voluntary movement, or that one remembers each such sensation (as it were, carrying around with one a catalogue of such sensations). Moreover, the fact that one may have a kinaesthetic sensation when one attends to the movement of one's limb does not imply that one has or need have any kinaesthetic sensations when one does not so attend. The fact that one cannot say how one's limbs are disposed when one's kinaesthetic receptors are numbed or damaged does not imply that when one *can* say how one's limbs are disposed one says so on the basis of any kinaesthetic sensations one might be supposed to have. The ability to describe how one's limbs are disposed and how one's body is oriented may well depend on the normal functioning of kinaesthetic receptors, but it does not depend on having sensations that provide one with the evidence for one's orientation or bodily disposition. Our normal knowledge of how we are oriented or our limbs disposed is non-evidential.

4.2.1.3 *Voluntary movement*

Wernicke introduces a flow diagram superimposed on an outline of the cortex for the first time, to show how voluntary movement occurs. Fig. 4.2a represents a sensation moving along the path EO to a point in the occipito-temporal lobe where it leaves a memory image. A stimulus may then proceed from O to a motor point in the frontal lobe F through some portion of the great fibre tracts connecting the occipito-temporal lobe with the frontal lobe. Once it has reached this point, the excitation in the centrifugal path FB causes movement which is voluntary. What makes it voluntary is that it is caused by a stored memory image of the kinaesthetic sensations that characterize this type of movement. Wernicke holds that 'the path EOFB suffices for a complete explanation of voluntary movement on the pattern of a reflex process' (p. 40). To this it should be objected that it makes no sense to speak of sensations travelling through the brain, let alone leaving sensory traces. It is nerve impulses that travel thus. The path EOFB does not suffice to give an explanation of voluntary movement, not only because the anatomy is incorrect, but more importantly because the explanation is incoherent.

Given the mechanistic description of voluntary movement in fig. 4.2a, how does a human being act freely? To try to explain this, Wernicke considers the scheme in fig. 4.2b, as applied to the voluntary movement of one's eyes. A visual sensation travelling from the retina at E excites the movement of the eye at B through a pathway involving the reflex centre X and the motor centre Y. However, there are accessory pathways, from X to O which allow the laying down at O of a memory image of the sensation from the retina, and from Y to F that lay down there an image of the movement of the eye. Wernicke places X in the corpora quadrigemina, connected to the optic pathway E. Because of the simultaneous excitement of O and F an association is set up between them: namely, the path OF, taken to be in the cerebral cortex. Henceforth the memory image of the sensation at O easily elicits the movement image at F, and so the voluntary movement over the pathway FYB. Wernicke presupposes that the genesis of all voluntary movements can now be understood. 'The scheme provides for the possibility of a choice of movements; the more memory images the individual has at his disposal, and the more practised he is in associating memory images, the greater is his choice' (Wernicke, 1874, p. 42). This provides 'a scientific definition of free will'. Wernicke's explanation, however, is defective. For being caused to act by a sensation is neither necessary nor sufficient for acting freely. To be caused to sneeze by a sensation in one's nose, *a fortiori* being caused to sneeze by the memory of such a sensation, is not to sneeze freely – far from being a voluntary act, it is a paradigm of an involuntary one.

According to Wernicke, voluntary movement is distinguished from reflex movement by two properties. First, 'it does not follow the stimulus instantaneously but rather owes its elicitation to memory images of earlier sensations which are reawakened only in response

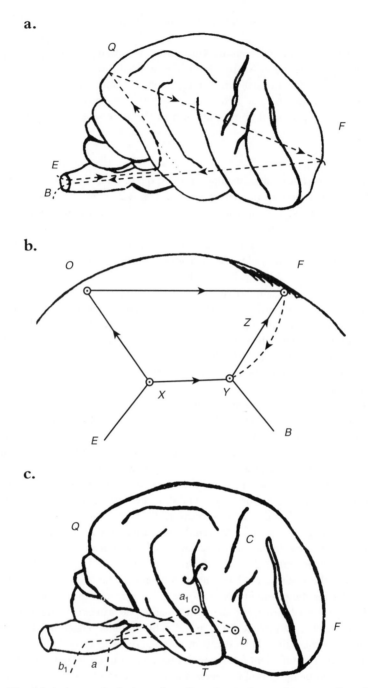

Fig. 4.2. Wernicke's theory of aphasia. **a:** flow diagram superimposed on an outline of the cortex showing how voluntary movement occurs. **b:** the network controlling the voluntary movement of the eyes. **c:** origins of a clonic aphasic syndrome. For description of the networks in **a** to **c**, see text. (Wernicke, 1874, figs 1–3.)

to an external stimulus' (p. 39). Second, it has a 'pre-formed pattern – polished, specific and adapted to the attainment of a goal. It is thus characterized by the presence of a representation of the movement to be carried out, and as was shown above, this representation also must be conceived as a residue of a sensation [a memory image]'.

To this it may be objected that voluntary movement is not movement caused by mental images of kinaesthetic sensations. Voluntary movements are movements that are constitutive of voluntary actions. Voluntary actions are actions that are under the agent's control, that he can do or refrain from doing at will. So they are actions that can be (but need not be) intentional, done for reasons, that sometimes follow decisions to act, that can be performed on request or to order. Wernicke's further claim that spontaneous (i.e. voluntary) movements possess a preformed pattern (i.e. are intentional) is mistaken. Not all voluntary movement is intended – not every gesture of one's hands as one talks is intended, but it is voluntary; i.e. the movements are under one's control.

4.2.1.4   *Sound images and language*

Wernicke now applies his theory of the genesis of voluntary movement, construed in the classical empiricist terms of Locke's representational idealism, to linguistic behaviour. As an 'image' of a sensation he offers 'a sound image' (representation, sense impression) of a word or syllable. In fact, that cannot be deemed to be an image of a *sensation*, for auditory perception does not involve sensations at all, save for sensations of being deafened. This image is taken to be transmitted in much the same manner as was envisaged for the supposed visual image, although whatever a visual image might be supposed to be, it is neither a sensation nor the image of a sensation. In fig. 4.2b, O now lays down a memory image of the sound, and F lays down an image of the movements involved in speech. Associations are now set up between the sound image (or representation) and the movement image (or representation) (OF). 'When later, the spontaneous movement, the consciously uttering of a word, takes place, the associated representation of movement is innervated (elicited) by the memory image of the sound' (p. 43). Now, as in the case of all voluntary movements, muscles are activated (along the path FYB in fig. 4.2b), in this case for speech. Wernicke supposes, then, that when one voluntarily and intentionally utters a word 'W', the movements of one's mouth and vocal chords are caused by a memory image of the sound of 'W' eliciting the memory image of the movements of one's mouth and vocal chords, which in turn cause the movements to occur.

This supposes that we all have kinaesthetic sensations corresponding to every single muscular movement that is necessary for the pronouncing of each phoneme of the language we speak. It supposes that we have the ability to conjure up memory images of such kinaesthetic sensations and to know which memory image corresponds to which phoneme. These claims do not rest on any empirical evidence. They are responses to the demands of a particular *picture*. The conception of speech that emerges from this strange picture is as follows: prior to saying something, the speaker must say to himself in his imagination whatever it is that he wishes to say aloud. The 'mental images (ideas or representations)' of the sounds he wishes to utter will then produce mental images (ideas or representations) of the kinaesthetic sensations of laryngeal movements and movements of tongue, lips, etc. associated with the utterance imagined. These will then conjunctively cause those very muscles to move. But it is not true that before we say what we want to say, we must always first say it to ourselves in the imagination. And it is surely mistaken to suppose that we have kinaesthetic sensations corresponding to every movement of larynx, tongue, lips, etc., the memory of which is involved in every act of speech.

How then does a classic aphasic syndrome arise? Wernicke explains such a syndrome by means of fig. 4.2c, in which F is the frontal, O the occipital, and T the temporal lobe (compare with fig. 4.2a). C designates the central fissure and 's' the Sylvian fossa. 'a_1' is the central termination of the acoustic nerve ('a' being the place where it enters the medulla, and 'b' stands for the representations of movement in the cerebral cortex which are alleged to be necessary for the production of sound, connected with a_1 by association fibres a_1b running in the insular cortex). The sound-producing motor nerves pass from b to the medulla (where they leave the brain). Interruption of the path aa_1bb_1 will cause aphasia, with the clinical syndrome varying according to the portion of the path affected. Consider, for example, that the path aa_1 has been interrupted; i.e. a pathological process has destroyed the acoustic nerve at some point in its central course. In adults, this produces deafness without any signs of aphasia, as long as these adults possess what Wernicke refers to as an extensive 'stock of sound images' acquired during childhood and capable of being reproduced at will. In childhood, deaf-mutism results if destruction of the acoustic nerve occurs before a 'stock of sound images' has consolidated in the cerebral cortex. This is explained within Wernicke's scheme, as due to the fact that the child 'has not acquired any representations of sounds from which representations of movement can be called into consciousness'.

However, Wernicke's conception of 'stocks of sound images' and 'representations of sounds' should be challenged. Speech is learnt imitatively as a normal child learns to mimic the mother (etc.), who trains him to reproduce sounds. But that is no reason to suppose that the child's sound reproductive abilities are dependent on his amassing a stock of mnemonic images of his own laryngal movements that are neurally associated with a corresponding stock of mnemonic images of phonemes. Abilities depend on neural structures, but these structures need not, and in these cases could not, contain copies of that which the abilities are abilities to do.

4.2.1.5 *Language acquisition, words and concepts*

Wernicke holds that thinking and speaking are two completely different processes, and that one must regard concepts and words as not only distinct but mutually independent. Consequently he supposes that the child's language acquisition is a dual process. On the one hand, the child must learn, by imitation, how to enunciate words. On the other hand, the child must connect the words it learns to pronounce with the concepts it has acquired through abstraction from sense experience.

According to Wernicke, the impact of sound waves upon the eardrums causes the child to have an auditory sense impression. This can be stored in memory in the form of a sound-image. The sound-image in turn has to be linked with the image of kinaesthetic sensations of the laryngeal movements associated with the reproduction of similar sounds. The integrity of the path aa_1b in fig. 4.2c is critical for the development of the child's linguistic abilities through imitation. Damage to it means that the child will not be able to reproduce the sound-images stored in memory, and so will be unable to enunciate words.

It is striking, however, that Wernicke holds that if a_1 (the cortex of the first temporal convolution) is destroyed, 'the sound images of the names of all possible objects will be destroyed from memory, although the concepts may still remain in full clarity' (p. 50). He believed this, since he held that the concept of an object O depends on the visual and tactile images of O from which it has been abstracted, and hence that possession of the concept of O may remain unimpaired, even though the use of the word 'O' has been lost.

Wernicke's account is indebted to the traditional empiricist conception of language and concept acquisition that is derived from John Locke. It is, unfortunately, mistaken. We shall point out only some of the more obvious confusions.

Our innate vocal imitative propensities are, no doubt, crucial to normal language acquisition. The child learns to reproduce the vocal sounds of the utterances of his parents, siblings, etc. What he imitates, however, is not a sense impression of a sound, let alone a mnemonic image of such a sense impression, but the sound itself. No doubt neural changes must occur for him to be able to do so. But what are imitated are the sounds he hears, not are images of the sounds. To do so, he must, no doubt, exercise his larynx, tongue and lips. But there is no reason to suppose that in order to do this the child must have stored a stock of mnemonic images of separate kinaesthetic sensations of laryngeal, etc. movements between which he chooses.

Concepts are not abstractions from sense impressions. The ability to call up mental images of X is neither necessary nor sufficient for possession of the concept of X. We possess numerous concepts to which no mental image could possibly correspond (e.g. concepts of numbers, of logical connectives (conjunction, alternation, conditionality, negation), of generality, of legal relations, of virtues and vices). Even if we *can* conjure up a mental image of X, we possess no concept of an X unless we can correctly use a word, phrase or other symbol that signifies X. If we use the word 'X' correctly, it matters not a whit whether, when we use it, an image of an X crosses our mind or not. A concept is something that can be applied or misapplied, introduced by a definition or explanation, that can be substituted for another, extended in various ways, can be grasped, understood or misunderstood, shared with others, mastered and possessed.

To possess a concept is to have a certain skill. It is, above all, to have mastered the use of a symbol. The criteria for whether a person possesses a concept are behavioural. They include the person's correct use of a symbol (word, phrase or iconic symbol) that expresses the concept, and the appropriateness of the person's behaviour in response to the use by others of symbols that express the concept. Concepts are not kinds of entity. To have grasped the meaning of the noun 'W', to have mastered its use, implies that one has acquired the concept of a W. But the concept of a W is no more *correlated* with the word 'W' or cognate phrase than is the meaning of the word 'W'. For neither meanings of words (i.e. their uses) nor concepts are kinds of entities that might be *correlated* with a word, any more than values are kinds of things that might be *correlated* with coins. Words are no more 'representations' of concepts than coins are representations of their values.

Wernicke notes that patients suffering from various forms of aphasia are commonly unable to remember a word, but are able to explain (roughly) what the word that they are striving to recollect means. He supposes that they retain the concept, but have forgotten its name, because the neural connection between the phonetic 'store' and the concept 'store' is damaged. But this is a misconception and a misdescription. Not only is the brain not a store, either for words or for concepts, but further, concepts are not the kinds of things that could be stored, in the brain or anywhere else – any more than one can store the meanings of words without the words. Words that express concepts are not names of the concepts they express (the word 'horse' is the name of a kind of animal, not the name of the concept of a horse, even though someone who has learnt what the word means can be said to possess the concept it expresses, a concept that is also expressed by the German noun 'Pferd' or the French noun 'cheval'). Someone who cannot recollect the word 'horse' but can say that the word he is trying to recollect is the name of the kind of animal people ride at racecourses can indeed be said to possess the concept of a horse but to be unable to recollect the word 'horse'. But that does not imply that he has a store of non-linguistic concepts at hand, which has become disconnected from the store of their names. It means that he can recollect the linguistic (paraphrastic) explanation of what the word he is trying to recollect means, but cannot recollect the word.

Wernicke avers that thinking and speaking are two completely different processes. In so far as this means merely that one can think without speaking and speak without thinking, then, of course, he is right. But in so far as it means that a person is able to think that *p* independently of having mastered the skill of expressing what he thinks in his behaviour, he is wrong. The horizon of a creature's thought is the horizon of its behavioural expressive repertoire. A creature *can* (in principle) think what it *can* (in principle) express in its behaviour. Of course, a person's speech centres may be damaged, and he may no longer be able to express the thought that *p*. But then he must have possessed the ability to do so antecedently, and the unverifiable supposition that he is thinking that *p* presupposes that were he to regain his powers of speech, he would be able to express that thought.

4.2.2   Lichtheim's concept centre

Lichtheim's (1885) development of Wernicke's confused psychological scheme is made without explicit reference to cortical structures. Like Wernicke, Lichtheim introduced a centre where concepts are stored in addition to a centre of auditory images and a centre of motor images. Fig. 4.1a shows the very influential diagram summarizing relations between these centres as conceived by Lichtheim. A is the centre for auditory images ('auditory word representations') and M the centre for motor images ('motor word representations'), equivalent to a_1 and b in Wernicke's diagram of fig. 4.2c. A reflex arc consists of an afferent branch of aA, which 'transmits the acoustic impression to A'; an efferent branch Mm, which conducts impulses from M to the organs of speech; and is completed by the commissure binding together A and M. B is the centre 'where concepts are elaborated'. It comes into play, when connections between A and B are activated, taken to be when there is intelligent consideration of the auditory images. The objections elaborated above (§§4.2.1.1–4.2.1.5) with respect to Wernicke's introduction of the idea of auditory images and motor images hold, of course, for Lichtheim's use of these phrases. The best that research could show is that brain areas exist that are causally implicated in the ability to recall spoken words, and that others exist which are causally required for different kinds of laryngeal, etc. movements. The idea of a 'concept centre' is entirely opaque, as is the meaning of 'concept elaboration'.

Lichtheim's observations of some aphasic patients showed that they could be grouped according to the following association of symptoms: loss of the abilities to speak at will, to repeat words, to read aloud, to write at will and to write to dictation, all without any loss of the ability to understand spoken words or written words or loss of the ability to copy. He suggested that this constitutes the true aphasia of Broca and the motor aphasia of Wernicke. It could be due to lesions at centre M in fig. 4.1a. Another set of symptoms belongs to patients who can no longer understand spoken or written language, or repeat words or write to dictation or read aloud, although they can write and copy words as well as speak. This, Lichtheim conjectured, could be due to lesions at centre A in fig. 4.1a. However, given that these centres cannot be centres for the storage of images of movement or images of sensations (see §§4.2.1.2–4.2.1.3), it is not clear that the letters M and B stand for anything more than the names of the two sets of syndromes.

4.2.3   Concepts and representations

Lichtheim holds that 'the mere excitation of the auditory representation (aA in fig. 4.1a) is not sufficient to secure correct speech (Mm), but this representation must enter into relationship with the concept (centre at B)'. These comments suggest that Lichtheim thought that words are names of concepts, and that to secure intelligent and intelligible speech, one must not only pronounce words, but also link them with the concepts they express. This would, it seems, be explained if, as Wernicke had suggested, one part of the brain stored the phonemes and another stored the correlated concepts. But, as we have seen, neither words nor concepts are stored, and concepts are not entities of a kind that can be correlated with words (here the word, there the concept, here the coin, there its value). Rather, certain neural structures at certain loci are causally essential for a person to remember words. Apparently they do not suffice for remembering what they mean, i.e. how they are to be used and how they are to be explained (for which other structures at other loci are necessary). But neither concepts nor meanings are entities, and certainly they are not storable in the cortex or anywhere else. A normal speaker needs to be able to pronounce the words of his language correctly, and to use them appropriately. Correct use involves mastery of their combinatorial possibilities in sentences, and a grasp of the appropriate circumstances of their use in utterances. The criteria of understanding are using a word correctly in utterances (including one-word sentences), explaining what one means by the use of a word in a sentence (including a one-word sentence), and responding intelligently to the use of the word by another person. Furthermore, as mentioned above (§4.2.1.5), to possess a concept is to have an ability. One cannot store abilities in the brain or anywhere else. But the normal functioning of the brain is a causal condition for possession of the ability. Students of the relationships between brain function and language skills can, at most, perform the valuable function of identifying precisely which parts of the brain are causally implicated in the possession and exercise of which ability. The startling discovery that emerges from the study of aphasic patients is how *composite* many of our linguistic abilities are, each presumably dependent upon distinct brain areas. But it is mistaken to suppose that one area stores a memory image and another stores a concept.

Lichtheim claimed that some of his aphasic patients were unable to 'find the auditory representation of a word' and that they were unable to tell the number of syllables in it. This was particularly marked with proper names, very rarely with verbs, adjectives and pronouns. But this simply means that the patient cannot remember the proper names, or cannot say the proper names to himself in his imagination. Lichtheim claimed that we can readily form a mental image of the nominatum in the case of proper names, but less readily in the case of other parts of speech. This cannot be right: we know who Hannibal, Hasdrubal and Hamilcar were, but may well be unable to form a mental image of them; most people can readily form mental images of colours that are correlates of colour adjectives. The fact is that mastery of the use of words has nothing (logically speaking) to do with one's eidetic powers. If there is any causal connection, it has to be shown, rather than assumed.

4.2.4   Conclusion

Wernicke's influential attempt to explain our linguistic abilities by transforming anatomical data into psychological form and to construct a theory out of such material was thought to have failed due to the use of erroneous anatomical data. However, later generations based their explanations on a largely uncritical acceptance of his ideas, stripped of their anatomical references. Here we have shown that the experimental psychology of the 1870s as applied by Wernicke is incoherent. But it has had profound repercussions in the twentieth century for both psycholinguistics and theories of the functional neuroanatomy of the brain on which linguistic skills depend, as we shall now show.

4.3   The Mental Dictionary and its Units: Treisman

In 1960 Treisman carried out experiments in which subjects were asked to 'shadow' a passage of prose given to one ear via earphones – i.e. repeat it aloud continuously as they heard it – while hearing a different passage in the other ear. In the course of the experiment, the two passages were switched. Subjects were able to make the switch without repeating more than one or two words from the wrong passage. Words were more likely to be repeated from the incorrect passage if it contained narrative prose, say from a novel, rather than statistical approximations to English. Thus the context of the prose was important in determining the accuracy of the switch. Treisman (1960) commented that 'Shadowing experiments suggest that there is a single channel system for analysing meaning, presumably comprising the matching of signals with some kind of dictionary and its store of statistical probabilities' (p. 246). She illustrated the role of this 'mental dictionary', with its dictionary units which are supposed to be utilized during the shadowing experiments, by means of fig. 4.3. When a passage is switched, two of these units, B and C, will be activated in the dictionary after the first word in the switched passage (A). B is the unit activated from the shadowed ear, and C is the unit activated both by its lowered threshold due to word A and the attenuated signal from the rejected ear. This leads to word C being sometimes repeated.

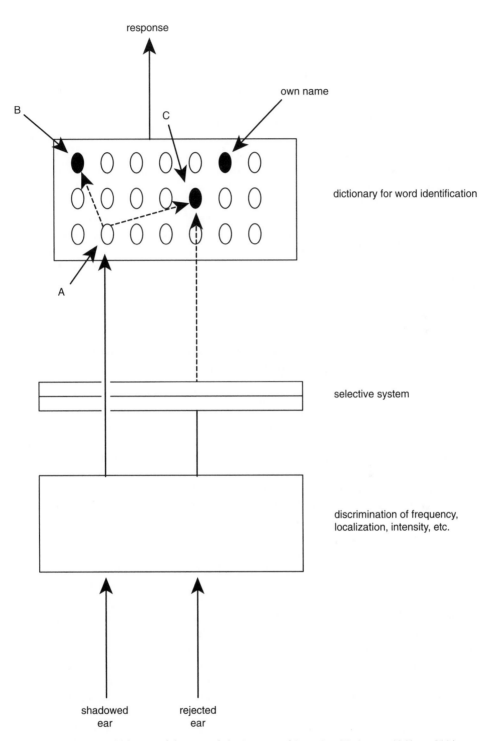

Fig. 4.3. Treisman's theory of the mental dictionary and its units. (Treisman, 1961, p. 211.)

Treisman (1961) also thought that there must be a 'concept store' in the brain because of the research of Wilder Penfield in Montreal. He had examined patients whose exposed brains were subjected to electrical stimulation in a search for the foci of epileptic discharges. Penfield observed patients who, although not able to name objects such as a knife, were able to describe a knife, for example, as 'something that cuts'.

The concept of a channel that *analyses meaning* does not make sense any more than does a 'dictionary' in the brain. Treisman could simply have said that shadowing involves comprehension, and switching is dependent on the subject's understanding of what he is attending to (but one could imagine shadowing a voice rather than a story). Treisman does not explain the phenomenon, but redescribes it in metaphorical terms that are presented as if they allude to something further. There is no matching of signals with a 'dictionary'. There is a normal human ability to comprehend and anticipate narrative continuity, which depends no doubt upon a neural structure about which we know very little. We can infer from the errors people make how the apparently simple ability is actually constituted of further subordinate abilities. We may suppose that different but connected neural structures are involved, and seek to identify these structures. But that is all.

4.4   The Modular Study of Word Recognition and Reading Aloud: Morton

4.4.1   The model system

Morton (1964a) took up Treisman's ideas of 'units' and 'conceptual stores' and elaborated them into a model system (fig 4.4a). He suggested that units exist for each word which they make available as a response, depending on whether the threshold of the unit is reached and the unit fires. A set of units constitutes a 'dictionary'. The dictionary receives a sensory input such as the presentation of a written word, which, if sufficient for a unit associated with a particular word, fires and makes the word 'available as a response'. The sensory input for a particular word will exceed its threshold depending on the number of visual characteristics (shapes, letters, etc.) the input, the written word, and the unit for the word have in common. If the threshold of the unit is reached, then its word is said to be 'perceived'. The activation threshold for each unit depends not only on the sensory input but also on the 'context' in which the sensory information is presented. An appropriate context for the utterance of the word lowers the unit's threshold, so increasing the probability that the unit will fire and make the word available. A number of unspecified 'sequential' processes operate to ensure that the context produces the threshold-lowering effect. The process of speaking a word involves a 'selection mechanism' which first chooses the word on the basis of the word's unit possessing a relatively high probability of firing. This probability is determined not only by the sensory input and the *context*, as defined above, but also by the nature of the 'previous responses' of the system – that is, the previous words uttered (Morton, 1964a; fig. 4.4a).

The units which make up the dictionary were later named 'logogens' by Morton and Broadbent (1967), so that each logogen corresponds to a word (fig. 4.4b). When the thresh-

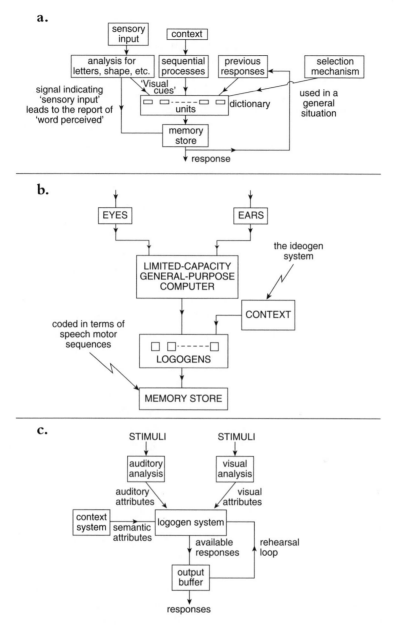

Fig. 4.4. **a:** a model for word recognition (Morton, 1969a, fig. 3). **b:** a model for speech recognition (Morton and Broadbent, 1967, fig. 1). **c:** the logogen model for word recognition (Morton, 1969a, fig. 1.)

old for the firing of a logogen is reached, the corresponding word is made available in the form of an appropriate motor sequence needed to utter the word, which is placed in a 'memory store'. Different sensory inputs are 'coded' in the form of different 'cues' which may lower the threshold for the firing of certain logogens. In addition, different contexts, which may be either verbal, i.e. the phrase or sentence in which the word is to be uttered, or non-verbal, i.e. the circumstance of utterance, may also change the threshold for the firing of different logogen units. The difference between reading a word (a 'recognition situation') and deciding to utter the word (a 'generation situation') is taken as one in which the logogen units have their thresholds lowered by a sensory input in the former case, but by a context in the latter case. Morton then supposes that the context in which words are used alters the firing threshold of the logogen units, so that in appropriate contexts less 'sensory information' is necessary to fire the unit. In reading, one not only uses the immediate sensory stimulus of the written word, but also the *context* of the word, in order to facilitate the use of the succeeding words. This was set out in Morton's (1969) logogen model in which a set of logogen units, making up a 'logogen system' or 'dictionary' receives input that changes the firing threshold of certain units in the dictionary (fig. 4.4c). The context in which the speech is heard or read also determine the threshold of the logogens. Those logogens which fire then send the appropriate motor sequences needed to utter the word(s) to a temporary memory store or 'output buffer' from which the 'response' – in the form of uttering the word or sentence – may ensue. On the other hand, reinforcement of the motor sequence held in the output buffer may occur by means of a rehearsal loop back to the appropriate units in the logogen system.

The time for which a logogen unit is above the threshold for a particular word must be relatively short (of the order of 1 second according to Morton), otherwise words would become available for use in a chaotic fashion. On the other hand, the 'context system' (fig. 4.4c) can determine that the threshold of appropriate logogens is lowered continuously so as to facilitate the use of these words, but not so much as to make the word available independently of the sensory input. Nevertheless, the input cannot produce a 'stimulus effect', which is 'recorded in some verbalizable form such as a three-syllable word', as this would act like a context and so, 'if the information were incorrect', lead to confounding speech. There is a continual 'exchange of information' between the context system, and the logogen system, which, however, does not lead to responses in the form of word utterance.

One should note here that Morton uses the word 'information' in two different ways. The first, in 'if the information were incorrect', uses the word 'information' in the ordinary sense. The second, in 'continual exchange of information', uses 'information' in the information-theoretic sense. Furthermore, it is not possible for a 'stimulus effect' to be recorded in some verbalizable form such as a 'three-syllable word'. Logogens do not speak English, write things down and remember things. The person reading may notice that the word is trisyllabic or that it begins with 'P', but the logogen could not. How, then, would the fact that the person so notices affect the putative logogen? And if we operate at the personal level, do we really need to descend to the logogen level at all? The answer would seem to be Yes, if Morton purports to be explaining personal behaviour or accomplishment by systems which, in humans, are neuronal. But in fact the hypothesized neural level of the assumed logogen is not doing any serious work. At most it redescribes, in misleading terms, the phenomenon to be explained.

4.4.2   The cognitive system

Morton (1980, pp. 119–20) now replaces the term 'context system' with 'cognitive system', which unlike the logogen system does not consist of units, but involves the 'computing of meaning' retrieved by 'accessing' the logogen system (figs. 4.5a and b). He argues that all the 'information' associated with a particular word is not 'located' with its logogen and therefore retrieved by ' "accessing" the logogen system'. The cognitive system also 'contains information associated' with the word. The single logogen system which was previously claimed to provide a mechanism for reading and listening to speech (see fig. 4.4c) is now replaced by three logogen systems (enclosed by the dotted line in fig. 4.5a; see also fig. 4.5b). These are the 'visual logogen system', the 'auditory logogen system', and the 'output logogen system'. Each of the input logogen systems carries out a categorization procedure. In the case of the visual system, this might take the form of noting the shape and position of letters in a word. Each of the logogen units in the 'output logogen system' possesses two thresholds. If the first of these is reached for a particular logogen, a 'code' indicating this is sent to the 'cognitive system' (previously called the 'context system' in figs. 4.4b and c); if the second threshold is reached, then a code is sent to the 'output logogen system'. Separation of word recognition by the input logogen system and speech ('word production') by the output logogen system then allows for priming. If one sees the word 'ball', hears it spoken, or sees a ball and then says 'ball', then the same output logogen unit is activated in all cases. As mentioned previously (see fig. 4.4c), the 'response buffer' temporarily stores the motor sequences needed to utter the word: namely, the 'phonological code'. There is a connection between the 'visual analysis system' and the response buffer. This is effected by a process that utilizes rules for 'grapheme to phoneme conversion': that is, between the smallest con-trastive units in the writing system (e.g. 't', 'e', ':' etc.) and the smallest contrastive units in the phonetic system. This conversion allows for the fact that one can 'read non-words aloud' (see Morton, 1980). The need for different logogen systems for word recognition during speech compared with the written word that is read is said to be necessitated by the obser-vation that there is no cross-modal priming; that is, hearing the word does not facilitate recognizing the written word (Morton, 1979).

There are many objections to this account.

(1) How can there be information (now not in the information-theoretic sense) some-where in the brain? In what language would it be written? If it is not in English, how could one understand it? If it is in neuralese, how would this help one? How could one obtain the information allegedly stored in the brain?

(2) Morton's descriptions amount to little more than the fact that we know how to use the words of our language; i.e. we know what they mean, and, if we have learnt to read, we are able to read instructions. These are abilities, and they do not involve dictionaries, neural or otherwise.

(3) We are told that 'sentence-meaning' is something to be computed. But it is mistaken to suppose that the meaning of a sentence is something we *compute* in order to understand

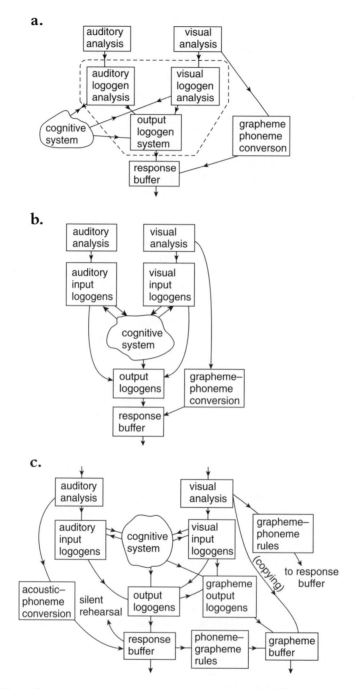

Fig. 4.5. Morton's more recent logogen models for language. **a:** the 1997 logogen model. **b:** a different arrangement of the model in **a**. **c:** the 1980 logogen model. (Morton, 1980, figs 1, 2 and 4.)

the sentence heard or read. Understanding, being an ability, is no process, *a fortiori* not a computational process. One can ask how far one has got in carrying out a complex multi-plication, but not how far one has got in understanding the sentence 'Jack and Jill went up the hill'. One can be interrupted in carrying out a computation, but not in understanding what is said by the use of a sentence.

(4) Humans who have learnt to read have learnt a multitude of rules for grapheme–phoneme conversion. It does not follow that their brain or part of their brain has learnt any rules at all, since brains and their parts are not rule-following beings. They display regu-larities, but not rule-governed regularities – that is something only human beings can display. So no neural process could possibly 'utilize rules for phoneme–grapheme conversion'. Rather, the human ability to read is dependent on unknown neural processes that, in some unknown manner, make it possible for human beings to follow appropriate phoneme–grapheme conversions.

(5) The idea that the 'response buffer' temporarily stores 'phonological codes' in speech production confuses human abilities with their postulated vehicles, and ascribes to the vehicles properties of the abilities and their exercise. Human beings have the ability to think and to express their thoughts in words. But that does not mean that they first think their thoughts and then translate the wordless thoughts into spoken words. To say that the response buffer is the system which temporarily stores phonological codes does no more than register the fact that human beings who have learnt to read to themselves are also able to read aloud, so they must be able to pronounce, aloud or *soto voce*, the graphemes they see. Postulating a 'response buffer' does not *explain* anything at all – it merely redescribes the interlinked abilities. Doubtless the abilities have a neural vehicle, but at present we have little idea what it might be or how it might function.

Morton (1980) further claims that inputs to the 'response buffer' come from the output logogen system in the normal production of speech and in reading aloud. There is also a route from the input analysis systems to the response buffer. These are the pathways which permit the reproduction of nonsense words. The input auditory and visual logogen systems in fig. 4.5 serve as 'passive categorization systems' which, in the case of vision, receive information from the visual analysis system concerning shapes of letters and their positions. The logogens 'collect evidence' from the input logogen systems. If, as a consequence of this, the first of two thresholds of a logogen unit is reached, it sends a code to the cognitive system; if the context is appropriate, the cognitive system can further lower the threshold so that the unit fires and activates the response buffer.

It is difficult to understand what a 'categorization system' is. If a logogen is a neuron or group of neurons, they can receive information about which letters are visible, in what positions, and what the word shape is, only in the sense that they receive impulses from the retinae that are caused by the visual stimulus of the written words. These impulses involve information only in the information-theoretic sense. Furthermore, logogens cannot be 'evidence collectors', since they can respond only to electrochemical impulses and are not homunculi that might collect evidence for anything. Their hypothesized activities may enable human beings to see what they see, and to apprehend what they see as such-and-such letters. But when one sees the word 'cat' on a piece of paper, one surely does not have any evidence that it is the word 'cat' (crumbs are evidence for bread, but a loaf of bread on the table is not evidence for bread). And neither one's brain nor parts of the brain could have. The idea that logogens are evidence collectors with thresholds, 'and as such it is not necessary for all letters to be recognizable in order for the word to be recognized' simply redescribes that datum under the guise of explaining it. It is true that most readers will realize that the second word in 'The c–t sat on the mat' is 'cat' (the only other candidate is 'cot' and cots cannot be said to sit on things). That is not because something in their brain has collected evidence in excess of its threshold, at which point it sends a code to the cognitive system. There is no such thing as a part of the brain collecting evidence. A neuron possesses a 'threshold' for firing impulses, and perhaps in some sense even a group of neurons may be said to have such a threshold. But for a neuron or group of neurons to fire is not for anything or anyone to 'send a code' to anything or anyone, let alone to a cognitive system.

It is interesting to note that we could reconstruct Morton's 'model' with homunculi: there is a visual homunculus VH. When a person has seen a written word, VH (who lives in his head) receives information about what the person is looking at. So he notes which letters are present and in what positions in the word; he carefully notes the shape of the word and other visual features, collecting evidence in order to find out what word is in view. Wonderfully, VH does not have to find out all the letters; at a certain point, he may realize what word it is, even though not all the evidence is in. So he immediately sends a coded message to his friend (CS), the cognitive system homunculus, who will then decipher the code and interpret what VH saw. And so on. This, to be sure, is risible – straight out of Walt Disney. But it is no less risible when the homunculi are replaced by logogens and logogen systems.

Morton (1980) modified the model of fig. 4.5b to allow for graphical output, as shown in fig. 4.5c with connections from the visual analysis system, the visual input logogen, and the response buffer. He believed that these changes were supported by observations on patients who can copy words, but cannot write to dictation, even though they understand and can repeat spoken words. These observations' can be met in the logogen model if a direct pathway exists between the visual analysis system and a grapheme output buffer (see fig. 4.5c). The need for a grapheme output logogen system is necessitated by the existence of patients who can write down words but not copy nonsense syllables or write them down to dictation. This logogen model is the same as fig. 4.5b, but has been adapted to allow for graphical output from the 'visual analysis system' (as in copying) and from the 'auditory analysis system' (as in dictation). There are now two logogen systems, one for speaking (as before) and now, in addition, one for writing (see Morton, 1980). The 'graphemic output logogen' is included to allow for patients who can write fluently, but not if there are nonsense words to be copied or written from dictation. The direct connection between the visual analysis system and the 'grapheme buffer' is to allow for the writing of nonsense words. A 'phoneme–grapheme rule system' is also included in the model to allow writing down nonsense words one has heard, as in dictation. There is a direct connection between the auditory analysis input system and the output buffer for word enunciation via an 'acoustic phoneme system', in order to accommodate one's ability to repeat heard non-words.

This new model (fig. 4.5c), like the earlier ones, is a misleading way of describing the decomposition of abilities into constituent abilities, not of explaining their exercise.

Certainly patients who can transcribe print into script irrespective of understanding (i.e. including nonsense words) have an ability to recognize letters in print and an ability to write those very same letters in script. Patients who can thus transcribe, but cannot write to dictation although they can repeat and understand spoken words, trivially, have the ability to transcribe, the ability to repeat spoken words, but have lost the ability to take dictation, i.e. to write down what they hear. But the model of fig. 4.5 does not explain anything. It merely describes the relevant abilities in a different (and misleading) way.

Morton's logogen model of fig. 4.5 budgets for the possibility of errors such as interchanging 'there' and 'their'. He notes that the rule-governed systems (presumably the logogen systems) have 'no notion of wordness'. But this is confused. As noted above, groups of neurons are not, and could not be, 'rule-governed systems', since only intelligent beings such as humans can *follow* rules. Only if one understands a rule can one act with the intention of acting in accordance with that rule. Following a rule presupposes understanding what it requires. Neurons can behave only in *regular*, not in rule-governed, fashion. There is no such thing as a neuron or group of neurons following rules. Morton now switches from talk of the logogen system knowing things (which is surely incoherent) to talk of the putative rules knowing things (which is equally incoherent). Rule systems are not agents with cognitive capacities, and they can neither be said to know, nor be said to be ignorant, of anything.

In considering rules of grammar and transformation, Morton (1964b) relies on Chomsky (1959). Morton endorses the derivation of a kernel string in Chomsky's grammar in which, for example, a sentence S consists of a noun phrase, NP, and a verb phrase, VP. The rule which expresses the analysis may be written as:

(1)   S → NP + VP (where the arrow indicates that we can write S as NP + VP).
      Other rules concerning grammar and vocabulary could be:
(2)   NP → T + N (where T and N are defined by rules 4 and 5).
(3)   VP → verb + NP
(4)   T → The
(5)   N → man, ball, etc.
(6)   Verb → hit, took, etc.

From these rules we could derive such sentences as 'The ball hit the man' and 'The man took the ball'. From these strings other sentences are derived by transformation rules. It is untrue however, that 'from these strings all other sentence-forms are derived by rules of transformation' (Chomsky, 1959, p. 27). All that has been shown by Chomsky is that they *can be* derived within his grammar. But, first, another grammar may be differently structured, permitting different derivations and transformations with the same results. Secondly, that a certain grammatical form can be derived within a grammar does not show that a speaker who uses that form has performed a kind of derivation. Indeed, all of the above has little to do with the subject of human speech, in which nothing is *derived*. Someone who says 'What a lovely day it is' does not *derive* the sentence uttered from anything. That it can be analysed in a certain way in Chomsky's grammar (and in another way in other grammars) does not show that the speaker *synthesizes* or *derives* it. Morton's model requires that 'If a word is to be analysed down to its neural basis or "kernel" (to retain Chomsky's term), then it must first be "recognized"' (p. 27). So words are analysed no longer into linguistic elements, but into their putative neural base. One can understand what is meant by analysing the word 'evening' into 'time of day prior to night', or 'vixen' into 'female fox'. Here the analysis of a word is given by specifying necessary and sufficient conditions for its application. But it is difficult to understand what is meant by analysing 'evening' into a neural something. Furthermore, the term 'kernel', which was introduced for sentences, has now been extended to words alone, and the 'kernel' of a word is said to be its neural basis. This makes scant sense. Morton suggests further that before a word can be 'analysed' (but why should it be analysed at all?), it must first be 'recognized', and this involves the firing of a unit. However, Morton has previously told us that to each word in a speaker's idiolect there corresponds a something (to be called a unit) that 'fires' when the word is seen (heard, about to be uttered?), which 'makes the word available'. These phrases and words are in need of explanation.

4.4.3   Thought units

Morton (1964b) develops the notion of 'thought units' through consideration of the following sentences:

> They went to see the new ——.
> We went to see the new ——.
> They did not go to see the new ——.
> You must see the new ——.
> They came to see the new ——.
> I would travel miles to see the new ——.
> They examined the new ——.
> The new —— was on view.
> Come to the exhibition of new ——.

These sentences, Morton holds, all have the same 'basic idea', which can be expressed by two or three 'thought units' such as 'regarding', 'newness' and 'travelling'. But this is insufficient explanation of what a thought unit is, and gives no criterion of identity for thought units. We are not given any explanation of what an 'idea' or 'basic idea' which can be expressed by the two or three thought units might be. Even brief examination of Morton's list suggests that something is awry. For surely 'they' has a different meaning from 'we'; the concept of a negation is involved in the thought (or proposition) expressed by the third sentence, but not in the others; the fourth sentence contains the modal term 'must', but the others do not; it is not obvious why the verb 'to see' expresses the same thought unit as the noun 'exhibition', and so on. It is therefore altogether unclear what is meant by the claim that these sentences have the same 'basic idea' which can be expressed by 'two or three thought units', and it is doubtful whether it could be made clear.

Thought units are said to link the 'syntactic and semantic systems'. Such units are also acted on by other processes, which are said to give rise to 'meaningfulness'. However,

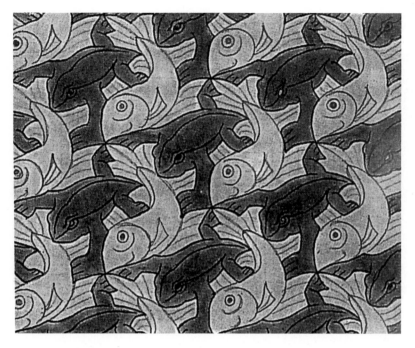

Plate 1.1. Maurits Escher's repeated pattern of fishes and frogs, 'Symmetry Drawing E50'. (From M. C. Escher, 1942: Cordon Art B.V., Baarn, Holland; © 2008 The M.C. Escher Company, Holland. All rights reserved.)

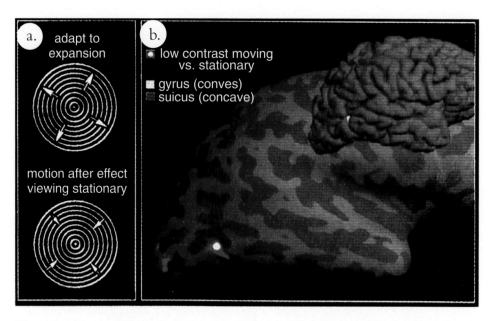

Plate 1.2. The part of the brain that is activated when experiencing a visual illusion. (Tootell et al., 1995, p. 140.)

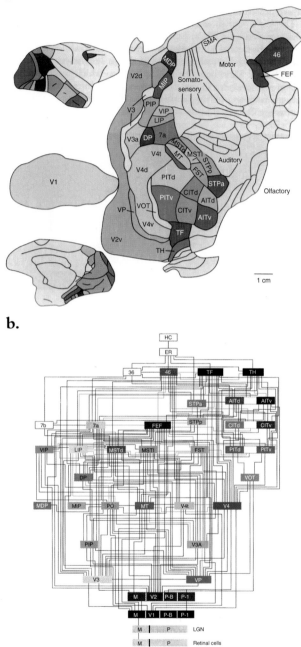

Plate 1.3. **a**: an unfolded map of the cortex of the monkey. The visual areas are colour-coded to distinguish them from cortical areas devoted to other functions (Felleman and Van Essen, 1991, fig. 2). **b**: the areas of the visual system shown in **a** are interconnected as shown in this schematic representation. (Felleman and Van Essen, 1991, fig. 4.)

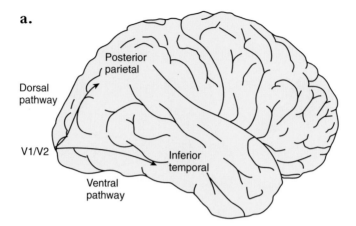

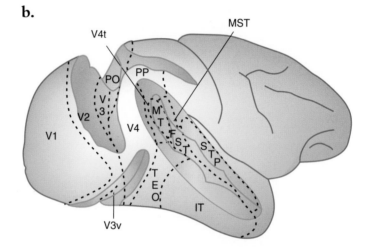

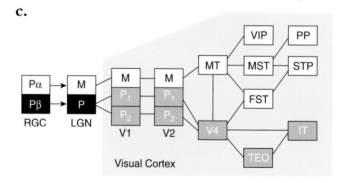

Plate 1.4. Cortical 'modules' that participate in the two visual streams constituting the 'where' and 'what' pathways. (Albright et al., 2000, figs 16B and C.)

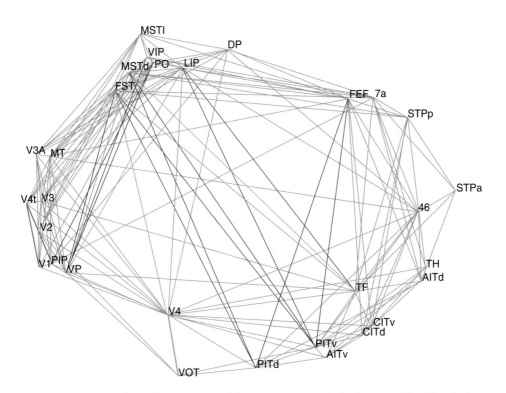

Plate 1.5. The topological organization of the macaque cortical visual system. The abbreviations for the different visual areas here and in Plates 1.3 and 1.4 are defined in the legend to fig. 5.13. (Young, 1992 fig. 1.)

a. Colour search

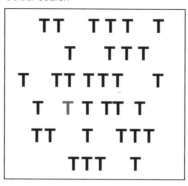

b. Conjunction search

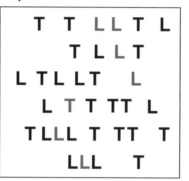

c. Colour search   Conjunction search

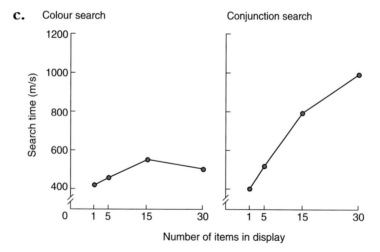

Plate 1.6. The search time for a unique item is faster when all items differ by only one attribute than if all items differ by two or more attributes. (Kandel et al. (2000; 4th edn, fig. 25.14), after Treisman et al., 1977, and Treisman, 1986.)

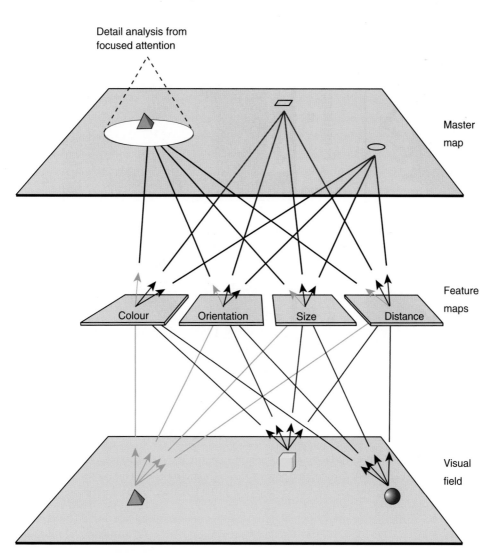

Plate 1.7. Treisman's (1986) hypothetical model purporting to show how 'different types of visual information processed separately are combined into a coherent image'. (Kandel et al. (2000; 4th edn, fig. 25.15), after Treisman, 1986.)

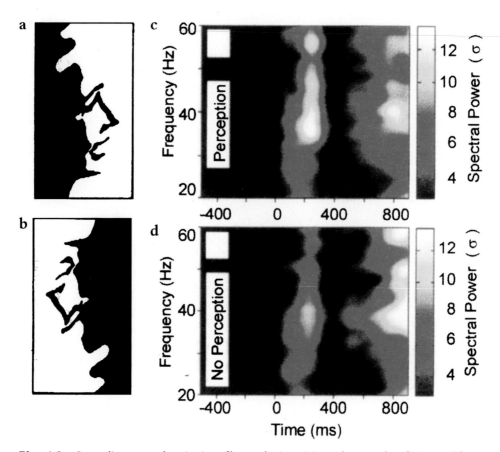

Plate 1.8. Long-distance synchronization of human brain activity. **a, b:** examples of 'Mooney' faces, (**a**) upright and (**b**) inverted; **c, d:** spectral power following stimulation, with the perception condition eliciting a significantly stronger gamma response (at 20–60 Hz) than the no-perception condition. (From Rodriguez et al., 1999, fig. 1.)

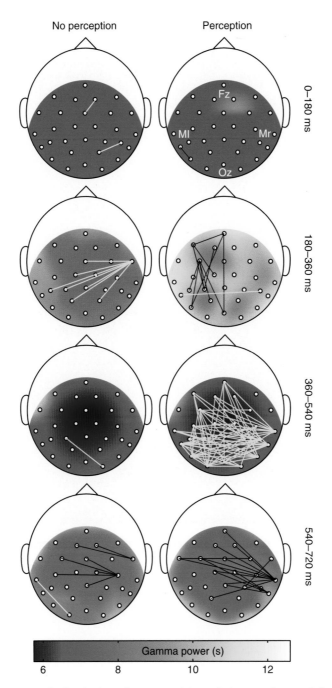

Plate 1.9. Average scalp distribution of gamma activity and phase synchrony. Colour coding indicates gamma power (averaged over 34–40 Hz) over an electrode from stimulation onset (0 ms) to motor response (720 ms). (From Rodriguez et al., 1999, fig. 3.)

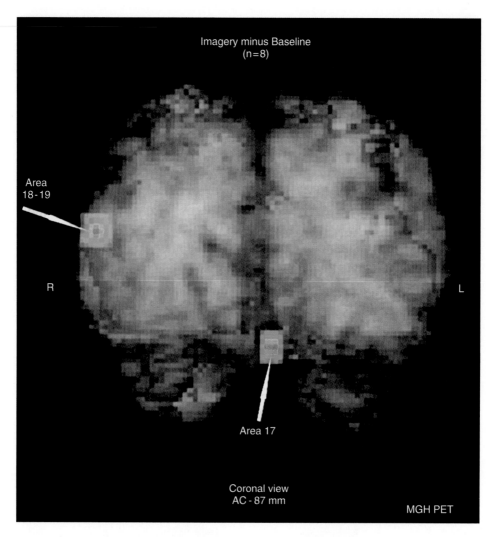

Plate 1.10.   Illustration of the stimuli used to determine the role of visual area 17 in visual imagery. (Kosslyn et al., 1999, fig. 1.)

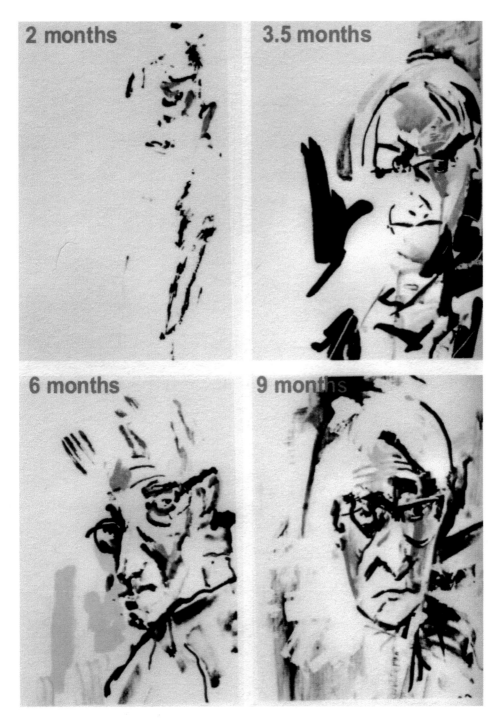

Plate 2.1. Self-portraits by the artist Anton Raderscheidt showing defects in his ability to attend to parts of his own body following a parietal stroke. (Bennett, 1993, fig. 7; © Anton Raderscheidt, Licensed by VISCOPY, Australia, 2008.)

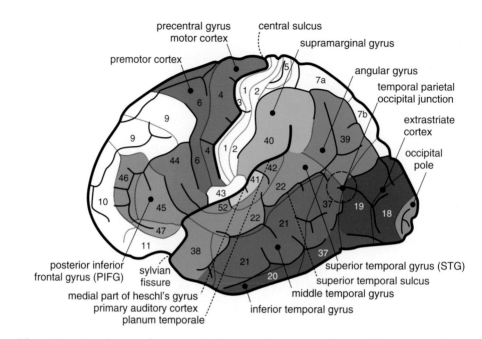

Plate 4.1. Lateral view of cortex with Brodmann's areas as indicated. (Demonet et al., 2005, fig. 6.)

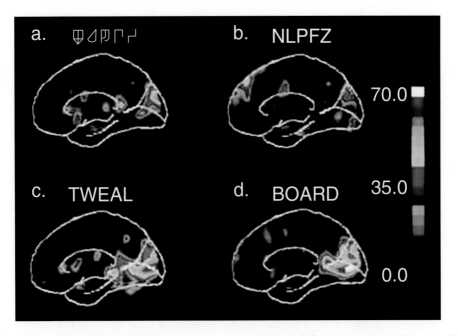

Plate 4.2. PET images of subjects when presented with four different sets of word-like stimuli. (Petersen et al., 1990, fig. 1.)

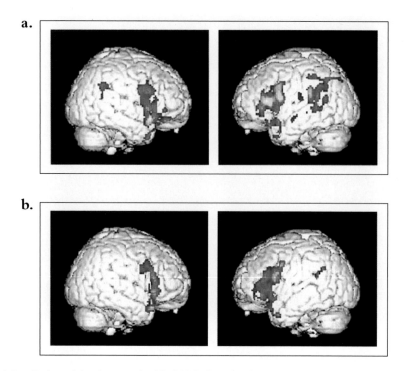

Plate 4.3. Brain activity (measured with fMRI) during judgements concerning the syntactic (**a**) or the semantic (**b**) aspects of a sentence. (Dapretto and Bookheimer, 1999, fig. 1.)

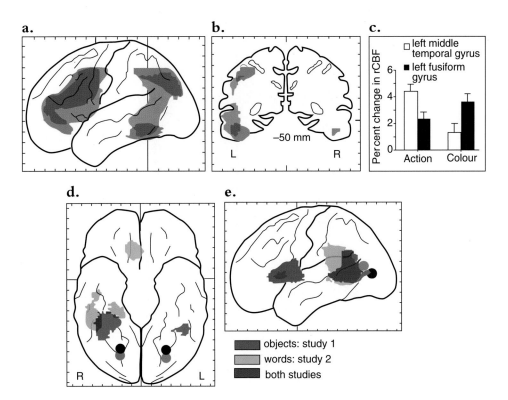

Plate 4.4. Discrete cortical regions active (according to PET) while speaking colour words and action words. **a:** lateral view of left hemisphere showing activated region for colour words (*green*) and action words (*grey*). **b:** coronal section (50 mm posterior to the anterior commissure) showing activation regions for colour words and action words. **c:** percentage changes in PET-measured regional cerebral blood flow (rCBF) for colour and action words in temporal and fusiform gyrus. **d:** ventral view of the brain, showing regions of increased regional cerebral blood flow when subjects uttered colour words rather than action words. **e:** lateral view of the left cerebral hemisphere showing regions of increased blood flow when subjects spoke action words in comparison to uttering colour words (*red* indicates activations in response to line drawings of objects; *yellow*, in response to the written names of the objects; *blue* in response to both; the *black* and *green* circles indicate previously reported locations of maximum activity during the perception of colour (**d**) and motion (**e**) fig. 4.10. (Martin et al., 1995, figs 1 and 2.)

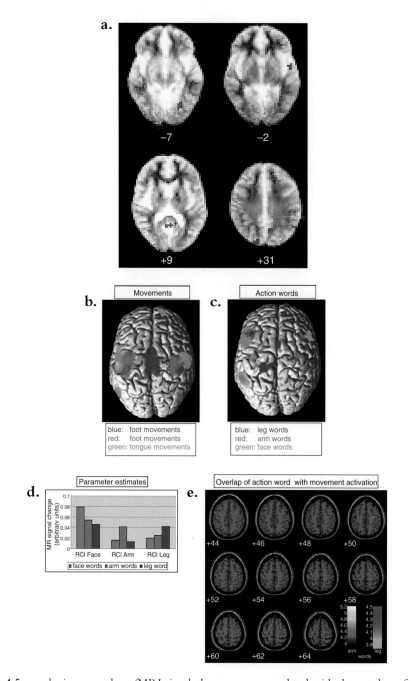

Plate 4.5. **a:** brain areas where fMRI signal changes were correlated with the number of words spoken in a set period (~20 sec); *red* voxels positive and *blue* voxels negative correlations; left side of the brain is shown on the right side of the image (Kircher et al., 2000, fig. 1.) **b–d:** brain areas activated (according to fMRI) by subcategories of action words are adjacent to and partly overlap activations produced by the corresponding movement types. **b:** activated areas during tongue, finger and foot movements; **c:** activated areas during reading action words related to faces, arm and leg movements; **d:** extent of differential activation by subgroups of action words in the left hemisphere. **e:** overlap of activation produced by 'arm' and 'leg' words with that produced by finger and foot movements, respectively (colour scales indicate *t* values for arm and leg word-related activation separately; these are difficult to distinguish in the figure). (Hauk et al., 2004, fig. 2.)

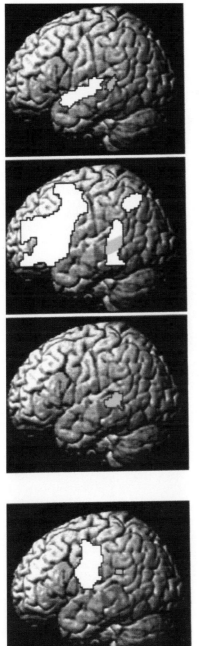

Experiment 1

Words – SCN

Experiment 2

Word retrieval from
semantic memory

Experiment 4

Word perception +
word retrieval

Experiment 3

Articulation without
perception of own
utterances

Plate 4.6.   Activation areas on the lateral surface of the left cerebral hemisphere, according to PET, correlated with the rate of hearing words (experiment 1: *yellow* highlights the superior temporal sulcus); activation correlated with 'semantically cued word retrieval' (experiment 2: *yellow* highlights superior temporal sulcus); activation correlated with perceiving a word and remembering ('retrieving') it (experiment 4: *yellow* highlights superior temporal sulcus); activation correlated with articulation without responding to one's own utterances (experiment 3: activation included the medial left temporo-parietal junction, highlighted in *yellow* and displayed, for illustrative purposes, on the lateral surface of the hemisphere). (Wise et al., 2001, fig. 8.)

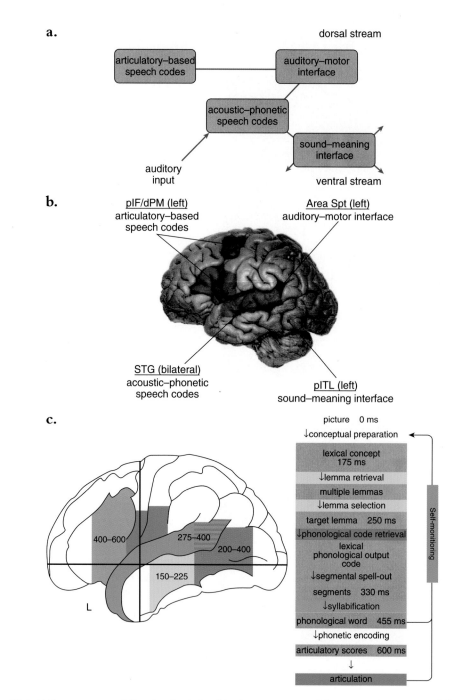

Plate 4.7. **a:** suggested functional relationships between areas of the cortex that support different components of a proposed 'language system'. **b:** lateral view of the brain showing the cortical areas in **a.** (Hickok and Poeppel, 2004, fig. 1.) **c:** suggested relationships between different cortical regions (*left*) and the Levelt model of speech (*right*), with identical colours indicating the relationships. (Indefrey and Levelt, 2004, fig. 5.)

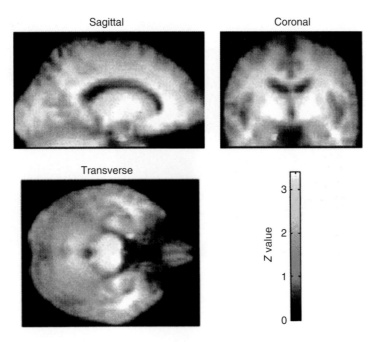

Sagittal

Coronal

Transverse

Z value

3

2

1

0

Plate 5.1. Neuronal responses in the left amygdala as measured by PET in a series of experiments by Morris et al. (1996).

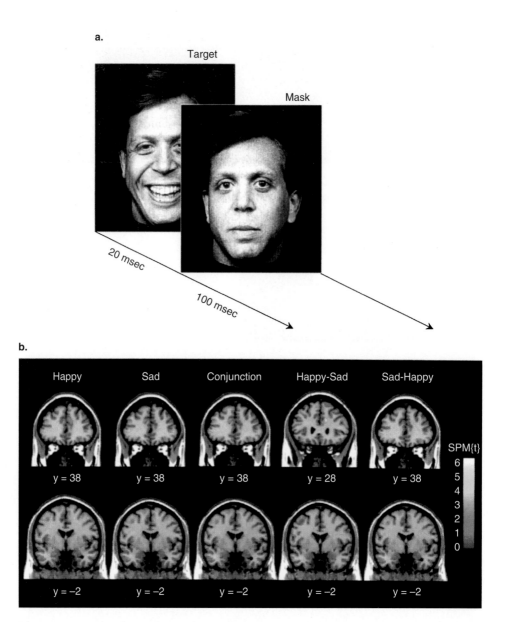

Plate 5.2. Results of experiments taken as showing enhanced bilateral activation within the amygdala and anterior cingulate gyrus (**b**), as measured with fMRI, when viewing happy face or sad face expressions for a short period (20 msec) before these were masked with neutral facial expressions for longer periods (100 msec) (**a**). The top row presents coronal views at the location of the anterior cingulate gyrus, and the bottom row a coronal view of the amygdala. Results labelled 'Conjunction', 'Happy-sad' and 'Sad-happy' have not been considered in the text but are described in Killgore and Yurgelun-Todd (2004) (for further description, see text). (Killgore and Yurgelun-Todd, 2004, figs 1 and 3.)

whether a sentence is meaningful depends on the conventions of use of the constituent words (including combinatorial conventions) and their mode of combination in the sentence, not on processes that act on thought units.

4.4.4   Computational studies

Modern theories of visual word recognition and reading aloud build on the ideas of Morton adumbrated above. For example, the model of 'language processing' due to Patterson and Shewell (1987) (see fig. 4.6a) follows the architecture of Morton's (1980) model for language involving single words and non-words. But the idea is abandoned that threshold-firing input and output logogens exist. These are now replaced by an 'auditory input lexicon' in the case of speech and an 'orthographic input lexicon' in the case of print (where 'orthographic' refers to the printed word), so that lexical entries corresponding to words are the elements and not logogen units. Components of the Patterson and Shewell (1987) model were retained by Coltheart et al. (2001) in order to give a computational account of the process of reading aloud, which they call the Dual Route Cascaded Model (fig. 4.6b). Coltheart et al. (2001) comment that 'The renaissance of cognitive psychology itself began . . . in the late 1950s and early 1960s, particularly with Broadbent (1958) and it is significant that one feature of this renaissance was a resumption of the use of box-and-arrow notation'. 'The renaissance of cognitive psychology' is arguably a misnomer, since what was introduced was not cognitive psychology at all, but *computational* psychology masquerading as cognitive, which was geared to the computer model *ab initio*.

We have briefly reviewed the development of the logogen model which forms the basis for so much contemporary modelling of word recognition and reading aloud. Our conclusions are very different from the claim that the model is based on empirical observations leading to hypotheses concerning mechanisms involved in reading, etc. One may concede that abilities may have a vehicle. One may further agree that if the vehicle of an ability is identified, then the exercise of the ability may be explained by reference to changes in, or operations of, the vehicle. But Morton has not identified a vehicle for the abilities that concern him; he has merely reified those abilities. Far from being able to explain the neural mechanisms the operation of which explain the exercise of the power to read, what Morton has done is merely to analyse the ability to read into subordinate constituent abilities and to assert that in cases of agnosia, the relevant ability is not exercised because its reification cannot be accessed. But that is tantamount to explaining why A does not V by reference to the fact that it cannot access its ability to V.

4.5   The Modular Study of Fluent Speech: Levelt

4.5.1   The model study

An influential model for fluent speech was developed by Levelt in the early 1990s. He first posed questions concerning how we 'access' words when we speak, and what the rate of lexical access is during normal speech, emphasizing that such access requires a system that

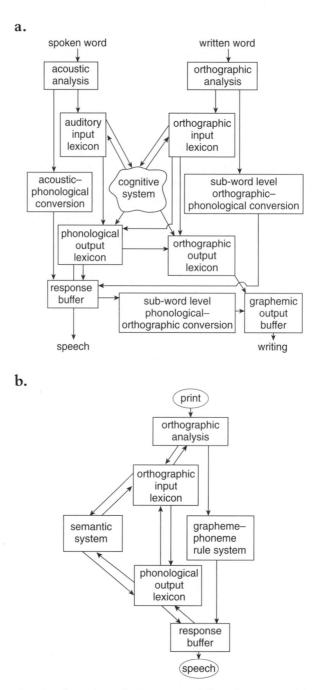

Fig. 4.6. Recent theories of speech. **a:** the Patterson and Shewell (1987) model of visual or auditory word recognition and writing or speech (from Patterson and Shewell, 1987, fig. 13.1). **b:** the Coltheart Dual Route Cascaded Model of visual word recognition and reading aloud (Coltheart et al., 2001, fig. 6.)

must follow certain design requirements. Levelt suggests that the process by which we retrieve a word, that is, the processing procedures that determine our capacity to use words we have learnt may be studied in a number of ways, including the study of slips of the tongue engineered in a laboratory setting. Observations of these have provided us, according to Levelt (1992), with the principal features of the 'processing architecture' that is required for speech. This includes 'lexical selection' (a part of 'grammatical encoding'), which he defines as the selection of a word from the mental lexicon of thousands of words, as well as 'phonological encoding', which involves determining from the word's 'phonological code' a 'phonetic shape' for the chosen word (fig. 4.7a). Levelt's (1992) model is detailed in fig. 4.7b. This consists of a number of modules, the first of which is concerned with 'conceptualization and intention' − that is, with the concepts to be expressed in the message and with the intention that it be communicated. This is akin to Lichtheim's (1885) concept centre in which concepts are supposedly stored (see fig. 4.1a). The *conceptual preparation module* feeds into a *lexical selection module* responsible for selecting the appropriate words from the mental lexicon for the concepts that are to be expressed. Such words, or lemmas, belong to particular syntactical categories (viz. nouns, verbs, etc.), with each of these words having to be placed in an appropriate syntactic sequence. The next set of modules is concerned with *morphological encoding* and *phonological syllabification*, which provide for each chosen word a sound form called a 'lexeme', specified in the lexicon, giving a phonetic program for the word. The *phonetic encoding module* gives the specification of the phoneme for the chosen word. In the *articulatory plan module,* the speech sounds to be articulated and the prosody of the utterance are said to be specified. *Self-monitoring* involves identification of errors in our speech, such as slips of the tongue, that we can then correct.

Levelt talks of the 'process' of accessing and selecting words when we speak. However, there is no *process* of retrieval of words when we use them. We may be skilled in formulating our thoughts in elegant, brilliant, precise ways, etc. (or not). The only *processes* are neural, and they are not processes by which we do anything, but processes that enable us to do the things we do. Furthermore, we don't *access* words. We use words that we have learnt. That is not to access anything. When I walk home, I know the route I use, but that does not imply that I have access to a map. When a painter draws a scene he saw yesteryear, he remembers the scene − but he does not have access to it, and to remember does not mean that one has access to a photographic album in the mind or brain. We remember words, can use the words we have learnt, but we certainly do not have a skill in *accessing* words, unless it is one exercised in looking up things in a dictionary. We have skills in using words, skills in the mastery of vocabulary and syntax, skills in forms of speech and writing. These do not involve accessing anything. As for 'selecting' words, we do not normally *select* from anything, unless we pause to choose between alternative phrasings. The idea of lexical selection − that one selects a word from amongst thousands of alternatives − is wrong. When I say at the bakery 'Could I have a loaf of white bread, please?', there are not thousands of alternatives to the word 'bread'. The fact that I know thousands of words does not mean that they are all alternatives, and it surely is not true that I run through all the words I know (unconsciously, of course, at the speed of electricity) until I come to the word 'bread'.

There is no such thing as a 'mental lexicon'. What there is, is the human being's mastery of a vocabulary, his ability correctly to use the words of any language he knows. That is a

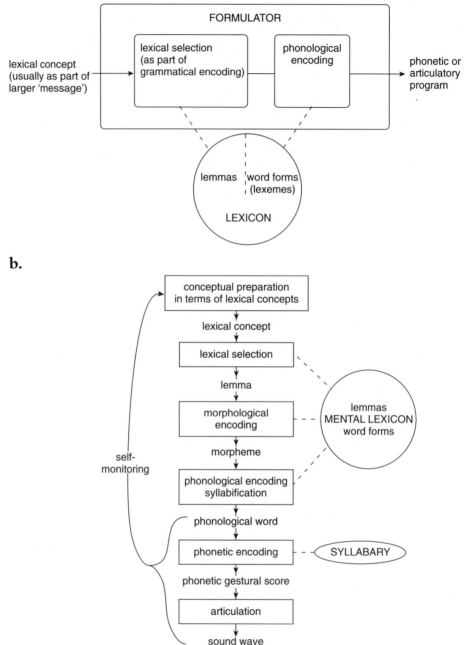

Fig. 4.7. The theory of Levelt for speech. **a:** Levelt's 1992 model of 'lexical access' in speech. (Levelt, 1992, fig. 1.) **b:** Levelt's 1999 model of 'lexical access' in speech (for description, see text) (Levelt et al., 1999, fig. 1.)

skill, but not a skill in looking up anything in a mental lexicon. How is the speaker supposed to know what lexical concept he wishes to express if he has not yet looked up the word for it? Assuming that he knows what concept he wishes to express, how does he find the word for it? Words are not words *for* concepts, although there are words that *express* concepts. The misconceived phrase 'preparation of the articulatory gesture' suggests that we first select the word from our mental lexicon to fit the concept that we want to express, and then find out how to pronounce it. 'Phonetic encoding', which involves, according to Levelt, speakers using a store of phonemes for frequently used syllables, simply means that speakers know how to pronounce numerous syllables in their native tongue. Far from explaining the exercise of this ability, it merely redescribes it in misleading terms. There is no articulatory plan, as we rarely plan our utterances, let alone their pronunciation, in advance. Of course, we usually say what we say intentionally, and often say something with the intention of producing a certain effect. But this does not mean that any planning goes on in advance. We do not, before saying something aloud, say to ourselves that *that* is the phonological form which our 'articulatory plan' takes.

The ability to correct slips of the tongue, etc., is misunderstood as self-monitoring. To monitor myself is to attend to my activities. But unless I am an actor rehearsing a play, I don't attend to my own speech. If I am a competent speaker, then I will doubtless notice the occasional infelicity in my speech. But that is not because I attend to what I say, but rather because I notice the mistakes I make. What I notice is what intrudes itself upon my attention, not what I deliberately attend to. The theory of Levelt is more a mythological redescription of the observed phenomena than an explanation of them. The various notions in Levelt's theory are based on an engineering approach to human speech, in which the human being is conceived on the model of a computer. Unfortunately, engineering terms and descriptions of the psychological attributes of humans are incoherently intermingled in this exercise.

4.5.2 Development of the model system

Infants (from the Latin 'infans', i.e. speechless) are human beings who cannot yet speak. Word production by children, according to Levelt (1992), 'emerges from a coupling of two initially independent systems, a conceptual system and an articulatory system'. Levelt suggests that, on the one hand, the 'primary notions of agency, interactancy, the temporal and causal structure of events, object permanence and location' are established, allowing for the 'creation of our first lexical concepts, concepts flagged by means of a verbal label'. On the other hand, a repertoire of babbles is initiated at about the seventh month when acoustic properties are perceived, leading to further exercises in their repetition and reorganization of their syllabic structure, with audiomotor patterns beginning to resonate, becoming tuned to the mother tongue (De Boyssan-Bavelies and Vihman, 1991; Elbers, 1982). 'Real word production begins when the child starts connecting some particular babble (or a modification thereof) to some particular lexical concept' (Levelt et al., 1999). Levelt (1994) holds that this duality of word production in speech holds throughout further development. At 1.6–2.6 years, words are processed by 'concatenations of phonological segments' (Elbers and Wijnen, 1992; Levelt, 1994). Phonetic encoding of words now has its foundation in phonological encoding, in which words are given as a pattern of phonemes that guides the phonetic encoding and the articulatory delivery. At these ages the relations between various lexical concepts determines the order of words in a sentence, so that 'agent might come first and location last'. Levelt (1992) comments that, at about 2.6 years, the child develops a system of lemmas, packages of 'syntactic information', one for each lexical concept. The mature system for producing a word in speech is then arrived at and, as already noted (see fig. 4.7b), consists of proceeding from the lexical concept to its lemma and from there to the word's phonological code in order to determine its 'phonetic-articulatory gesture' – presumably its significant utterance.

Levelt's description of the way in which children learn to speak is not acceptable. One cannot couple a 'conceptual system' with an 'articulatory system', for one cannot couple concepts to words. We can give words a use, and we can teach children how to use the words of their language. When they have mastered the use of a word, they can be said to have acquired the concept expressed by that word. To suppose that concept acquisition is a matter of the child attaching babbles to particular lexical concepts is therefore a dire confusion. It is akin to supposing that in order for a coin to be worth five pounds, it has to be attached to the value of five pounds – here the coin, there the value!

It is equally misguided to suppose that concepts are flagged by means of a verbal label. Words are not labels – if they were, then sentences would be lists. But sentences are not lists. One performs a speech-act by means of a sentence, but one cannot perform a speech-act by means of a list. Concept words, like proper names, can be used as labels – but not as labels of concepts, only as labels of exhibits, or of bottles, boxes, files and so forth.

Levelt's suggestion that prior to mastery of the use of any words the child has to acquire the primary notions of agency, interactancy (*sic*), the temporal and causal structure of events, object permanency and location is altogether unclear. Levelt does not explain what a *notion* is or tell us what the criteria for possession of a notion are. Once the child has mastered the rudimentary skills of movement and locomotion, he becomes a voluntary agent who can bring about changes around him by manipulation, pushing and pulling. Has he then acquired the notions of agency? If so, then, to be sure, cats and dogs likewise acquire such notions. Do babies have a notion of the temporal and causal structures of events? It is wholly unclear what this means – but if babies have it, then so do cats and dogs. For it seems that all that is required for possession of such a notion is to be able to bring about change at will. But then why introduce the idea of a notion and of possession of notions at all?

Levelt's suggestion that words are 'processed' at 1.6–2.6 years is problematic. We can explain what it means for our machines – word-processors – to process words. But until an acceptable explanation is offered, we do not know what it means for the brain or its parts to process words. Analogies between the brain and the machinery we devise for our purposes are ancient. Early in the last century the favoured analogy was with the operator in a central telephone exchange. It is not evident that word-processors offer a better analogy than the telephone system, and the onus of proof lies upon those who invoke it. Nor is it clear what is meant by phonetic or phonological 'encoding' of words. We know what it is to encode words in an agreed code, such as the Morse code or a secret cypher. But we do not know what it is to encode words, phonologically or phonetically, in the brain. *A fortiori* we know of no evidence to support this recent form of trace theory. The theory rests not on evidence, but on a preconception that there must be a brain-trace, otherwise we would not be able to do what we can do. Encodings in the brain are engrams by another name, and smell no sweeter. That there are neural changes corresponding to the acquisition of the abilities to pronounce a word and to recognize a spoken word when heard is plausible – we would be bewildered if there were none. Talk of phonological and phonetic encodings adds nothing to that truism.

Finally, it is incoherent to ascribe to a child, who can barely utter a sentence, possession of a system of syntactic information, and even more incoherent to suppose that such a system *develops* in the child. Information does not develop; it has to be acquired. To possess information is to know something to be so. To possess syntactic information is to know something about the syntax of expressions in a language. A small child that can barely speak a sentence cannot be said to know anything about syntax. It is no doubt beginning to learn how the words it has learnt can be meaningfully ordered in a significant utterance. If that rudimentary skill is described as knowledge of syntax, it has to be sharply distinguished from the knowledge of syntax possessed by grammarians and learnt from grammar books.

4.6 The Functional Neuroanatomy of Language Comprehension

4.6.1 Attention to visual compared with semantic aspects of words

In 1990, Petersen and his colleagues, using PET, showed that areas in the left medial extrastriate visual cortex were activated by visually presented pseudo-words that obey English spelling rules (e.g. FLOOP, TOGLO), as well as by actual words. They were not activated during presentation of nonsense strings of letters (e.g. NLPFZ) or letter-like forms. Plate 4.2 shows such PET images, indicating areas of increased blood flow through a slice of the brain given by the vertical dashed line in fig. 4.8a, when subjects were presented with four different sets of word-like stimuli. (Each slice is taken from the same sagittal location 2 cm left of the midsagittal plane; anterior is at the left of each image; at the top of each section is a sample from the stimulus set that produced the activation.) These stimuli are indicated above the images and show false font (Plate 4.2a) and letter string (Plate 4.2b) presentations for which there is little activation in the inferior or posterior parts of the image. This is to be contrasted with PET scans following presentation of pronounceable non-words (fig. 4.8a) as well as real word stimulus presentations in which each produce clear activations in three identifiable loci. These are shown in fig. 4.8a located in the medial extrastriate area (BA18/19) in the case of real words (filled squares) and pronounceable non-words (shaded area). The other identifiable locus is in the left inferior frontal area (inferior frontal gyrus (IFG); BA44,45,47) (fig. 4.8b) which is activated during presentation of real words but not by pronounceable non-words. The filled circle in fig. 4.8b indicates a site which was excited when people were asked to associate a word with the word they read; the shaded circle indicates a site which was excited when they simply read a word. This study indicated to Petersen et al. (1990, p. 1043) that:

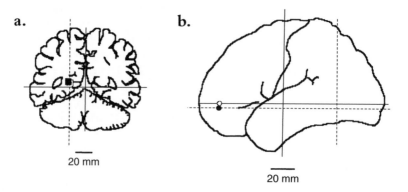

Fig. 4.8.   **a:** the medial extrastriate area activated by real words (filled square) and pronounceable non-words (pseudo-words; shaded square that is not observable on the original figure. (Petersen et al., 1990, fig. 3.) **b:** lateral view of the left hemisphere showing inferior frontal areas activated by visual presentation of real words (circle) or by asking the subject to consider a semantic association for the visually presented word (filled circle). (Petersen et al., 1990, fig. 3.)

> The presence of a left-lateralised area in posterior, extrastriate cortex that distinguishes between letter strings that do not conform to English spelling rules argues that access to information specific to English orthography is present very early in the visual processing stream. These areas may represent the neural mechanism underlying the perceptual advantage that words and pseudowords show over irregular letter strings.

This area in the posterior extrastriate cortex therefore seems to be active when one reads familiar words. Patients with lesions in this area are unable to read words even though other aspects of their linguistic abilities are intact. The activation of a left inferior frontal area (IFG; within BA45,47) when recognizing written words and when associating words with them (fig. 4.8b) allegedly indicates that this area is active during 'semantic computation of single words'. These observations using PET were the first imaging studies to claim that 'separate cortical areas are active during attention to visual as compared with semantic aspects of words' (Petersen et al., 1990, p. 1041).' Petersen et al. (1990) considered this research as identifying areas concerned with the *complex computations* made on letters which potentially join these into a word unit and involve frontal regions concerned with semantic *computations* on single words.

It is not clear that the conclusions Petersen has drawn from his investigations are warranted. Neither the brain nor its parts have access to any information whatsoever, let alone to information about English orthography. There is no reason to suppose that reading involves computation, let alone complex computations, on letters. No doubt reading involves the ability to recognize words, which in turn involves the ability to recognize letters. But no fluent reader calculates the words he reads from the letters of which it is composed. The fact that little children who are learning how to read may in some sense do so does not show that adults do. Little children may learn to multiply 3 × 3 by counting 1, 2, 3–4,

5, 6–7, 8, 9, but it does not follow that an adult does so too, only much more quickly. And the brain itself is not in the business of calculating or reading. No doubt someone who can read can also recognize incorrect orthography (at least in a society in which orthography is rigorously determined). Petersen's experiments were not necessary to tell us that. It is true that a competent reader normally understands what he reads. But that does not imply that anything that can be deemed a semantic computation on words takes place. All that can be concluded from these experiments is that different cortical areas are involved in reading meaningless strings of pseudo-words from those that are involved in reading proper words with understanding.

4.6.2   Auditory compared with visual presentation of words

The above work of Petersen and colleagues involved determining those parts of the brain which are active when words are read. What parts are active when words are heard? Petersen and Fiez determined these in 1993, using PET scanning again. They showed that different regions of the brain were activated when real words are heard and understood: namely, the left temporo-parietal cortex (BA39) as well as the left anterior superior temporal region (BA22). This is shown in fig. 4.9a, which presents PET studies of sagittal slices like those in Plate 4.2 when words are read (left slices) and when words are heard (right slices), with the upper set of slices taken 25 mm left of the midline, and the lower slices 53 mm left of the midline. The upper left image shows extrastriate visual cortex activation posteriorly for words read (compare with Plate 4.2c and d) with no activation in the corresponding slice (upper right) for words heard. The opposite holds true for the more lateral slices (i.e. 53 mm left of the midline rather than 25 mm left of the midline). The principal area active for words heard is shown in the left temporo-parietal cortex (BA39).

Petersen and Fiez (1993) consider this work on determining the parts of the brain that are active when words are heard as contributing to an understanding of 'language- and information-processing' in the brain. The difficulty with this proposition is that the brain does not receive information but neural stimuli, such as results from the action of photons on the retinal photoreceptors. The 'processing' of single words can, in the end, only mean understanding these words, something which brains do not do. Rather, what was discovered was that when words are read with understanding, the left temporo-parietal cortex is involved.

4.6.3   Attention to the semantic as compared to the syntatic aspect of a sentence

Dapretto and Bookheimer (1999) used fMRI to determine those parts of the brain which are active during the comprehension of pairs of sentences which differed from each other as a result of substituting one word for another. The substituend could be either synonymous or not synonymous. For example,

(1)   East of the city is a lake.
(1′)   East of the city is a river.

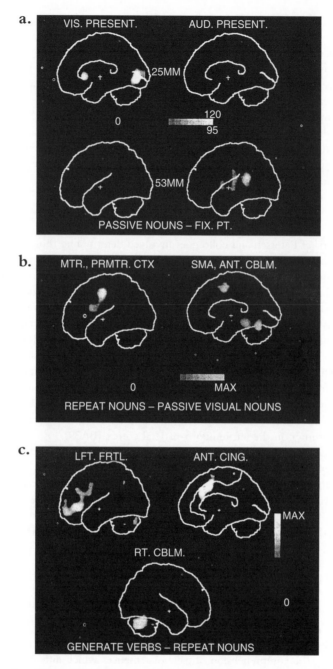

Fig. 4.9. **a:** activated areas of the brain, ascertained with PET, during passive visual (left) and auditory (right) presentations of words. (The upper slices are taken 25 mm left of midline, and the lower slices are taken 53 mm left of midline.) **b:** activated areas of the brain when subjects repeat aloud visually presented words with a control condition of visual presentation (the left image is 40 mm left of midline and shows activation in primary motor cortex (MTR) and premotor cortex (PRMTR)); the right image is taken near the midline and shows activation in supplementary motor cortex (SMA) and midline cerebellum (CBLM). **c:** activated areas of the brain when subjects spoke verbs appropriate to visually presented nouns (*upper left*, 40 mm from midline, activation in left prefrontal (LFT, FRTL); *upper right*, near midline and shows activation in anterior cingulate (ANT, CING); *lower* image, 25 mm right of midline, shows activation in lateral cerebellum (RT.CBLM). (Petersen and Fiez, 1993, figs 1–3.)

This was compared with pairs of sentences which differed as a result of an active/passive transformation. For example,

(1) The teacher outsmarted the pupil.
(1′) The teacher was outsmarted by the pupil.

The former types of pairs are referred to as 'semantic' cases, the latter as 'syntactic' ones.

Subjects were asked to listen to such pairs of sentences and decide whether the sentences in a given pair had the same literal meaning. Plate 4.3 shows fMRI scans of brain activity observed when judgements were made about the meanings of the sentences. Plate 4.3a shows the 'syntactic' case as compared with the rest, and Plate 4.3b the 'semantic' case compared with the rest. It will be noted that during the judgements involving the 'syntactic' cases part of Broca's area (BA44, the pars opercularis) is active, whereas during the judgements involving the 'semantic' cases the lower portion of the left inferior frontal gyrus (BA47, the pars orbitalis) is involved. Dapretto and Bookheimer (1999) suggest that their work shows:

> Two aspects of receptive language, semantic and syntactic analysis of sentence meaning, appear to have distinct neural substrates within the IFG (inferior frontal gyrus; BA44,45,47). This conforms to the general principle of functional segregation in the human cerebral cortex, according to which local ensembles of strongly interconnected cells share input and/or output properties that differ from the input and/or output properties of other ensembles. These functionally segregated local collectives are then functionally integrated through recursive and parallel processing (Edelman, 1993). The breadth of deficits observed in patients with Broca's aphasia – including phonological awareness, articulation, naming, syntactic comprehension, strategic semantic priming and word generation – are best explained by damage to distinct functional brain regions with specific linguistic processing affinities, rather than to a single undifferentiated linguistic module (p. 431).

It is not clear what 'semantic and syntactic analysis of sentence meaning' means. A person who listens to speech does not (normally) *analyse* anything. (In abnormal cases one might: e.g. 'John, where the teacher had had "had had", had had "had"; "had had" had won the day.') It is equally unclear what 'analysis of sentence meaning' is supposed to signify, for sentence *meanings* are not obviously the kinds of things that lend themselves to analysis without more ado, any more than *values* of commodities do. It is less clear why the two kinds of case are described respectively as 'semantic switch' and 'syntactic switch', since the syntactic switch is *also* a semantic one in the case of the pair

> The teacher outsmarted the student.
> The teacher was outsmarted by the student.

But it is not in the case of

> West of the bridge is the airport.
> The airport is west of the bridge.

It may well be that to grasp that

> The teacher was outsmarted by the student

has a different meaning from

> The teacher outsmarted the student

requires a moment's reflection on who did what to whom; whereas to recognize that

> East of the city is the lake

means something quite different from

> East of the city is the river

requires no reflection at all, but only the knowledge that a lake is not a river. It seems to us far from evident that the experiments support the conclusion that Broca's area is causally implicated only in syntactical skills, and the left inferior frontal gyrus in semantic ones. A much clearer classification of what counts as a semantic skill and what counts as a purely syntactic one is needed before experimentation can commence.

Dapretto and Bookheimer's suggestion that the deficits associated with Broca's aphasia are to be explained by reference to damage to parts of the brain involved in linguistic processing is surely a misdescription. In order to use computer jargon with regard to the brain, one must first explain what 'to process language' means, what it would be for a human being to process language, and what it would be for the brain of a human being to do so. At the moment, all that can be discerned is that damage to different parts of the brain causes the loss of certain aspects of a human being's linguistic abilities.

4.7   The Functional Neuroanatomy of Speech

4.7.1   Speech

Petersen and Fiez (1993), using PET on subjects required to read the words presented to them, reported increased activity in and around Broca's area (BA44,45), as well as the supplementary motor area (superior BA6) and areas of motor cortex representing mouth and lips. Fig. 4.9b shows the results of PET scans on sagittal slices when subjects read the words before them aloud as compared with when they saw them but did not read them aloud. The left image (taken 40 mm left of the midline) shows activation in primary motor (upper activation; BA4) and premotor cortex (lower activation; BA6). The right image (taken near the midline) shows activation in the supplementary motor cortex (SMA, upper activation) and midline cerebellum (lower activation). Fig. 4.9c shows that when subjects specify a verb corresponding to a noun which they read with a control condition of simply repeating the noun, there is activation of prefrontal regions some of which are associated with Broca's area (upper left-hand image, taken 40 mm left of midline; BA44,45). Other areas activated are the anterior cingulate (BA24 anterior; upper right-hand image taken near the midline) as well as the lateral cerebellum (lower image taken 25 mm right of the midline).

4.7.2 Spoken action words and colour words

In 1995, a landmark PET study was made concerning areas of the brain that are active during the use of words describing pictured objects (Martin et al., 1995). Achromatic line drawings of common objects were presented. During PET scans, subjects were required to name each object, then to name a colour associated with each object (e.g. a subject might say 'yellow' when shown a picture of a pencil) and to name an action associated with each object (e.g. 'write' when shown a picture of a pencil). In these studies, the spoken colour words were associated with activation of a region in the ventral temporal lobe just anterior to the area involved in the perception of motion (BA22, 21 posterior). These observations are illustrated in Plate 4.4a and b. Plate 4.4a shows a lateral view of the left hemisphere with active areas when subjects specified colours (region shown in green) and action words (region shown in grey) in comparison to naming objects (dark blue regions show areas of overlap). Plate 4.4b (coronal section 50 mm posterior to the anterior commissure) shows the location of bilateral fusiform and left parietal lobe activation when colour words were uttered, and left temporal and parietal activations when action words were uttered. The percentage change in PET-measured regional cerebral blood flow (rCBF), during the naming of objects in the drawing, is given in Plate 4.4c at the site of peak activity in the left middle temporal gyrus (open bars; BA21) and left fusiform gyrus (closed bars; BA19). It is clear that action words are accompanied by maximum activity in the left middle temporal gyrus (BA21), whereas colour words are associated with the left fusiform gyrus (BA19).

In a separate experiment, Martin and his colleagues (1995) presented the written names of objects, rather than line drawings. In this case the subjects read the written name of each object and then specified either a colour word or an action word associated with the named object. Plate 4.4a–e shows that despite the change in stimulus from line drawings of objects to their written names, the areas of activation of the brain were similar to those in the first study. Relative to specifying an appropriate action, increased activity when a colour was attributed to an object was seen in the ventral portion of the right temporal lobe (Plate 4.4d). By comparison with uttering colour words, specifying action words involved increased activity in the left temporal lobe (posterior middle and superior temporal gyri; posterior BA21/22) and left inferior frontal lobe (Broca's area; BA44, 45), as was the case for match-ing action words to drawings of objects (Plate 4.4e). In Plate 4.4d–e red indicates activations in response to line drawings of objects; yellow indicates activations in response to the written names of the objects; and blue indicates regions activated in both studies. Also shown are black and green circles centred on previously reported locations of maximum activity during the perception of colour (Plate 4.4d) and of motion (Plate 4.4e).

The perception of something moving is dependent on a region which is dorsal to that for colour (posterior BA39 or V4). Action words generate peak activity in the middle tem-poral gyrus, 1–2 cm anterior to the site of peak activation for motion perception (anterior

BA39 or MT), and in a region which, it is suggested, might be a site for 'stored knowledge about the visual patterns of motion associated with the use of objects'. From this research, Martin et al. (1995) conclude that 'The ability to retrieve information about a specific attribute of an object can be selectively disrupted by a focal lesion. These findings suggest that object knowledge is stored in the brain as a distributed network of discrete cortical areas' (p. 102). What this actually suggests is that the abilities of which this knowledge consists are dependent upon a distributed network of discrete cortical areas.

4.7.3   Naming animals and tools

In 1996 Damasio and her colleagues carried out PET studies on a large number of patients with different brain lesions. This work indicated that specific brain regions are associated with the exercise of the abilities to name tools, animals and persons. Furthermore, these regions are located outside the classic language areas of Broca (BA44,45) and Wernicke (at the junction of BA21,22,42). Damasio and her colleagues (1996) suggest that

> A central question in the neurobiology of language concerns the neural structures that become active when the word that denotes a person or object is recalled, and is either silently verbalized or vocalized; that is, when an item from the lexicon of a given language is retrieved and explicitly represented in the mind. The traditional answer, based largely on more than a century of aphasia studies involves a set of left cerebral hemisphere structures around the Sylvian fissure, among which the Broca and Wernicke areas figure prominently. (p. 499)

What these PET studies show is that the ability to call to mind and use proper names of specific people and common nouns for animals and tools is dependent on the integrity of regions in the left temporal lobe.

Fig. 4.10 summarizes the results of Damasio and her colleagues (1996) for subjects with defects in recollecting a person's name (lesion in the most anterior sector of left temporal pole; BA38); recollecting a common noun for an animal (lesions in the anterior sector of left inferior temporal region overlapping minimally into the posterior part of the left temporal pole; BA20/21); recollecting a common noun for a tool (lesion in the very posterior sector of the inferior temporal region and the most anterior part of the lateral occipital region (posterior inferior temporal; BA37,19). Fig. 4.10 shows the naming scores for each word of three groups of subjects with lesions in the temporal pole TP (BA38) only; the posterior inferior temporal IT (BA20,21) only; the inferior temporal pole, IT (BA37,39) (with outer borders overlapping in some instances into either TP or posterior IT). The scores were, for personal names, posterior IT > IT > TP; for names of animals, TP > posterior IT > IT; for names of tools, IT > IP > posterior IT. Thus the words for persons, animals and tools show best correlations with TP (BA38), IT (BA20,21) and posterior IT (BA37,19) respectively. These correlations were confirmed for normal subjects. It is important to note that Damasio et al. (1996) made sure in these studies that the patients with these severe difficulties in recollecting such names could still talk about many of the properties relevant to the thing specified by the name. For example, they could describe a skunk as a small black and white animal that makes a nasty smell, but could not actually name it. So the

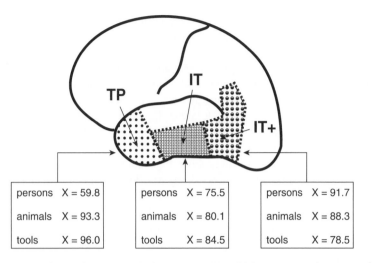

Fig. 4.10. The capacity of patients with damage in temporal lobe (TP) or inferior temporal sector (IT) or posterior temporal sector (IT+) to name items in photographs of well-known people, animals and objects. The naming scores are shown, which for persons were lowest in TP, for animals in IT, and for tools, in posterior IT+. (Damasio et al., 1996, fig 2e.)

brain regions identified above (IT, posterior IT and TP) that were lesioned in these patients are necessary for the ability to recollect such a noun and use it.

Damasio et al. (1996, p. 503) comment: 'We suggest that the regions identified in our study play an intermediary or mediational role in lexical retrieval. For example, when the concept of a given tool is evoked (based on the activation of several regions which support pertinent conceptual knowledge and promote its explicit representation in sensorimotor terms), an intermediary region becomes active and promotes (in the appropriate sensorimotor structures) the explicit representation of phonemic knowledge pertaining to the word form which denotes the given tool.' Or, more appropriately, that neurons in the intermediary region are involved in the retention of the phonemic ability associated with a word – that is, the ability to pronounce it.

Damasio et al. (1996) go on to say that 'An individual's learning experience of concepts of a similar kind (such as manipulable tools), and their corresponding words, leads to the recruitment within the available neural architecture, of a critical set of spatially proximate microcircuits'. However, as we have suggested, words are not matched to, and are not names of, concepts. What should be said is that to master the use of a word, one must be able to say what it means. Sometimes, with age and lesions, one may be able to remember that there is a word that means such-and-such, but be unable to remember the word.

Caramazza (1996, p. 485) interpreted the observations of Damasio et al. (1996) as showing that 'lexical knowledge is organized by category in distinct areas of the left temporal lobe'. He poses the question, 'How is knowledge of a word organized in the brain? However, as knowledge is an ability or complex of abilities, it makes no sense to ask how knowledge is *organized* in the brain, unless one first clarifies what if anything is meant by 'organizing knowledge in a part of the body'. An appropriate question is what parts of the brain are required to function normally for different aspects of the ability to use different categories of words to be possessed and to be exercised. Three neural networks in the brain seem to be involved, according to Caramazza's interpretation of Damasio et al. (1996). One representing, i.e. correlated with knowledge of, the conceptual content or meaning of certain types of words; one representing, i.e. correlated with knowledge of, the phonological (sound) elements that compose words – that is, knowing how to pronounce the word; and a third one investigated by Damasio et al. (1996), mediating between the first two, that, it is claimed, represents modality-independent lexical knowledge, which specifies words of the language without directly providing information about their phonological forms. This conception is summarized in fig. 4.11a, which shows these three levels claimed to represent the word knowledge necessary for speech. For example, the semantic features (carnivorous, furry, domesticated, pet) activate lexical nodes (the word CAT), which, in turn, activate their corresponding phonological features (k, ae, t); that is, the word can be enunciated (see fig. 4.11ai). The difficulty with this interpretation is that neural networks cannot specify words or provide information. At best the experiments show that there are three areas linked with distinct abilities involved in the intelligent use of a limited range of nouns.

Caramazza (1996, p. 485) finally comments that 'Representations at the conceptual level are initially used to select modality-independent lexical representations; these lexical representations are then used to select phonological representations. In other words it is thought that there are abstract lexical representations mediating between conceptual knowledge and the phonological form of words.'

This conclusion is premature. The term 'representation' thus used signifies no more than a part of the brain that is causally implicated in the possession and exercise of an ability that is partly constitutive of the mastery of the use of a word. So a representation, thus understood, cannot be used, but only activated. It can be activated, but it cannot select anything. It can only activate another part of the brain that is causally necessary for a speaker to utter a word with understanding.

What does the research of Damasio et al. (1996) on these patients with different brain lesions actually show? It shows no more than that a subject's ability to read a text with understanding involves, as component abilities, the ability to recognize written letters, written words, and the knowledge (itself an ability) of what the words mean. Different parts of the brain are implicated in the exercise of the abilities. In order for a subject to use words for persons, animals and tools, they must possess certain cortical areas in an intact state: namely, TP, IT and posterior IT respectively (fig 4.10).

It has been known for some time that patients with damage to the ventral temporal cortex are significantly more impaired at naming and recollecting information about animals than about tools and other manipulable man-made objects (see Sartori et al., 1993; Gainotti et al., 1995). Chao et al. (1999) have now shown, using fMRI scans, that pictures or written names of animals and tools are associated with activation in lateral (superior and middle temporal gyri; BA21,22) and ventral (fusiform gyrus) regions respectively of the posterior temporal lobes. Fig. 4.11b gives the amplitude and time course of category-related modulation of activity in a time series for lateral fusiform gyrus (i; BA37), medial fusiform gyrus

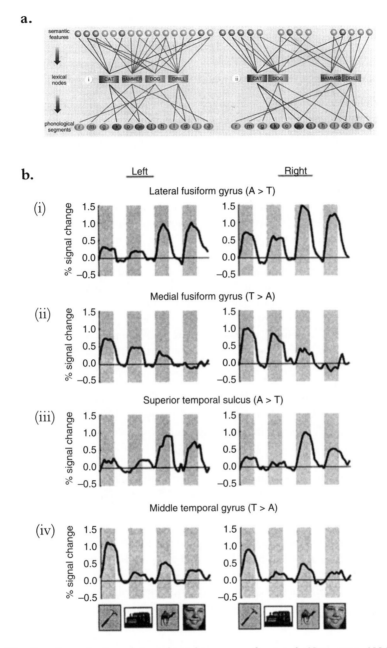

Fig. 4.11. Speech. **a:** the knowledge of words necessary for speech (Caramazza, 1996, p. 485). **b:** perceiving animals (A) or tools (T) accompanied by activity in different areas of temporal cortex (Chao et al., 1999, fig. 2.)

(ii; BA37), superior temporal sulcus (iii; Ba21/22) and middle temporal gyrus (iv; BA21) when viewing animals (A) and tools (T). The grey bars indicate presentation of meaningful stimuli, indicated by the pictures below them, and intervening white areas indicate presentation of control stimuli (phase-scrambled images of the objects that are not shown). It is clear from fig. 4.11b that the more lateral aspect of the fusiform gyrus responds more to pictures of animals than to pictures of tools, the medial fusiform gyrus to pictures of tools (and houses). The results expand on the degeneration studies of Damasio et al. (1996) in showing the importance of the posterior temporal lobe in responding to pictures of animals and tools (compare fig. 4.10 with fig. 4.11b). However, there is also more response to pictures of animals than to pictures of tools in the posterior superior temporal sulcus and of pictures of tools rather than of animals in posterior middle temporal gyrus (fig. 4.11b). So there is a bilateral increase in activity for pictures of animals as opposed to pictures of tools (fig. 4.11b). Chao et al. (1999, p. 918) comment: 'In summary, the results of these studies suggest that object knowledge is stored as a distributed network of cortical regions that prominently includes the posterior regions of the ventral and lateral temporal cortex. Our ability to think about and identify different categories of objects may depend on the activation of stored information about the critical sensory- and motor-based properties that define an object and distinguish it from other members of the same category.' However, as pointed out above, to know something is to possess an ability or complex of abilities and therefore cannot be 'stored'. Similarly, what is known – the information acquired – cannot be *stored* in the brain, although areas of the brain are causally implicated in a human being's retaining information acquired.

Perani et al. (1999) came to many of the same conclusions as Chao et al. (1999), using PET. Perani et al. (1999) found that the left fusiform gyrus (BA37) and lingual gyrus were activated when considering pictures of living things compared with pictures of tools; in contrast, the fusiform gyrus and the inferior occipital gyrus (BA18) were activated when considering visually presented words for living things rather than tools.

A summary of the work of Perani et al. (1999), and that of others working prior to 1999 on this topic, is given in fig. 4.12, which shows PET studies for picture (a) and word (b) stimuli displayed on lateral and medial brain projections (left and right cerebral hemispheres are shown from lateral and medial views, with tick marks on the y and z axes separated by 20 mm increments; the axis originates at the anterior commissure). Foci related to names or pictures of living things are displayed with outline symbols, whereas foci related to those of inanimate things are displayed with full symbols. It is clear from fig. 4.12 that in general both stimuli produce most activation in the posterior temporal lobe, with that for inanimate objects placed at a more superior position to that for living things.

4.7.4   Speaking with strings of words compared with single words

Kircher et al. (2000), in a recent fMRI study, determined the regions of the brain that are active when subjects were asked to speak about whatever came to their mind on viewing a Rorschach inkblot over a 3-minute period. The number of words spoken over that period was positively correlated with increased activation in the left superior temporal (BA22) and supramarginal (BA39/40) gyri. Plate 4.5a shows these brain areas where signal changes were

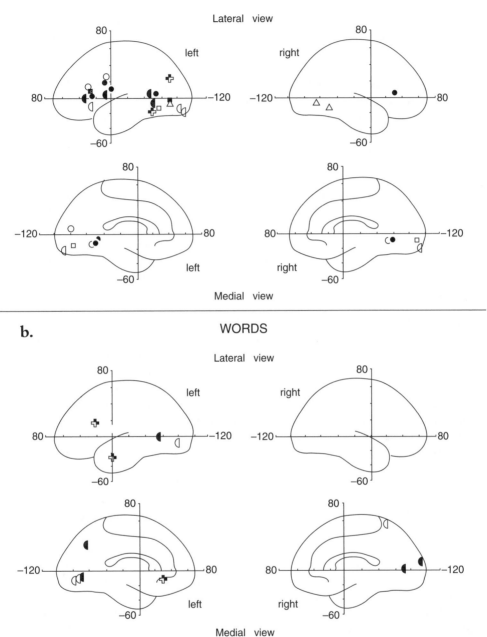

Fig. 4.12. **a:** summary of the sites of cortical activation, according to PET, during experiments in which subjects were asked to discriminate (as similar or different) between drawings of pairs of meaningless shapes, pairs of animals, or manipulable tools. **b:** summary of the sites of cortical activation during experiments in which subjects were asked to discriminate between visually presented pairs of non-words (same or different), pairs of words for animals, pairs of manipulable objects, all given in a variety of fonts. In **a** and **b**, foci related to living stimuli are displayed with outline symbols, whereas foci related to non-living stimuli are displayed with full symbols. (Perani et al., 1999, fig. 4.)

correlated with the number of words spoken (Talasrach Z coordinates are shown at the bottom of each slice). Red voxels indicate positive, and blue voxels negative correlations. The left side of the brain is shown on the right side of the image. The rate of articulation is positively correlated with activation in the left superior and supramarginal gyri. In contrast, negative correlations were found with the fusiform gyri (BA19) and superior occipital gyrus (BA19) bilaterally as well as the posterior cingulate (BA30). Thus continuous speech is accompanied by activation of areas in the left temporal and inferior parietal cortex, which is quite different from the areas that are active when uttering single words; this is associated more with left parietal activation, as noted above.

Kirchner et al. (2000) consider these experiments in the light of their conception of what a subject must do in order to speak. 'Conceptual preparation' involves the subject's selecting the relevant information and ordering this in such a way that it allows development of a plan for the expression of what they want to say. 'Grammatical encoding' involves the selection of appropriate word forms from the 'mental lexicon' and their grammatical inflection and somatic ordering. 'Phonological and phonetic coding (lexical retrieval)' is a process in which the 'phonetic codes' of the words are obtained from memory, and their syllabification, intonation and metrical structure determined. Finally, 'articulation' involves speech itself through the execution of suitable motor commands to muscles.

This sketch of the process involved in speech is misconceived. It confuses the description of the complex abilities involved in intentional speech with a mythical tale of things that have to be done before one speaks. It is true that the ability to speak can be decomposed into multiple constituent abilities. It is an important neuroscientific discovery that many different parts of the cortex are causally involved in speech and comprehension, and that lesions deprive one of different aspects, different constituent abilities, of that highly complex ability. But it does not follow that in order to speak, one must first do all manner of preparatory things, as before starting a car one must open the door, sit down in the driver's seat, close the door, put on the safety belt, put the key in the starter, turn it, depress the clutch, engage the gears, release the brakes, etc. *Sometimes* one may think carefully before speaking – but not usually. *Sometimes* one may rehearse in one's imagination what one is going to say before saying it out loud – but not often. Normally, one makes a remark, responds to what another has said, asks a question, makes a request, etc. without rehearsing anything. A large number of distinguishable abilities are involved in spontaneous speech. These, as has been discovered, are dependent upon coordinated activity in many different parts of the cortex. But those neural activities are not preparatory cognitive ones. Neither the brain, nor parts of the brain, can *order information*. That is something a person may do. *Sometimes* one orders information by writing down a series of points and then arranging them. Sometimes one may tell a tale, and one must order the incidents to produce a coherent story. This one typically does without any rehearsal – it is a skill acquired in the course of increasing linguistic and intellectual skill that accompanies maturation. The fact that it is typically done without rehearsal does not mean that it is actually rehearsed by the brain and its parts.

The supposition that the speaker, prior to utterance, has to engage in conceptual preparation is incoherent, since it recapitulates, *in foro interno*, the very phenomena that are to be explained. If the speaker has to order the information he possesses, then he will have to rehearse it to himself *sotto voce* and decide which item of information should be stated first.

But how is he to rehearse it to himself? Rehearsing it to himself presents the very same array of questions (barring explicit vocalization) to neuroscience as rehearsing it out loud. If he has to develop a plan for the expression of what he wants to say, how does he know what it is that he wants to say? If he has to encode grammatically what he wants to say by selecting words from a mental lexicon, how does he read the mental lexicon, and how does he know what word he wants to retrieve from it? Does he first find it in another lexicon – perhaps a lexicon of concepts that he possesses? And what would a wordless lexicon of concepts look like? Once he has the stock of words, how does he know how to order them into the correct sentence? Does he consult the order of the concepts in the thought he is thinking. (A nineteenth-century French politician once remarked on how wonderful French is – the order of words uniquely matches the structure of the thought expressed!) In phonological and phonetic encoding, how exactly are words 'encoded'? Are words entered non–phonologically and correlated with a phonological entry. What would verify the hypotheses that such-and-such a neural configuration is an *entry*? This conceptual framework is completely incoherent.

According to Hauk et al. (2004), the experiment illustrated in Plate 4.5b–e supports the idea that brain areas activated by reading subcategories of verbs referring to face, arm or leg actions (e.g. to lick, pick or kick) are adjacent to and partly overlap activations associated with the corresponding actions themselves. Plate 4.5b shows the fMRI signal measured during tongue, finger and foot movements. This should be compared with Plate 4.5c, which gives the fMRI signal changes that occur when reading verbs related to facial (green), arm (red) and leg movements (blue). Plate 4.5d gives the fMRI signal change estimates for clusters differentially activated in the left hemispheres by subgroups of verbs. Finally, Plate 4.5e shows the extent of activation produced by 'arm' and 'leg' words with that produced by finger and leg movements respectively (numbers below separate slices label Z coordinates in space, and the colour scales indicate *t* values for arm and leg word-related activation separately). The results show that whereas tongue movements elicit activation in premotor areas just posterior to the inferior frontal patch activated by face words, the other word types and their related body movements produce significant overlapping activity in the motor cortex (see Plate 4.5e). Activation for finger movements overlap with arm word-related blood flow increases in left precental gyrus and in right middle frontal gyrus. Activation for foot movements overlapped with activation produced by leg words in dorsal premotor areas on the midline and in left dorsal pre- and postcentral gyri. These results, then, show that reading words referring to actions performed with different body parts is associated with the motor and premotor cortex in a somatotopic fashion.

4.7.5   Word repetition

Wernicke's area has for more than 100 years been taken to occupy part of the left superior temporal gyrus (STG; BA42/22,22,21). Lichtheim (1885) took this area to be a region in the cortex necessary for one to be able to remember, or recall, familiar heard words, and that parts of the brain necessary for our being able to understand the meaning of a word or for speech are connected to the parts of the cortex required for recall. In a recent PET study, Wise et al. (2001) have shown that the STG is central for long-term memory of new

words. In particular, the posterior left superior temporal sulcus is active during the generation of phonetic sequence, whether heard or rehearsed silently. Their PET results for four
different kinds of experiments are shown in Plate 4.6, with projections of activated voxels
shown on the magnetic resonance image template of the lateral surface of the left cerebral
hemisphere. In experiment 1, subjects heard either bisyllabic nouns or signal-correlated
noise; there was correlation between activity and the rate of hearing words, but not with
the signal-correlated noise. Voxels located within the posterior left superior temporal sulcus
are shown highlighted in yellow in Plate 4.6, and all other voxels are shown in white. In
experiment 2, the subjects had to think (without vocalization) of as many verbs as they
could (in the available time), in response to concrete nouns (e.g. SHIRT: wash, iron, mend,
etc.); alternatively they had to think of nouns in response to hearing a superordinate noun
(e.g. FISH: cod, salmon, perch, etc.); regions of activity elicited during these experiments
are shown. In experiment 3, subjects either repeatedly said the phrase 'buy Bobby a poppy'
out loud (with the place of articulation for the consonants at the lips), or mouthed the
phrase without saying it (with lip movements but no voicing or adduction of the vocal
chords), or used a single, voiced vowel sound ('uh') to replace the words in the phrase
(without movement of the articulators), or thought of the phrase repeatedly. This produced
the activation pattern given by the voxels for articulation but not those responding to
hearing utterances in the medial left temporo-parietal junction, highlighted in yellow and
displayed, for illustrative purposes, on the lateral surface of the hemisphere in Plate 4.6. In
experiment 4, subjects were asked to think of nouns after hearing a superordinate noun
cue; immediately following the scan the subjects performed the task again out loud, with
their responses recorded to give an estimate of the number of nouns they could think of
per minute; regions of enhanced brain activity associated with the sum of activity for word
perception and word recollection are shown in Plate 4.6. Wise and his colleagues comment:
'The results are compatible with an hypothesis that the posterior superior temporal cortex
is specialized for processes involved in the mimicry of sounds, including repetition. Mimick-
ing both words and non-speech sounds requires that an analysis of the sound structure of
the percept is used to direct the muscles of respiration, et cetera' (2001, p. 38).

     This hypothesis can be challenged. Neither the brain nor the person (unless he is a
phonologist) analyses sound structures. The person must be sensitive to the sounds he wishes
to mimic, and he must be able to reproduce them at will. Doubtless specific localized neural
activity is necessary for both the perceptual sensitivity and the reproductive ability and its
exercise. But neither the person nor his brain *directs* the muscles.

4.8   The Functional Neuroanatomy that Underpins Psycholinguistic Accounts of Language

To what extent do the descriptions given of the functional neuroanatomy that subserves
language comprehension (§4.6) and speech (§4.7) cohere with psycholinguistic accounts
of language? The most comprehensive recent claims concerning this issue have been made
by Indefrey and Levelt (2004) in the context of Levelt's (1994) model of speech that we
discussed in §4.5.1 (see fig. 4.7b). Plate 4.7 summarizes their suggestions, with the terms

defined in §4.5.1, and should be compared with figs. 4.7a and b. 'Conceptually driven lexical selection' occurs between 175 and 250 ms after asking the subject to name a picture and is dependent on activity in the midsection of the left middle temporal gyrus (BA21). This is followed by 'lexical phonological code retrieval', which is accompanied by activity in the posterior sections of the middle and superior temporal gyrus (BA21 & 22) of the left hemisphere over a period of 250–330 ms. Next, between 330 and 455 ms, syllabification takes place with activity in the left posterior inferior frontal gyrus (BA45). 'Phonetic encoding' and 'articulation' require the support of a number of areas, including the right sensorimotor cortex (BA3,4,43) and the right supplementary motor area (BA6) and occurs between 455 and 600 ms. 'Self-monitoring', which involves any necessary corrections to one's own speech, is dependent on the superior temporal gyrus (BA22).

Cortical 'processing' then appears to divide from the superior temporal gyrus into two 'streams' after heard speech (Hickok and Poeppel, 2004; see Plate 4.7a and b). One of these, the ventral stream, is probably involved in 'lemma selection', and consists of the middle temporal gyrus (BA21), the inferior temporal gyrus (BA20), and the temporal sulcus (the STG in Plate 4.7b). This is roughly in agreement with Indefrey and Levelt (2004; Plate 4.7c). The other stream is dorsal and involves syllabification and word articulation (Plate 4.7c). It is said to 'map sound onto articulatory-based representations' and projects to posterior inferior frontal regions (pIF in Plate 4.7b; BA45) for syllabification and to parts of Broca's area, the frontal operculum/insula and the motor–face area (BA4) for word articulation. Comparison of Plate 4.7b and c shows that the account of Hickok and Poeppel (2004), on the one hand, and that of Indefrey and Levelt (2004), on the other, concerning this functional neuroanatomy are in reasonable agreement.

Hickok and Poeppel (2004, p. 67) conclude their review with the comment that the 'functional anatomy of language' they present has strengths and weaknesses, such as 'What are the computations involved in mapping sound onto meaning, or auditory onto motor representations?' Indefrey and Levelt (2004, p. 94) conclude their comprehensive review with the upbeat comment that they have been able to specify 'region and time windows of activation for the core processes of word production: lexical selection, phonological code retrieval, syllabification and phonetic/articulatory preparation'.

These conclusions incorporate all the errors that we have found in the history of neuroscientific and neurological investigations of linguistic abilities. The fact that the ability to identify a picture of an X as a picture of an X, and to say that it is, doubtless can be decomposed into a multitude of subordinate abilities: e.g. the ability to use the word 'X', to identify things that are X, to pronounce the word 'X' correctly, to explain what it means, and to notice whether one accidentally mispronounces it. These various linked abilities are dependent on the normal functioning of many different cortical regions. It does not follow that these various regions are exercising these abilities. Nor does it follow that these abilities are exercised consecutively. All that follows is that the ability conjunctively to exercise them depends on the successive activation of the various regions.

5

Emotion and Cortical-Subcortical Function: Darwin to Damasio

5.1   Introduction

Fruitful research on the emotions requires clarity with regard to the category of the emotions and the differentiation of emotions from feelings that are not emotions at all, although commonly confused with them. So before recounting some of the salient advances in research over the past century or so, we shall endeavour to provide a schematic map of the conceptual terrain.

Feelings (disregarding feelings that are hunches, thoughts or inclinations, as in 'I feel like going to the cinema tonight', or 'I feel we should tell him'.) must be differentiated into sensations, tactile perceptions, appetites and affections (fig. 5.1). Pains, tickles and tingles are bodily sensations with a more or less determinate bodily location. They are felt *in* a part of the body, but not *with* a part of the body. Unlike perceptions, sensations are not correct or incorrect, and are not susceptible to cognitive error. There is no such thing as thinking one is in pain but being mistaken. Phantom pains or reflected pains may lead one to judge that one has an injury where there is none, but what is erroneous is neither the sensation nor its felt location – it is the judgement concerning the somatic location of the pain or injury. Localized bodily sensations must be distinguished from sensations of overall bodily condition, such as feelings of weariness or lassitude. Feeling the heat, solidity, elasticity or dampness of an object are forms of tactile perception – exercises of a cognitive faculty that inform one how things are in one's environment in respect of perceptible qualities such as warmth, cold, hardness, softness, wetness, dryness and so forth. Like all perceptions, they may be correct or incorrect, and we distinguish between things feeling thus-and-so to one and things being thus-and-so. Natural appetites are such things as feelings of hunger, thirst or animal lust. Non-natural (acquired) appetites are addictions.

An appetite is a blend of desire and sensation. Sensations characteristic of appetites have a bodily location (sensations of hunger are located in one's midriff) and are forms of unease that dispose one to action to satisfy the desire. The desire that is blended with sensation is characterized by its formal object: hunger is a desire for food, thirst for drink, lust for sexual intercourse. The intensity of the desire is typically proportional to the intensity of the sensation. Satisfying an appetite leads to its temporary satiation and so to the disappearance of

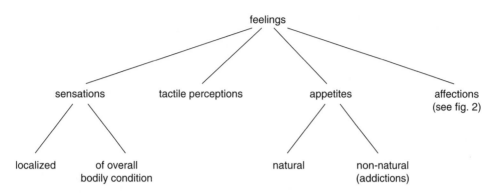

Fig. 5.1.   Types of feelings distinguished. (Bennett and Hacker, 2005, fig. 1.)

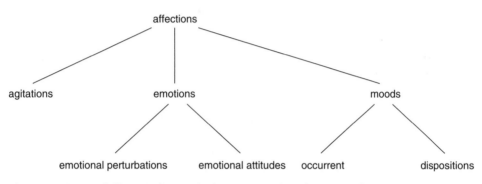

Fig. 5.2.   Types of affections distinguished. (Bennett and Hacker, 2005, fig. 2.)

the sensation. Appetites are not constant, but recurrent, typically caused by bodily needs or hormonally determined drives.

Affections too are felt. The feelings that are affections can be distinguished into agitations (e.g. astonishment, excitement), moods (e.g. cheerfulness, depression) and emotions (e.g. fear, love) (fig. 5.2). Unlike sensations, affections do not inform one about the state of one's body, though they are sometimes linked with sensations. One does not feel pride in one's chest, even though one's chest may swell with pride, or fear in one's mouth, even though one's mouth may be dry with fear. One's blush of embarrassment does not inform one of the state of one's facial arteries, although it may inform one that one is more embarrassed than one thought, and one's tears of grief do not inform one of the state of one's lachrymal glands, although they may inform one that one is grieving more than one had anticipated. Unlike feelings that are perceptions, the affections do not inform one of the state of the world around one. Paradigmatic emotions are love, hate, hope, fear, anger, gratitude, resentment, indignation, envy, jealousy, pity, compassion, grief, as well as emotions of self-assessment such as pride, shame, humiliation, regret, remorse and guilt.

Agitations are short-term affective disturbances, commonly (but not only) caused by something unexpected, e.g. being and feeling excited, thrilled, shocked, convulsed, amazed, surprised, horrified, disgusted, delighted. They are caused by what we perceive, learn or realize. Because they are disturbances, caused by unanticipated disruptions, they are not motives for action as emotions may be, but temporarily *inhibit* motivated action. One's agitations are manifested in expressive behaviour *because* one is, for example, excited, surprised or shocked, but one does not act *out of* excitement, surprise or shock as one may act *out of* love, pity or gratitude. Agitations are modes of *reaction*: one cries out *in* horror, recoils *with* revulsion, is convulsed *by* laughter, or is paralysed *with* shock. Occurrently felt emotions, as opposed to longer-standing emotional attitudes, often bear a kinship to agitations – for example, in the perturbations of rage, fear and grief.

Moods are such things as feeling cheerful, euphoric, contented, irritable, melancholic or depressed. They are states or frames of mind. They may be occurrent or longer-term dispositional states (one may feel depressed for an afternoon, or one may be suffering from a depression that lasts for months – being then prone to feel depressed during one's waking hours). Moods are less closely tied to specific objects than emotions – one can feel cheerful without feeling cheerful about anything in particular, but one cannot love without loving someone or something in particular. They are not linked to specific patterns of intentional action, since, unlike emotions, they do not afford motives for action. Moods colour one's thoughts and pervade one's reflections. So they are linked to manners of behaviour, demeanour and tone of voice.

It is important, especially in the study of human emotions, to distinguish between episodic emotional perturbations and emotional attitudes. Emotional perturbations resemble agitations in certain respects. Some, e.g. fear or anger, have characteristic somatic accompaniments, both sensations that are felt and physiological reactions that are measurable. Others do not, e.g. feelings of pride, humility, compassion and gratitude. They are manifest in *expressive behaviour* that may take various forms. It may be behaviour that is not action, such as blushes, perspiration, pallor. It may be voluntary (utterances of love and affection, hope or pride), partly voluntary (raised voice of anger, which can be suppressed) or involuntary action (cry of terror). It may be exhibited only in the manner of acting (e.g. tone of voice, impatient gestures).

Emotional attitudes, such as love, hate, pride, shame and remorse, may last for long periods of time and motivate action done for reasons. One may love or hate a person, activity, cause or place for years. One may be proud of the achievements of one's youth for the rest of one's life, and one may respect or detest, be jealous or envious of, someone for years. One may be ashamed or guilty of one's misconduct for decades, and one's regrets for one's follies may never cease. One's judgement may be clouded not only by emotional perturbations but also by one's long-standing resentments, envies or jealousies. The emotions of love, hate or envy, for example, consist above all in the manner in which the object of one's emotion matters to one and the reasons one has for holding it to be important, and hence too in the motives it affords one for acting (for one acts *out of* love, hate or envy). One's emotions are then evident in the reasons that weigh with one in one's deliberations, in the desires one harbours in respect of the object of the emotion, and in associated thoughts and fantasies.

Emotions have objects as well as causes. What makes one afraid (a noise downstairs at night) need not be what one is afraid of (a burglar, who may not even exist). What one is frightened *by* is the cause of one's fear; what one is frightened *of* is its object. What makes one feel ashamed, e.g. someone's indignant tirade, is not the same as what one is ashamed of: namely, one's own misdemeanour. A person need not know the cause of his emotion, but, save in pathological cases, he cannot be ignorant of the object of his emotion, i.e. whom he is angry with, what he is ashamed of, what he is afraid of.

It is obvious that the intensity of one's emotions is not proportional to the intensity of whatever sensations may accompany their occurrent manifestations. One's pride in one's children's achievements cannot be measured somatically, but may be manifest in one's behaviour, in the way one praises them and how one talks about them. One's fear of heights may be manifest above all in the lengths one goes to avoid them, rather than in any per-turbations – given that one avoids heights at all costs. Emotions do not display the same pattern of occurrence, satiation and recurrence as appetites. They have a cognitive dimension absent from appetites. For the frightened animal is afraid of something it knows or believes to be dangerous or harmful; a mother is proud of her offspring, believing them to be meri-torious, and the repentant offender is remorseful, knowing or believing himself to have done wrong and wishing to make amends. Human emotions, rooted though they are in our animal nature, are nevertheless run through, as mere animal emotions are not, with thought and belief, wish and want, fantasy and imagination – as is to be expected of language-using, concept-exercising creatures.

5.2   Darwin

In 1872, Charles Darwin published his book *The Expression of Emotions in Man and Animals*. The scope of the book was wider than suggested by the title, since Darwin investigated expressive behaviour in general, studying not only the expressions of fear, anger, grief, etc. but also behaviour expressing pain, assent, dissent, puzzlement and helplessness, which are not emotions. Expressive behaviour can be differentiated into facial expression, movements of the body and limbs, posture and voice. Darwin concentrated upon facial expression, but also discussed gesture and mien.

The argument of the book was that the mode of expression of the emotions, at least in the range of the more primitive emotions, is innate. It is common to the whole of mankind, and so supports the hypothesis of the descent of all races from a common progenitor. Fur-thermore, it shares common features with the modes of manifestation of emotions by other animals, in particular the apes, thus supporting the evolutionary hypothesis that man is continuous with the rest of animate nature. So Darwin's enterprise gave oblique support to evolutionary theory. It is very surprising that Darwin paid hardly any attention in his theory to the communicative role and evolutionary benefit of regular, determinate and readily recognizable manifestations of basic emotions among animals in general and man in particular.

Of course, his researches were pursued also for their intrinsic interest. The question of *what* facial expression gives expression to *which* emotion had been raised by others. So too had the question of how these specific expressions are physiologically produced. Darwin relied upon Sir Charles Bell's physiological researches (see *Anatomy and Philosophy of Expres-sion*, 1806) into facial musculature and its employment in the expression of the emotions, upon the work of Pierre Gratiolet (see *De la Physiognomie et des Mouvements d'Expression*, 1865) and G. B. Duchenne de Bologne (see *Méchanisme de la Physiognomie Humaine*, 1862)

a.   **b.**

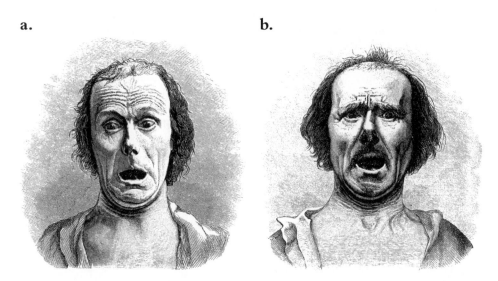

Fig. 5.3.   Facial expressions illustrating the manifestations of emotion. **a:** terror. **b:** horror and agony. (Darwin, 1872, 1965, figs 20 and 21.)

– in particular making use of the latter's methods of using photographs of facial expressions to illustrate the manifestations of emotion (see fig 5.3a, showing terror, and fig. 5.3b, showing horror and agony, both being wood engravings made for Darwin's book from Duchenne's photographs). What was novel was Darwin's investigation into the question of *why* these innate forms of expression of emotion should have evolved, why just these specific muscles should be used to exhibit fear, anger, grief, etc., respectively.

The strategy he employed was to appeal to three distinct principles. The first was his Principle of Serviceable Associated Habits. According to this principle, expressive behaviour that is directly or indirectly useful in relieving or gratifying desires or feelings associated with an emotion will tend to be repeated whenever that emotion recurs (no matter how feebly) even if the behaviour is pointless. The second was the Principle of Antithesis, according to which contrary emotions tend to induce diametrically opposed expressive behaviour. The third was the Principle of the Direct Action of the Nervous System, as exhibited in blushing, perspiring, raised breathing and pulse rates, differential glandular secretions, etc. associated with specific emotions. Darwin hoped to be able to explain all of the forms of expressive behaviour by reference to these three principles and their interplay. Moreover, if they could also be invoked successfully to explain the expressions of emotion among primates and other animals, this would reinforce the argument for common evolutionary origins.

Darwin's first principle was supported by a great deal of illustrative data. It has won considerable backing in recent years, although Darwin's surprisingly Lamarckian explanation of its transmission is rejected. The second principle is generally thought to be more questionable. The third can hardly be challenged, but it is the one for which Darwin, as he admitted, had least explanation to offer.

Darwin's book, although an immediate bestseller, became forgotten in the course of the first half and more of the twentieth century. Its central doctrines of the *universality* and *innateness* of the fundamental forms of emotional expression were rejected. This was due partly to the rise of highly relativist forms of anthropology (the leading protagonists of which were Margaret Mead, Gregory Bateson and Ray Birdwhistell), and partly to the dominance of dogmatic behaviourism among experimental psychologists until the early 1960s. It was only with the repudiation of behaviourism and the questioning of Mead's anthropology that Darwin's theories received fresh consideration.

Darwin's evidential methods were, by later standards, excessively anecdotal, and his questionnaires often tended to suggest a bias in the answers. But his ideas were put to systematic tests meeting current standards of evidence by Paul Ekman in the 1960s and 1970s, and received powerful confirmation (Ekman, 1971, 1972). Ekman and his colleagues showed that there are distinct patterns of facial expression of the emotions corresponding to such primary emotions as fear, anger, happiness (presumably satisfaction, or being pleased, or contented) and disgust. These patterns appear to be behavioural universals, characteristic of literate and preliterate cultures alike, irrespective of the availability of specific emotion names in the language or of exposure to imagery in mass media. So, for example, in this research, data were gathered in New Guinea by telling the subjects a story (without mentioning any emotion terms) and asking them to select a face from a set of three photographs which was appropriate to the events recounted. Table 5.1 shows the results appropriate for the stories listed in the first column. Within each row, the percentage of subjects who gave the correct response differentiating between three emotions was calculated across all subjects (regardless of whether the photographs used to represent them differed). The table shows that the appropriate face was chosen at a significant level for all discriminations (rows) except the differentiation of fear from surprise (last three rows). This demonstrates universality in emotion *recognition*. Other experiments demonstrated comparable universality in primary emotion *expression*. Of course, this does not imply that the expression of emotion is not subject to differential forms of social constraint and socially conditioned forms of behaviour.

5.3   Cognitive versus Precognitive Theories for the Expression of Emotions

Scientists have differed over the relation between emotion and cognition. Zajonc (1984) has been a main proponent of the view that 'affect and cognition are separate and partially independent systems and although they ordinarily function conjointly, affect could be generated without a prior cognitive process'. Thus, according to Zajonc, affective judgements may be made on first meeting a person even though very little of what he refers to as 'cognitive processing' has taken place. Evidence which is taken to support this view has been provided by Murphy and Zajonc (1993) by means of the following experiments. Comparisons were made between the effects of what are called affective and cognitive priming under extremely brief, 4 millisecond (suboptimal) and longer 1 second (optimal) exposure conditions. Subjects were told they would be presented with an assortment of

Table 5.1 Table purporting to show that there are distinct patterns of facial expressions corresponding to different emotions

	ADULT RESULTS		
Emotion described in the story	*Emotions shown in the two incorrect photographs*	*No. of subjects*	*Per cent choosing correct face*
Happiness	Surprise, disgust	62	90**
	Surprise, sadness	57	93**
	Fear, anger	65	86**
	Disgust, anger	36	100**
Anger	Sadness, surprise	66	82**
	Disgust, surprise	31	87**
	Fear, sadness	31	87**
Sadness	Anger, fear	64	81**
	Anger, surprise	26	81**
	Anger, happiness	31	87**
	Anger, disgust	35	69*
	Disgust, surprise	35	77**
Disgust (smell story)	Sadness, surprise	65	77**
Disgust (dislike story)	Sadness, surprise	36	89**
Surprise	Fear, disgust	31	71*
	Happiness, anger	31	65*
Fear	Anger, disgust	92	64**
	Sadness, disgust	31	87**
	Anger, happiness	35	86**
	Disgust, happiness	26	85**
	Surprise, happiness	65	48
	Surprise, disgust	31	52
	Surprise, sadness	57	28[a]

*p < .05.

**p < .01.

[a] Subjects selected the surprise face (67 per cent) at a significant level (p < .01, two-tailed test).

Source: Ekman and Friesen, 1971, table 1.

Chinese characters that they were to rate on a 5-point scale, where 1 indicated they did not like the ideograph at all and 5 indicated they liked the ideograph quite a lot. Subjects were then shown slides of 45 target Chinese ideographs. Four priming conditions, two control and two experimental, were investigated. The series of 45 trials began with 5 control trials having no prime at all (subsequently referred to as the no-prime control). The remaining 40 trials consisted of 20 control trials that had random polygons as primes (subsequently referred to as the irrelevant prime control) interspersed with 20 experimental trials that had facial primes. Of the 20 experimental trials, 10 of the target ideographs were shown twice, once primed with positive affect (i.e. preceded by an image of an individual smiling) and once primed with negative affect (i.e. preceded by an image of the same individual scowling). The results of these experiments are shown in fig. 5.4. Clearly the liking ratings were significantly influenced by the affective primes when these were presented for 4 mil-

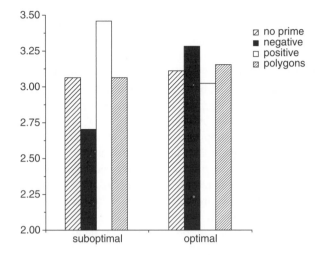

Fig. 5.4. Results of experiments taken as showing that affect and cognition are separate and partially independent systems (for description, see text). y-axis: mean like ratings on a scale from 1 to 5 for the ideographs when preceded by positive as opposed to negative primers. (Murphy and Zajonc, 1993, fig. 1.)

liseconds but not when they were presented for 1 second. The explanation suggested is that participants in the 1 second condition had sufficient time to reflect that their affective reaction, taken as a reflex response, was produced by the priming stimulus, and so they were able to discount this when reacting to the second stimulus. A further study by Murphy and Zajonc (1993) forced subjects to make a cognitive judgement by asking them to rate Chinese ideographs for femininity after being presented with male or female priming faces. In this case the ratings were influenced by the priming faces if these were presented 1 second before the ideographs but not 4 milliseconds before. According to Murphy and Zajonc (1993), these results indicate that the neural activity underpinning affective processing can sometimes occur faster than the neural activity required for cognitive processing and so lend support to the hypothesis that the neural networks involved in affect and those required for cognition are separate and partially independent systems.

It is difficult to know what to make of such experiments. In the first place, they concern attitudes – in particular, attitudes of liking and not liking – rather than emotions. Secondly, the object of the attitude, a hitherto unencountered shape of a Chinese ideograph, is so anomalous as to cast doubt on the nature of the judgements the subjects were being asked to make or what liking or not liking them showed. It is, after all, not unlike being asked whether Monday is fat or thin, or whether Wednesday is green or blue. Thirdly, it is interesting that the priming affected the arbitrary judgements of liking when exposure was suboptimal, but there is no reason whatsoever to explain the difference between these cases and the cases of judgements preceded by optimal exposure by reference to the subjects' having time for so-called 'cognitive processing', given the complete unclarity about what 'cognitive processing' is supposed to mean. To suggest that subjects had time to discount the positive priming presupposes that the subjects were aware of the influence of the positive priming upon their (arbitrary) judgements. But is that evident? The supposition that the neural networks responsible for affective response differ from those responsible for knowledge may or may not be true, but in the case of many cognitively laden emotions, the component of knowledge or belief cannot, logically, be prized off the emotion, since without the element of knowledge or belief, the identity of the emotion evaporates, leaving no more than somatic agitation of one form or another.

Lazarus (1982) has argued the opposite point of view: namely, that what he calls 'cognitive appraisal' is an important ingredient in emotional experience. Experiments alleged to support his case have been carried out using anxiety-evoking films presented to subjects with different accompanying sound tracks (Speisman et al., 1964). Such a film might involve a workshop accident in which a board is caught in a circular saw which rams with considerable force into a worker, who then dies in terrible pain on the floor. Another film showed a Stone Age ritual involving adolescent boys having their penises deeply cut. Skin conductances of subjects were taken during the film, as indicative of their stress response, when the film was not accompanied by any sound track ('silent' condition) and when it was accompanied by the following sound tracks: one in which it is indicated that the workshop film only involved actors or that the incision film did not involve any operation (constituting a 'denial' condition); another sound track appealed to the viewer to consider the workshop accident in an objective way and to view the incision film from the point of view of an anthropologist viewing native customs (constituting an 'intellectualization' condition); finally, a sound track was presented which heightened the trauma produced by the visual presentation by emphasizing the horror, cruelty and pain associated with the film (the 'trauma' condition). Fig. 5.5 shows skin conductance of subjects taken during the film. The different conductance values are given for the three different sound tracks that accompanied the film. These are the trauma track, which pointed up the threatening aspects of the film, and gives the greatest increase in skin conductance; the intellectualization sound track, which was accompanied by the smallest increase in skin conductance whilst watching the film; the denial sound track, which gave a skin conductance increase marginally greater that that of the intellectualization process; and finally, no sound track at all, which was accompanied by skin conductance changes intermediate between those for the threatening sound track and the denial sound track. Lazarus and his colleagues interpreted these results as pointing to the fact that denial and intellectualization both produced substantial reductions in stress. Thus by changing what they took to be the cognitive appraisal of the subjects witnessing the traumatic events the physiological indicator of their state of stress could be significantly altered. Lazarus and his colleagues have taken this to imply that cognitive appraisals play an important role in determining emotions (Folkman and Lazarus, 1990; Lazarus, 1991).

Unlike the previous experiments, the bearing of the experiment on the conclusion derived from it is clear. What is unclear is why it should be necessary to conduct experiments to show that thought and reflection can influence one's emotional responses. That is arguably a priori evident, inasmuch as reasons are involved in many emotional reactions, and reflection, by definition, can affect the weight and balance of reasons.

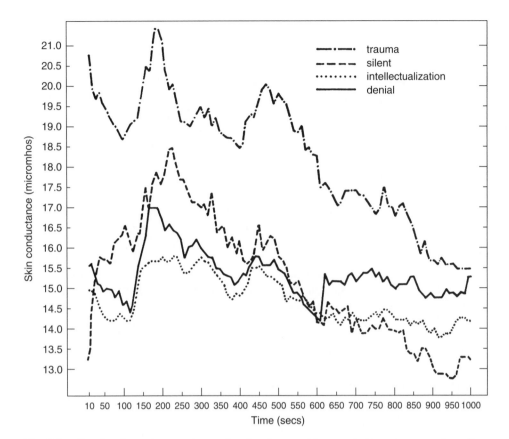

Fig. 5.5.   Results of experiments taken as showing that cognitive appraisal is an important ingredient in emotional experience (for description, see text). (Speisman et al., 1964, fig. 1.)

5.3.1   On physiological measurements of emotional responses

It is important to realize that neither the subjective nor the objective somatic accompaniments of an emotion, such as changes in skin conductance, are by themselves sufficient conditions for the identification and ascription of a given emotion such as that associated with stress. For one's bodily state, subjectively experienced in terms of sensations or objectively determined in physiological terms, is not an emotion. It is only part of the syndrome of an episode of an emotional perturbation in appropriate circumstances, given the appropriate knowledge, beliefs and concerns of the agent. The measurements taken of skin conductance during the film provide only part of the somatic reaction of the individual, and the appropriate knowledge, beliefs and concerns of the viewer must be carefully controlled for − no easy task! Whether these reactions are manifestations of one emotion or another, or have nothing to do with an emotion, depends upon the circumstances and on what the agent knows or believes of the circumstances in which he finds himself and upon what he cares about. We shall elaborate this point further below.

5.3.2   Involvement of the amygdala and the orbitofrontal cortex in the emotional responses to faces

Both animal and human studies indicate that the amygdala of the brain is involved in emotional reactions to faces (Rolls, 1995; Le Doux et al., 1990; Le Doux, 1993a, b). Monkeys that have had their amygdala ablated are tame (Kluver and Bucy, 1939; Weiskrantz, 1956), and no longer make appropriate responses to signals of danger or threat. Radiotelemetry recordings of amygdala activity in monkeys during social interactions show the highest responses to ambiguous or threatening situations (e.g. threatening face displays), and the lowest to tension-lowering behaviours (such as grooming and huddling; Kling and Steklis, 1976; Kling et al., 1979). Furthermore, lesions of the human amygdala are accompanied by changes in recognitional responses of fearful facial expression (Calder et al., 1996) as well as in fear conditioning (Bechara et al., 1996). All these observations point to the necessity of intact neural networks in the amygdala if animals and humans are to be able to respond fearfully in appropriate circumstances.

The orbitofrontal cortex of the brain is also involved in emotional reactions to faces and objects, for if it is damaged in primates there is considerable reduction in the normal aggression associated with fear at the sight of a human or a snake (Butter and Snyder, 1972). The orbitofrontal cortex is located in the ventral prefrontal cortex, whereas the amygdala is a subcortical region in the anterior part of the temporal lobe. These areas are best identified with respect to the numbers on the cytoarchitectural map of the human cortex due to Brodmann (1909), shown in fig. 5.6 (see also Plate 4.1). In this figure, **a** shows the lateral surface of the brain and **b** shows the medial surface. As the amygdala has a subcortical location, it is not provided with Brodmann numbers for its location, whereas the orbitofrontal cortex does and is located in Brodmann areas 11,12, 13 and 14, which are delineated in a lateral view in fig. 5.6.

There is much experimental research on the role of the amygdala and the orbitofrontal cortex in emotional responses to faces. We shall therefore examine this in some detail below in order to best elucidate recent developments in the study of emotion and neural activity. Activity in the amygdala and/or the orbitofrontal cortex, often occurs in conjunction with enhanced activity in the anterior cingulate cortex as will be noted below. The next sections focus on the properties of the amygdala and orbitofrontal cortex.

5.4   The Amygdala

5.4.1   Faces expressing different emotions and the amygdala: PET and fMRI

There is direct *in vivo* evidence for a differential neural response in the human amygdala that accompanies facial expressions of fear and happiness – presumably the latter are expressions of pleasure or of being pleased (Morris et al., 1996). Positron emission tomography (PET) measures of neural activity were made while subjects viewed photographs of fearful or happy faces varying systematically in emotional intensity. This work showed that the

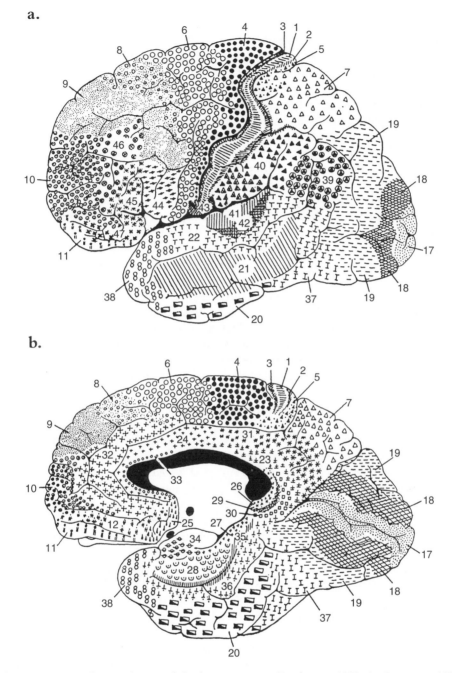

Fig. 5.6. Cytoarchitectural map of the human cortex. (Brodmann, 1909, in Carpenter, 1976, p. 286.)

neuronal response in the left amygdala is significantly greater when viewing fearful photographs as opposed to those showing happy expressions, of pleasure or satisfaction and contentment. Furthermore, this response showed significant changes that were correlated with the intensity of emotion indicated by the expression displayed in the photographs (increasing with increasing fearfulness, decreasing with increasing contentment). The faces used in these experiments are shown in fig. 5.7a. Faces i and v are prototypical neutral and fearful expressions respectively. Faces ii–iv are interpolated between these extremes. Computer morphing techniques were used to shift the shape and pigmentation of the neutral prototype towards the fear prototype. ii purportedly involves 25 per cent fear (and 75 per cent neutral), iii 50 per cent fear (and 50 per cent neutral) and iv 75 per cent fear (and 25 per cent neutral). Face vi is an enhanced 125 per cent fear expression, created by shifting the shape of the fear prototype 25 per cent away from neutral (increasing by 25 per cent any difference from neutral). Fig. 5.7b shows the results of these experiments. In 5.7b are shown the extent of regional cerebral blood flow (rCBF) values, indicating the extent of activation of the left amygdala in the interaction of emotional category and intensity (Plate 5.1). The x-axis of the graph represents the proportion of the prototypical expression in the face stimuli, with fearful being positive (100 per cent = 1.5) and happy negative (100 per cent = −1.5). A regression line has been fitted to the data (with broken lines representing 95 per cent confidence intervals for the gradient of the slope). This work has been taken to provide direct evidence that the human amygdala contains neural networks that function during the emotional salience of faces, with a specificity of response to fearful facial expressions. Functional magnetic resonance imaging (fMRI) studies support these PET results in showing that there is a differential neuronal response in the amygdala to the presentation of fearful faces compared with that of happy faces (Breiter et al., 1996). It is unclear, however, what this differential response to facial expressions out of any relevant context means. Perhaps it signifies a greater sensitivity to expressions of fear of one's kin than to their expressions of contentment.

Increased neuronal activity occurs in the amygdala as well as the anterior cingulate when subjects view photos of facial expressions indicating various degrees of sadness, as shown in fig. 5.8a(A)–(F) (Blair et al., 1999). In this figure, face (A) is taken as the 0 per cent face expressing the neutral prototype, whilst face (F) is the 100 per cent prototype for sad expressions. Increasing intensity of sad facial expressions (fig. 5.8a(A)–(F)) was associated with enhanced activity in the left amygdala and right temporal pole as determined by PET (fig. 5.8b). Results are also presented for increasing expressions of anger (fig. 5.8a(G)–(L)) in fig. 5.8c(A) and (B). This figure shows views of the brain for orthogonal slices at the pixel of maximal activation within (A), the left amygdala and (B) the right temporal pole with significant areas of activation displayed on mean MRIs produced from the co-registered structural MRIs from all subjects.

In a separate study using fMRI, Killgore and Yurgelun–Todd (2004) sought to determine the relative activity in the anterior cingulate gyrus and the amygdala when viewing sad or happy faces. They asked subjects to view sad and happy faces, with each stimulus trial consisting of two rapidly presented stimuli (Plate 5.2A): a 'target' face depicting either a sad or a happy emotional expression from one of eight posers and a 'mask' face consisting of a photograph of the same poser expressing neutral emotion; during each trial, the target face

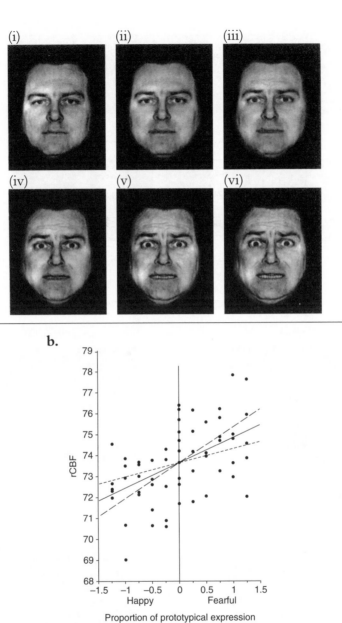

Fig. 5.7. Results of experiments taken as showing that neuronal responses in the left amygdala, as measured with PET (**b**) are significantly greater when viewing fearful photographs as opposed to those showing happy (contented) expressions (**a**) (see text for further description). (Morris et al., 1996, figs 1 and 3.)

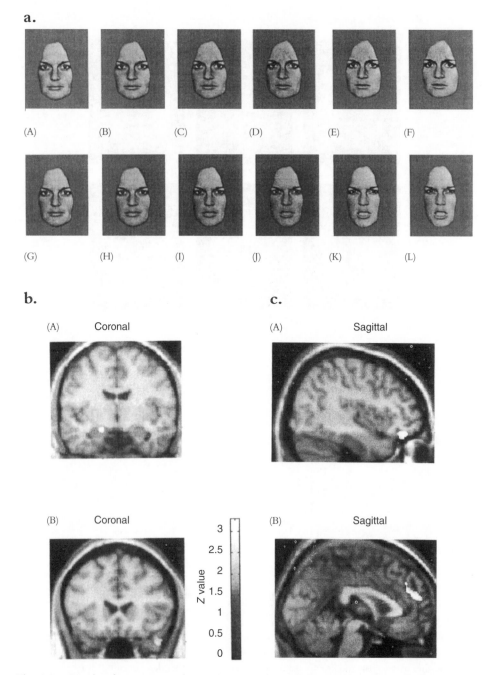

Fig. 5.8. Results of experiments taken as showing enhanced neuronal responses in the left amygdala (**b**), as measured with PET, are significantly greater when viewing increasingly sad expressions (A–F) whereas neuronal responses are enhanced in orbitofrontal cortex and anterior cingulate (**c**) when viewing increasing intensity of anger expression (G–L) (see text for further description). (Blair et al., 1999, figs 1, 2 and 3.)

was presented visually for 20 milliseconds and then immediately replaced by the neutral mask photograph for 100 milliseconds. Each trial was separated by a 3 second inter-stimulus interval. Due to the brief duration of the target and its temporal proximity to the lengthier mask presentation, subjects lacked explicit awareness of the mask. The results are shown in Plate 5.2b in which the top row presents coronal views at the location of the anterior cingulate gyrus (areas 24 and 32 in fig. 5.6b), and the bottom row a coronal view of the amygdala. The fMRI showed that masked happy faces were associated with significant bilateral activation within the amygdala and anterior cingulate gyrus, whereas masked sadness yielded only limited activation. On the other hand, masked sad faces are associated with significant activation within the left anterior cingulate gyrus (area 32 in fig. 5.6b), but no significant activation within either amygdala (Plate 5.2b). Killgore and Yurgelun-Todd (2004) conclude that the amygdala and the anterior cingulate are 'important components of a network involved in detecting and discriminating affective information presented below the normal threshold of conscious visual perception (*that is, neural networks in the amygdala and the anterior cingulate are active when subjects view happy faces for such short periods of time that they are unable to recall viewing them at all*)' (p. 1215).

5.4.2 Behavioural studies involving face recognition following damage to the amygdala

Contextual fear conditioning in rats involves the hippocampus, as well as the subiculum which projects to the B and AB nuclei of the amygdala (see fig. 5.9), for if these are destroyed, such fear conditioning is lost (see Frankland et al., 1998). This contextual fear conditioning is evident when rats exhibit fear not only in response to a particular conditioning stimulus (such as a tone) but also on being returned to the box in which the tone and the unconditioned stimulus (such as a shock) are paired.

Bilateral removal of the amygdala in primates leads to dramatic changes in behaviour, including a lack of emotional responsiveness, tameness and eating inappropriate food (Weiskrantz, 1956). In general, such damage leads to impairments in the ability to learn associations between, say, a visual stimulus and a reinforcer such as pain. 'Emotional memories', sometimes referred to as 'implicit memories', are said to involve remembering what one felt in a similar situation without recollecting the previous occasion on which one experienced the emotion. 'Declarative memories', sometimes referred to as 'explicit memories', are those in which the details and circumstances of a previous occasion are recollected. Given these definitions, then [our explanatory interpretations are given in italics]:

> In humans, damage to the amygdala interferes with the implicit emotional memories but not explicit memories about emotions, whereas damage to the medial temporal lobe memory system [*including the hippocampus*] interferes with explicit memories about emotions but not with implicit emotional memories (Bechara et al. 1995, LaBar et al. 1995). Although explicit memories with and without emotional content are formed by way of the medial temporal lobe system [*that is, are dependent on the integrity of the system*], those with emotional content differ from those without such content. The former tend to be longer lasting and more vivid (see Christianson 1989, Cahill & McGaugh 1998). At the same time, the medial temporal lobe

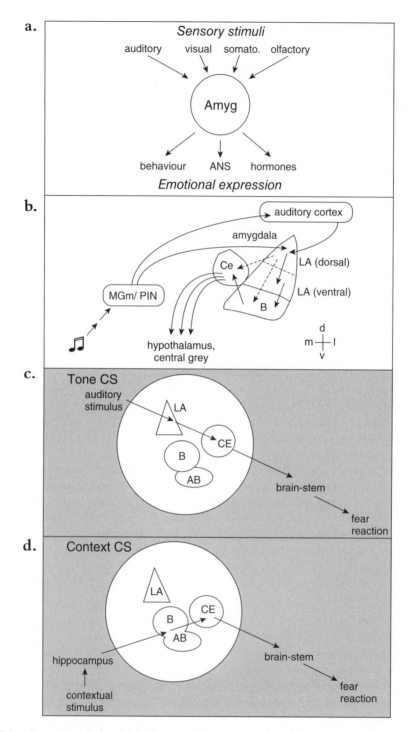

Fig. 5.9. Arrangement of nuclei in the amygdala and their relationship with other brain structures (for further description see text). Figs. 5.9**a** and **b** are from Quirk et al., 1996, figs. 1; figs 5.9**c** and **d** are from LeDoux, 2000, fig. 4.

memory system projects to the amygdala (Amaral et al., 1992). Retrieval of long-term memories of traumatic events may trigger fear reactions by way of these projections to the amygdala [*that is, remembering traumatic events in the distant past may be accompanied by fear and this is dependent on the connections between the medial temporal lobe and the amygdala*]. (Le Doux, 2000, p. 175)

5.4.3   Fear conditioning and the amygdala

The amygdala is important in some kinds of classical fear conditioning. Le Doux has determined in detail many of the pathways involved. These require some knowledge of the arrangement of nuclei in the amygdala (see fig. 5.9b–d). They include an output nucleus (CE, the central nucleus), together with the lateral nucleus (LA) which uniquely receives auditory input from the auditory cortex and the medial geniculate nucleus (MGn/PIN) of the thalamus as well as other sensory inputs and the basal (B) and accessory basal (AB) nuclei which receive input from the hippocampus (fig. 5.9c and d; Le Doux et al., 1990). Thus the lateral nucleus is thought to be the means by which 'sensory information' reaches the amygdala, after which this is sent to some of the other nuclei such as the basal and the accessory basal and to the central nucleus. The amygdala then projects from the central nucleus to areas of the nervous system which are involved in different responses associated with emotion such as those involving the autonomic nervous system (e.g. hypothalamus and blood pressure) and the central (peraqueductal) grey (motor freezing response) (see fig. 5.9a, b).

Le Doux has worked out the subcortical inputs that project to the amygdala through the medial geniculate nucleus which are necessary if conditioned fear stimuli are to affect an animal (see fig. 5.9b). The paradigm for his research follows that of Pavlov (1927). In this a conditioned stimulus (CS) which is initially neutral is temporally paired repeatedly with a stimulus which is not neutral, as it produces a physiological response, the unconditioned stimulus (US). This pairing leads to a correlation between the conditioned stimulus and the unconditioned stimulus such that the physiological response is eventually evoked by the conditioned stimulus alone. In LeDoux's work the physiological measures are changes in heart rate, blood pressure and motor freezing, which he interprets as indicating fear. This research, carried out mostly on rats, shows that if the conditioned stimulus is a tone and the unconditioned stimulus an electric shock to the legs, then the amygdala is implicated in the development of the conditioned stimulus fear response. Similar evidence for the amygdala being involved in fear responses is now available for primates (e.g. see Rolls, 1992).

5.4.4   Is cognitive appraisal an important ingredient in emotional experience? LeDoux's interpretations of his experiments on the amygdala

LeDoux has proposed that his work on the functioning of the amygdala in the conditioned fear response can help resolve the question as to whether cognitive appraisal is an important ingredient in emotional experience, as held by Lazarus (1982), or whether affect and cognition are separate and at least partially independent systems, as proposed by Zajonc (1984).

LeDoux regards the neural networks of the amygdala as essential to any animal's responding emotionally to a particular stimulus, and he uses the unfortunate phrase 'emotional computer' to characterize the workings of the amygdala (LeDoux, 1992a, b; 1996). The neural networks of the amygdala are necessary for an animal to feel and exhibit an emotion, and the neocortex together with the hippocampus are responsible for 'cognitive processes', which is to say that their networks must be functional for the appraisal of the situation that elicits an emotional response. LeDoux proposes that 'sensory information' about a stimulus that arouses an emotion is relayed simultaneously from the thalamus directly to the amygdala as well as to the cortex, which then completes a circuit back to the amygdala (fig. 5.9b). The direct pathway is relatively fast-acting and is based on simple stimulus features (such as intensity). It allows rapid response to threatening situations and therefore provides for the animal's survival. The indirect pathway through the cortex is slow-acting and allows the animal to assess the situation. LeDoux suggests that the direct pathway from thalamus to amygdala provides for preconscious and precognitive 'emotional processing'; that is, the integrity of this pathway is required for us to experience an emotion without remembering the circumstances of the occasion in which the emotion was previously experienced. On the other hand, the indirect pathway through the cortex to the amygdala supports a post-cognitive 'emotional processing'; that is, one which does involve recollecting such experiences. Accordingly both Lazarus (1982) and Zajonc (1984) are correct.

To what extent is the direct thalamic pathway involved in the normal fear behaviour of an animal? Rolls argues that:

> It is unlikely that the subcortical route for conditioned stimuli to reach the amygdala, suggested by LeDoux (1992, 1995[a], 1996), is generally relevant to the learning of emotional responses to stimuli. Animals do not generally want to learn that a particular pure tone is associated with reward or punishment. Instead, it might be a particular complex pattern of sounds such as vocalization (or, for example, in vision, a face expression) that carries a reinforcement signal, and this may be independent of the exact pitch at which it is uttered. This LeDoux system (with the medial geniculate) may not reflect the way in which auditory-to-reinforcement pattern associations are normally learned. (Rolls, 1999, p. 104)

5.4.5 'Fear' is unrepresentative of the emotions

Although fear is a ubiquitous aspect of the animal, and hence too human, condition, it is a poor representative of characteristic human emotions. For there are many emotions which typically involve little, if any, emotional perturbation or disturbance; for example, humility, respect, admiration, contempt and gratitude. Indeed, not all instances of fear need involve fearful agitation, not because the fear is slight, but because of the character of the object of fear. What one is afraid of may preclude any particular, or at least any intense, fearful perturbation. Fear of imminent physical danger obviously involves perturbation. But fear of global warming need not – even though the ensuing motivation may be powerful, and the effect on the agent's mood may be substantial. Similarly, the depth of a person's remorse may be exhibited not in a syndrome of sensations and perturbations that he feels, but rather in his strenuous endeavours to make amends for his past actions and in his obsessive thoughts about his offence. Furthermore, it would be mistaken to suppose that the sole, or even privileged, measure of intensity of fear (or other emotions) is the intensity of emotional perturbation, expression or neural stimulation caused. For this would wholly obscure the motivational force of the emotions. The intensity of an acrophobe's fear of heights is exhibited above all in the lengths he will go to avoid heights. The intensity of a person's hatred is much more likely to be shown in the actions he plans to harm the object of his hatred than in the emotional perturbations he feels or the neural concomitants in his brain when in the presence of the object of his hatred.

Emotions evolved as animal responses to features of the environment apprehended as affecting in one way or another the good of the animal. Neither brain states (which are essential for feeling an emotion) nor somatic responses (which may characterize an emotional perturbation) are emotions. They lack the intentionality, or 'directness towards an object', which is constitutive of most emotions. One cannot individuate an emotion by reference to either brain states or somatic reactions independently of the circumstances of their occurrence and the knowledge or beliefs, as well as the desires or wishes, of the creature.

5.5   The Orbitofrontal Cortex

5.5.1   Behavioural studies involving face recognition following damage to the orbitofrontal cortex

As noted above, damage to the orbitofrontal cortex in primates leads to reduced aggression to sighted objects that would normally produce fear, such as a human being or a snake (Butter and Snyder, 1972). Furthermore, neurons that fire maximally when the animal sees a face are found in the orbitofrontal cortex, as shown in fig. 5.10. This figure shows the firing rate of impulses for the neuron recorded from the orbitofrontal cortex in the left-hand column when the macaque monkey was presented with one of the four images in the right-hand column at time zero. It is clear that the neuron responds best when the macaque looks at a face (a), responds to a lesser degree to the other face presented (b), and does not respond to non-face stimuli, such as those in (c) and (d) (results from Rolls et al., 1998). Following injury to this area of the brain in humans, social conventions are ignored, and patients are unable to make appropriate plans for future action. These changes occur without impairment of intellectual functions or of memory and learning (Bechara et al., 2000).

5.5.2   The orbitofrontal cortex and face recognition: PET and fMRI

To investigate the possible significance of the effect of observing faces on the firing of orbitofrontal visual neurons described above, humans with damage to the ventral part of the frontal lobe have had their responses to faces tested. Impairments in the identification of facial emotional expression were demonstrated in a group of patients with ventral frontal lobe damage who had socially inappropriate behaviour (Hornak et al., 1996). Fig. 5.11a

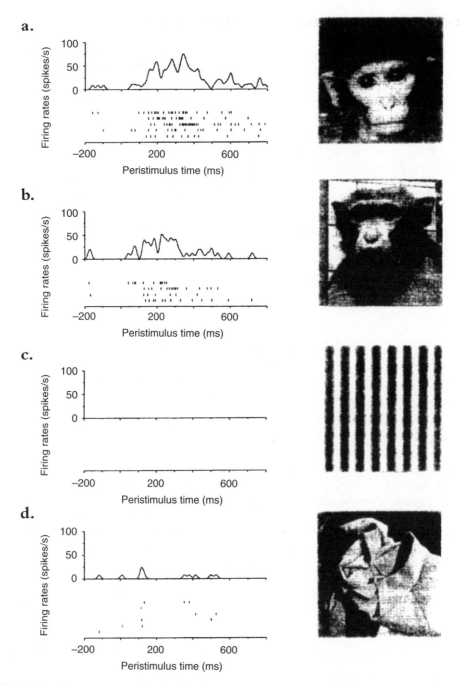

Fig. 5.10. Neurons exist in the orbitofrontal cortex of macaque monkeys that fire maximally when the monkey sees a face (for description see text). (Rolls, 1999, fig. 4.2b)

a.

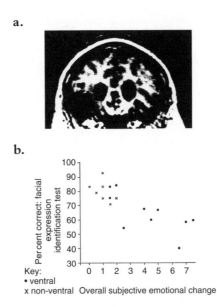

b.

Fig. 5.11. Evidence that the orbitofrontal cortex of humans possesses neurons whose integrity must be intact for a human correctly to identify a facial expression. **a:** fMRI scan of a patient with a right orbitofrontal lesion. **b:** graph showing changes in patients' ability correctly to identify facial expressions (for further descriptions, see text). Hornak et al., 1996, fig. 1, and (Rolls, 1999, fig. 4.23.)

shows an fMRI scan of the lesion in such a patient, with the dark patch on the left of the figure centred at just 43 mm anterior in the right orbitofrontal region. The impairments in expression identification could occur independently of perceptual impairments, as the following experiments showed. These consisted of presenting photographs of the following expressions: sad, angry, frightened, disgusted, surprised, happy (i.e. pleased) and neutral. Patients were asked to choose from a list the adjective best describing the facial expression in each photograph. In order to then obtain evidence on whether there was a relation between problems in identifying facial expression and subjective emotional changes since their illness or injury, patients were asked whether there was any general change in their ability to experience emotion, in particular the intensity or frequency of the following emotions: sadness (or regret), anger (or frustration), disgust (physical revulsion), excitement or enjoyment. Positive scores were given for changes in either direction. Fig. 5.11b shows that in such patients there is gradual decrease in their capacity correctly to identify facial expressions with an increase in their assessment of their own capacity to experience emotion. The demonstration that the identification of facial expression may be impaired independently of any difficulty in recognizing the identity of faces is also consistent with what has been found in other studies.

5.5.3   The orbitofrontal cortex and the satisfying of appetites: Rolls's interpretation of his experiments on the orbitofrontal cortex

Rolls suggests that the neural networks of the orbitofrontal cortex are implicated in the ability of animals to determine what he calls the 'reward value of food'. He and his colleagues have shown that if monkeys are gradually fed to satiety, then the firing of taste neurons in their orbitofrontal cortex is gradually reduced to zero (Rolls et al., 1989). This is interpreted as showing that 'primates work to obtain the firing of these neurons, by eating food when they are hungry' (Rolls, 1999, p. 32). However, it is evident that the primates can know nothing about these neurons. Rather, as the animals feed less, the firing of such neurons declines, showing that interest in eating the food, taken as indicating the 'reward value' of the food, is correlated with the activity of neurons in the orbitofrontal cortex. Rolls suggests that this idea is supported by experiments in which electrodes are placed in the orbitofrontal cortex of a primate which is then allowed to stimulate these at will. If the animal is gradually fed to satiety, the extent of self-stimulation gradually falls away, indicating to Rolls and his colleagues that there must be neurons in this part of the cortex that fire in relation to the extent of satiety (Mora et al., 1979; Rolls et al., 1980). Experiments like these also indicate the existence of neurons which, according to Critchley and Rolls (1996), are involved in the 'reward value' of visual stimuli, such as the sight of food; that is, they

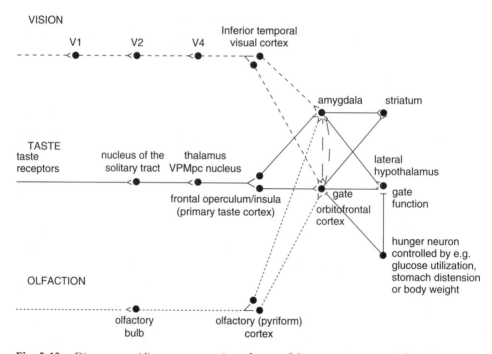

Fig. 5.12.   Diagram providing a representation of some of the connections to and from the orbitofrontal cortex. (Rolls and Treves, 1998, fig. 7.2.)

fire maximally under suitable conditions involving the sight of foods. The projection of the ventral visual pathway to the orbitofrontal cortex, together with that from the primary taste cortex in the insular, is required for this linkage to be possible (see fig. 5.12.).

5.5.4   Misconceptions about emotions and appetites

The research of Rolls described above does not distinguish between emotions and appetites. Rolls considers, as indicated above, that paradigmatic examples of emotions for experimental research are to be found in thirst, hunger and lust. These are appetites and not emotions. In what sense are appetites unlike emotions? First, emotions are not linked to localized sensations in the same way. Some emotions are associated with sensations (fear, rage), others are not (pride, remorse, envy). One does not have a feeling of pride in one's stomach or in one's chest, and although there are sensations characteristic of occurrent anger, such as throbbing temples and tension, one does not feel anger in one's temples or stomach muscles as one feels hunger in one's belly. Second, emotions not only have formal objects, in the sense that what one fears is what is thought to be frightening or harmful, they have specific objects, as when one fears tomorrow's examination or feels remorseful about lying to Daisy. Third, the intensity of emotions is not proportional to the intensity of whatever sensations may accompany their occurrent manifestation. How much one fears heights may be manifest in the lengths one goes to avoid them. Fourth, emotions do not display the pattern of occurrence, satiation and recurrence characteristic of the appetites described by Rolls, for the obvious reason that they do not have the same kind of physiological and hormonal basis as the appetites. Fifth, the emotions have a cognitive dimension absent from the appetites. The hungry animal wants food, the thirsty animal wants drink; but no particular knowledge or beliefs are essentially associated with these appetites. By contrast, the frightened animal is afraid of something it knows or believes to be dangerous. Finally, many human emotions are exhibited by characteristic facial expressions and manifested in typical tones of voice – as in the case of fear, anger, love and affection. Appetites are not.

5.6   Neural Networks: Amygdala and Orbitofrontal Cortex in Vision

In this section we shall consider the networks of connections of the amygdala and orbitofrontal cortex. In the overview of these networks provided in fig. 5.13, connections are shown to the amygdala and the orbitofrontal cortex from the ventral visual stream, including V1 to V2, V4 and the inferior temporal visual cortex, as well as connections from the primary taste and olfactory cortices. In addition, connections are shown from the somatosensory cortical areas 1, 2 and 3 that reach the orbitofrontal cortex directly as well as via the insular cortex.

5.6.1   Amygdala

The principal reciprocal projections from the cortex to the amygdala, a subcortical region in the anterior part of the temporal lobe, are shown in fig. 5.14. Note in par-

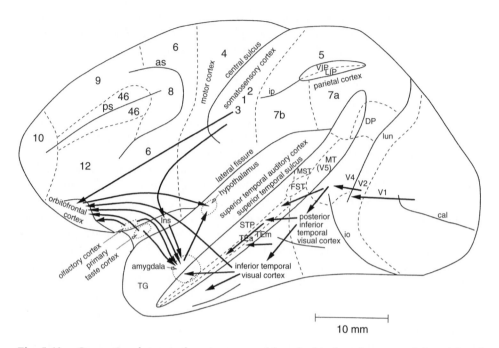

Fig. 5.13. Connections between the primate amygdala and orbitofrontal cortex and the origins of projections to these centres. The abbreviations are as follows: as, arcuate sulcus; cal, calcarine sulcus; cs, central sulcus; lf, lateral (or Sylvian) fissure; lun, lunate sulcus; ps, principal sulcus; io, inferior occipital sulcus; ip, intraparietal sulcus (which has been opened to reveal some of the areas it contains); sts, superior temporal sulcus (which has been opened to reveal some of the areas it contains); AIT, anterior inferior temporal cortex; FST, visual motion processing area; LIP, lateral intraparietal area; MST, visual motion processing area; MT, visual motion processing area (also called V5); PTI, posterior inferior temporal cortex; STP, superior temporal plane; TA, architectonic area including auditory association cortex; TE, architectonic area including high-order visual association cortex, and some of its subareas TEa and TEm; TG, architectonic area in the temporal pole; V1–V4, visual areas 1–4; VIP, ventral intraparietal area; TEO, architectonic area including posterior visual association cortex. The numerals refer to architectonic areas and have the following approximate functional equivalence: 1, 2, 3, somato-sensory cortex (posterior to the central sulcus); 4, motor cortex; 5, superior parietal lobule; 7a, inferior parietal lobule, visual part; 7b, inferior parietal lobule, somatosensory part; 6, lateral premotor cortex; 8, frontal eye field; 12, part of orbitofrontal cortex; 46, dorsolateral prefrontal cortex. (For further description, see text.). (Rolls, 1999, fig. 4.1.)

ticular the reciprocal connections from the anterior cingulate (area 24) and the orbito-frontal cortex (areas 11, 12, 13 and 14). Principal outputs of the amygdala include those to the periaqueductal grey in the brain-stem, which controls defensive and aggressive behaviour; the hypothalamus, which is involved in the control of blood pressure and other autonomic activities; the basal nucleus of Myenert concerned with startle responses and the ventral striatum (fig. 5.9b). There are outputs from the central nucleus of the

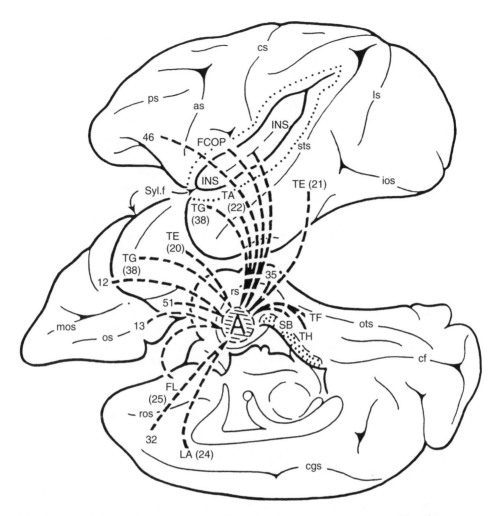

Fig. 5.14. Principal reciprocal projections from the primate cortex to the amygdala. Abbreviations are: as, arcuate sulcus; cc, corpus callosum; cf, calcarine fissure; cgs, cingulate sulcus; cs, central sulcus; ls, lunate sulcus; ios, inferior occipital sulcus; mos, medial orbital sulcus; os, orbital sulcus; ots, occipito-temporal sulcus; ps, principal sulcus; rhs, rhinal sulcus; sts, superior temporal sulcus; lf, lateral or Sylvian fissure (which has been opened to reveal the insula); A, amygdala; INS, insula; T, thalamus; TE (21), inferior temporal visual cortex; TA (22), superior temporal auditory association cortex; TF and TH, parahippocampal cortex; TG, temporal pole cortex; 12, 13, 11, orbitofrontal cortex; 35, perirhinal cortex; 51, olfactory (prepyriform and periamygdaloid) cortex. (For further description, see text.) (International Symposium, 1981, fig. 10.)

amygdala, which if damaged leads to a loss of virtually all manifestations of conditioned fear, such as changes in heart rate and blood pressure, in hormone release and freezing behaviour.

There are neurons in the primate amygdala which respond to visual, auditory, olfactory, somatosensory and gustatory stimuli (fig. 5.9a; see Sanghera et al., 1979). It is not surprising, then, that direct inputs to the amygdala are from the most sophisticated areas of sensory integration, such as the inferior temporal visual cortex, the cortex in the superior temporal sulcus (see arrows in fig. 5.13), as well as from the superior temporal auditory cortex (not shown in fig. 5.13). The amygdala also receives important inputs from cortical areas concerned with touch in the somatosensory cortex via the insula as well as concerned with taste, such as the primary taste cortex and the secondary taste cortex in the orbitofrontal cortex (fig. 5.13). In addition, there are a number of subcortical inputs to the amygdala, such as the hippocampus, the subiculum which carries the output from the hippocampus, the hypothalamus, thalamic nuclei, as well as the nucleus of the solitary tract, which is an important centre for control of the autonomic nervous system.

Whilst there are neurons in the amygdala that respond to a range of sensory stimuli, as noted above, there are no neurons in this part of the brain that are excited solely by what Rolls calls 'reward stimuli' (for elucidation of this concept see below); for neurons that do respond to such stimuli also respond to sensory stimuli. However, as described below, the orbitofrontal cortex does possess neurons that are exclusively excited by reward stimuli.

5.6.2   Orbitofrontal cortex

The orbitofrontal cortex receives input from the ventral or object–identifying stream in the inferior temporal cortex, the primary taste and olfactory cortex in the insula, and the somatosensory cortex (Brodmann areas 1, 2 and 3). It receives connections from a wide range of cortical and subcortical regions of the brain, including the olfactory, auditory, somatosensory, taste and visual cortices, as well as the amygdala. Fig. 5.15 shows the cortical connections to the orbitofrontal cortex of the monkey brain, with lateral, ventral and medial views presented (the abbreviations in this figure are the same as those for figs 5.13 and 5.14). Fig. 5.16 shows the reciprocal connections between orbitofrontal areas and the anterior cingulate (area 25). These various inputs to the orbitofrontal cortex reflect, in part, the kinds of neurons which single unit studies reveal in the orbitofrontal cortex. Thus taste and olfactory neurons are found in medial and anterior parts of the primate orbitofrontal cortex, with some neurons activated by both olfactory and gustatory stimuli (see fig. 5.12), indicating that they might be excited by the flavour of food (Rolls and Baylis, 1994). Furthermore, many of the neurons here are excited by visual stimuli as well as olfactory or taste stimuli (Rolls and Baylis, 1994). This might reflect the fact that 'the orbitofrontal cortex has developed greatly in primates in learning about which visual stimuli have the taste and smell of food [*that is, the neural networks of the relatively large orbitofrontal cortex of primates may be necessary in order for such animals to be able to learn which visual stimuli have the taste and smell of food*]' (Rolls 1999; our rephrasing in italics).

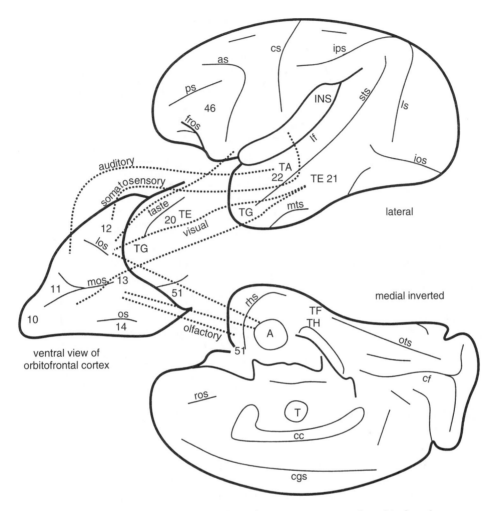

Fig. 5.15. Principal reciprocal projections from the primate cortex to the orbitofrontal cortex are shown (the abbreviations are the same as those in figs 5.13 and 5.14). (Rolls and Treves, 1998, fig. 7.8.)

5.7 The Origins of Emotional Experience

5.7.1 The claims of LeDoux

The concept of 'working memory' plays an important part in LeDoux's ideas on the relation between activity in the brain and emotional experience. Goldman-Rakic and her colleagues argue that the neural networks involved in working memory support the capacity to remember something for several seconds, so that it may be related to immediate sensory experience. Such networks in the prefrontal cortex possess neurons which exhibit sustained

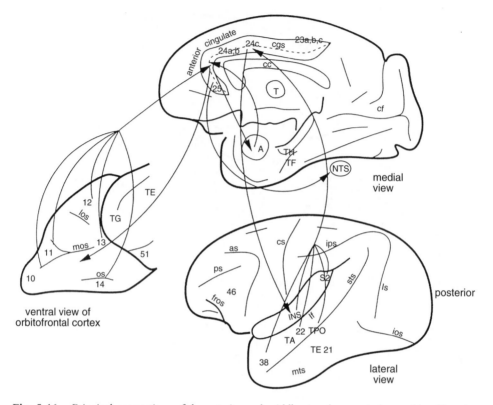

Fig. 5.16.   Principal connections of the anterior and middle cingulate cortical areas (the abbreviations are the same as those in figs 5.13 and 5.14). (Rolls, 1999, fig. 4.24.)

tonic impulse activity when triggered by the brief presentation of a stimulus, in contrast to sensory neurons that fire only during presentation of the stimulus. This integration involves interaction between the dorsolateral prefrontal cortex (taken as areas 12, 45 and 46; see fig. 5.6, also figs 5.14–5.16) and the anterior cingulate (area 24) as well as areas (such as those in the inferior temporal cortex) required to identify an object visually. Other areas involved include the inferior parietal cortex (in order to enable the animal to discern the spatial arrangement of objects) together with the hippocampus of the temporal lobe (required in order for the animal to retain long-term memories) (Fuster, 1998; Goldman-Rakic, 1996; Levy and Goldman-Rakic, 2000; Braver et al., 1997; Carter et al., 2003).

   LeDoux suggests that the activity in the neural networks involved in working memory is modulated by an animal's experiencing affectively charged events, such as those involving fear and hunger. This requires the integrity of projections from the amygdala and the orbitofrontal cortex to, for example, the anterior cingulate. In this way, 'working memory will become aware of the fact that the fear system of the brain has been activated [*that is, the neural networks involved in "working memory" receive inputs that are activated by those parts of the brain whose integrity is required for an animal to feel fear*]' (LeDoux, 2000, p. 176; our rephrasing in italics). LeDoux further claims that: 'you can't have a conscious emotional feeling of being afraid without aspects of the emotional experience being represented in working memory. Working memory is the gateway to subjective experiences, emotional and non-emotional ones, and is indispensable in the creation of conscious emotional feeling [*that is, the neural networks which underpin "working memory" must be active for one to have an emotional experience such as being afraid*]' (LeDoux, 1998, p. 276; our rephrasing in italics).

5.7.2 The claims of Rolls

Rolls suggests that 'the likely places where neuronal activity is directly related to the felt emotion' (Rolls, 1999, p. 73) are the orbitofrontal cortex, in addition to the amygdala, together with those parts of the brain that receive connections from them. For example, he suggests that after identification of an object, which is dependent on the inferior temporal cortex, the amygdala and orbitofrontal cortex are required in order for the animal to associate the object with a punishment or a reward. Once this is done, there is alteration in the activity of other parts of the brain by the output from these structures to the anterior cingulate (causally responsible for working memory) and to regions involved in determining autonomic responses in the hypothalamus and brain-stem (Rolls, 1975, 1993). This idea is similar to LeDoux's, except for the emphasis on reward and the functioning of the orbitofrontal cortex, rather than on fear and the functioning of the amygdala.

5.7.3 The claims of Damasio, following James

William James, both in his *The Principles of Psychology* (1890) and in his subsequent book *The Emotions* (1922), written together with C. G. Lange, propounded a highly influential theory of emotions. James asserted that one could not attribute fear, for example, to a person if that person did not have a heightened pulse rate, were not breathing shallowly, trembling, exhibiting gooseflesh and visceral stirring. Focusing exclusively upon emotional perturbations accompanying occurrent episodic emotion, James held that what excites an occurrent emotion is the *direct* cause of bodily changes, and the emotion is our own *perception* of those changes while they occur. Contrary to our common conceptions, it is not that we lose our fortune, are sorry and therefore cry, or meet a bear, feel afraid and therefore tremble; but rather we lose our fortune and cry and *therefore* feel sorry, meet a bear, tremble and *therefore* feel afraid. An emotion, according to James, is not the bodily and physiological perturbation consequent on apprehension of 'an exciting fact', but rather the person's *perception* of these somatic perturbations. We feel *emotions* because we perceive our bodily reactions. He therefore suggested that there are three essential steps in the production of an emotion. The first of these involves the initiation of particular visceral, vascular or somatic activities: for example, changes in the movement of the intestines, of blood pressure and heart rate and of skeletal muscles involved in locomotion and the defence reaction. In the second step, these changes are detected by peripheral sense receptors associated with each of these organs and muscles, and signals from these receptors transmitted to the brain. Here, in the third step, the brain generates activity which is necessary for feeling an emotion. For the emotion *is* the subjective apprehension of the relevant somatic changes.

Damasio (1994) built on the Jamesian theory in his 'somatic marker hypothesis'. He conceives of an emotion as the collection of bodily changes in response to 'thoughts'. His conception of thoughts is rooted in the empiricist tradition. In his view, thoughts are visual or auditory mental images. The images constituting thoughts are comparable to the images that, according to him, constitute perceptions, differing from them primarily in being fainter. An emotion, he claims, is simply 'a collection of changes in a body state connected to particular mental images [thoughts] that have activated a specific brain system' (p. 145). But he sharply distinguishes between *an emotion* and *feeling an emotion*. Feeling an emotion is a cognitive response to the cause of the emotion (namely, the image or thought that excited the bodily response) coupled with the realization of the causal nexus between the 'image' and the resultant somatic state (or the 'image' of such a state). So, feelings of emotion 'are first and foremost about the body, they offer us *the cognition of our visceral and musculoskeletal state* as it becomes affected by preorganized mechanisms and by the cognitive structures that have developed under their influence' (Damasio, 1994, p. 159). Such feelings give us a glimpse of what is going on in our body in association with specific mental causes of those feelings: namely, thoughts or images of other objects or situations. Accordingly, Damasio propounds his somatic marker hypothesis. The hypothesis is that somatic responses to 'images' serve to increase the accuracy and efficiency of decision processes, screening out certain options and allowing the agent to choose from among fewer. Further, 'When a negative somatic marker is juxtaposed to a particular future outcome the combination functions as an alarm bell. When a positive somatic marker is juxtaposed instead, it becomes a beacon of incentive' (Damasio, 1994, p. 174). The disposition to respond to 'images' (thoughts, perceptions, etc.) somatically in these ways was, Damasio suggests, 'probably created in our brains during the process of education and socialization, by connecting specific classes of stimuli with specific classes of somatic state' (Damasio, 1994, p. 177). Roughly speaking, culturally inculcated 'gut-reactions' provide the basis for rational decision making. In summary:

> When subjects face a situation for which some factual aspects have been previously categorized, the pertinent dispositions are activated in higher-order association cortices. This leads to the recall of pertinently associated facts which are experienced in imagetic form. At the same time, the related ventromedial prefrontal linkages are also activated, and the emotional disposition apparatus is competently activated as well. The result of those combined actions is the reconstruction of a previously learned factual-emotional set. (Bechara et al., 2000, p. 297)

The somatic marker hypothesis leads Damasio to conjecture that the decision-making and executive deficiencies in patients suffering from lesions in the prefrontal cortices is explicable by reference to lack of somatic markers to guide them. More generally, emotions are essential for rational practical reasoning.

5.7.4   Misconceptions concerning the somatic marker hypothesis of James/Damasio

Damasio's theory of the emotions is a modification of James's. But James's theory is sorely defective from a conceptual point of view, and cannot serve as the conceptual framework for the experimental and neurological investigation of the emotions.

James screens out all consideration of the emotions as long-standing attitudes, focusing exclusively upon occurrent emotions – passing episodes of emotional perturbation. This narrowing of focus led him to overlook crucial conceptual links that would perhaps have been more evident had he also examined emotional attitudes with their patent connection with motivation. He did not distinguish between the object of an emotion and its cause, failing to see that what makes us frightened (e.g. a noise in the night) need not be what we are frightened of (e.g. a burglar); hence too, he failed to see that while we may often not know the cause of our emotion (e.g. what made us angry), we must, at least in non-pathological cases, know the object of our emotion (who we are angry with or what we are angry about). Failing, as he did, to discriminate the object from the cause of an emotion, James also failed to see that there are not only causes of an emotion, but also reasons for an emotion – these being bound up with the character of the object of the emotion (if what we are frightened of (a snake) is indeed dangerous, then our fear is well-founded, i.e. is supported by good reasons; if what we are frightened of is harmless (a mouse), then our fear is unwarranted). Human emotions can be reasonable, justifiable or unjustifiable – for they characteristically involve an element of judgement and appraisal. But apprehension of involuntary somatic perturbations can be neither reasonable nor unreasonable.

James made much of the alleged fact that one cannot feel an emotion without apprehending somatic perturbation. This is doubtful – feeling proud of an achievement involves no distinctive apprehended perturbations; feeling respect for another person entails no bodily agitations; and feeling gratitude to another for a favour done does not imply racing pulses or melting bowels. But even if we grant James the fact that typically episodic emotions involve somatic perturbations, it nevertheless remains true that he completely overlooked the fact that one cannot (logically) feel an emotion the object of which is something about which one is altogether indifferent. Our emotions, in particular our emotional attitudes, show what we care about. That is why they are also logically bound up with our character traits (a loving disposition, a compassionate nature, an irascible temperament).

It should be evident that the mere apprehension of somatic changes consequent upon the perception of 'an exciting fact' is neither necessary nor sufficient for feeling an occurrent emotion. It is not sufficient , since to feel seasick in response to the perceived motion of the ship in which one is travelling is not to feel any emotion. It is not necessary, since to feel proud of one's children need involve no somatic perturbations. Having overlooked the essential difference between the cause and the object of an emotion, James cannot differentiate between emotions that may differ *only* with respect to their objects, e.g. shame and embarrassment, resentment and indignation, or remorse and regret. The somatic perturbations that accompany resentment may be identical with those accompanying indignation, but one feels resentful at the infringement of one's own rights, indignant at the infringement of the rights of others.

James screened out emotions understood as long-standing attitudes, focusing exclusively on emotional episodes and obscuring the connection between emotion and motivation. This is anything but a trivial and readily remediable oversight. For emotional attitudes are not mere dispositions to feel occurrent (episodic) emotional perturbations. To love another is not to have a disposition to feel one's heart melt in their presence, but to have an abiding protective concern for their welfare. To fear heights is not merely to have a disposition to feel the agitation of fear of heights, but to have a powerful motive for avoiding heights. Our long-standing emotional attitudes are primary springs of action. Our emotions are bound up with what we care about, and what we care about is the source of the reasons that move us to action. Finally, our somatic perturbations are not normally objects of much thought and reflection (save perhaps in the case of hypochondriacs). But our emotions colour our thoughts and stimulate our imagination, inform our fantasy life, our wishes and our longings.

Damasio's theory inherits the defects of its Jamesian ancestor. There are extensive conceptual confusions involved in his somatic marker hypothesis. A very general misconception that runs through Damasio's theory is the idea that to think is a matter of having certain visual or auditory images. That is mistaken. Mental imagery is neither necessary nor sufficient for thinking. One can have mental images without thinking – as when one counts sheep in one's imagination or recites a mantra in one's imagination to *prevent* oneself from thinking. One can think without having any mental images, as when one talks thoughtfully to another, or when one engages in an activity with thought and concentration. (When a surgeon operates, he is thinking about what he is doing – but that does not mean that mental images are going through his mind.) To have or feel an emotion typically involves a *variety* of cognitive and cogitative components – but having mental images is not a necessary accompaniment of having an emotion; nor is it uniformly a cause of any somatic perturbation that may be involved in the emotional episode. Damasio's theory is open to the following objections.

(1) An emotion is not an ensemble of somatic changes caused by a mental image of (i.e. a thought about) an object or an event. If a mental image of the swaying deck of a ship in a storm makes one's stomach turn, that does not mean that one is feeling an emotion – it means that one can induce seasickness by association.

(2) There is no difference between having an emotion and feeling an emotion, just as there is no difference between having a pain and feeling a pain. There is a difference between having (feeling) an emotion and realizing what emotion one is feeling – one can feel jealous without realizing it. But realizing what emotion one is feeling is not a matter of apprehending somatic changes as caused by images or thoughts. This conceptual error is a consequence of a further conceptual oversight.

(3) Damasio, like James before him, fails to distinguish between the causes of an emotion and its object. (What made Othello jealous was Iago's tale; what he was jealous of was Desdemona's apparent love for Cassio.) Suppose that a certain emotional perturbation involves a given array of somatic changes. What makes those sensations sensations of jealousy as opposed to envy, of fear as opposed to anger, of remorse as opposed to indignation, is not the mental image (or thought), if any, that *caused* them, but the *object* of the emotion, the agent's beliefs and desires concerning that object, and the circumstances in which the agent finds himself. What may make one afraid may be a noise in the night, but what makes one's racing pulses into sensations *of fear* is that one *believes* a burglar is in the house, and that one *apprehends* the (supposed) presence of a burglar as a *danger* (and, of course, it may just have been the cat – but that is not what one was afraid *of*).

(4) If emotions were essentially ensembles of somatic changes caused by mental images, then learning the meaning of emotion words, and hence learning how to use them, would be a matter of learning the names of complexes of bodily changes with specific causes –

akin' to learning the meaning of an expression like 'giddiness' or 'seasickness'. But we do not learn the use of emotion words by learning sensation names or names of overall bodily conditions. Rather, we learn what are appropriate *objects* of the relevant emotions, e.g. of fear (what is dangerous or threatening), of anger (what is annoying, offensive or in some way wrong), or pride (worthy achievement or possessions). Hence we learn how to use these terms ('afraid', 'angry', etc.) in the expression of our feelings towards the appropriate objects and in the description of the feelings (emotions, but not sensations) of others.

(5) Damasio, like James, screens out the reasonableness or unreasonableness of many emotions, the justifiability or unjustifiability of many emotional responses (both occurrent emotional perturbations and long-standing emotional attitudes). This is a consequence of his failure to distinguish the cause of an emotion from its object, since the rationality or irrationality of an emotion depends (among other things) upon the agent's beliefs concerning the object of the emotion, the rationality of those beliefs, and the proportionality of the emotional response to its object. His Jamesian account is quite incapable of budgeting coherently for this aspect of emotion. For if emotions were simply somatic changes caused by mental images (or indeed, the apprehension of such changes as so caused), then one could not have good reasons for feeling a certain emotion, and would not be answerable for one's emotions in the manner in which mature human beings are. For although there may be *a* reason (i.e. an explanation) why one has a headache, or why one's breathing rate or heartbeat (of which one is aware) rises, one cannot *have* a reason (i.e. a ground or warrant) for such things. By contrast, given appropriate circumstances, we can say that someone ought to, and has good reason to, feel proud or ashamed of himself. But we cannot say (save in a merely predictive sense) that his pulse rate ought to rise, or that his psycho-galvanic reflex reactions ought to change.

(6) It should be noted that there are many emotions, even episodic emotions, that involve or that need involve, no somatic disturbance. One may feel gratitude towards a person for a favour done, and continue to feel grateful to that person for the rest of one's days, without perspiring or blushing or feeling one's pulse rate increase, etc. One may be proud of one's children or of one's work without any somatic perturbation. And one may hope that tomorrow's party will be a success without feeling one's blood pressure rise or fall.

(7) One's feelings of emotion are not 'first and foremost about the body'; nor do they essentially 'offer us the cognition of our visceral and muscoskeletal state' (Damasio, 1994, p. 159). It is mistaken to suppose that 'the essence of feeling an emotion is the experience of such changes [in body state] in juxtaposition to the mental images that initiated the cycle' (Damasio, 1994, p. 145). One's emotions do not inform one either of the state of one's body or of the state of the world around one. But one's emotional perturbations may inform one of one's emotional attitudes. A pang of jealousy may indicate to one that one is falling in love with a person; a blush of embarrassment may bring home to one that one is ashamed of such-and-such; one's tears of grief may make one realize how much one loved the deceased. Far from one's emotions informing one of the state of one's body, the state of one's body informs one of one's emotions. Feeling grief does not inform one of the state of one's lachrymal glands, but one's hot tears may show one just how intensely one grieves for so-and-so.

(8) Damasio's somatic marker hypothesis is misconceived. Bodily reactions are not ersatz guides to what to do, and do not inform us of good and evil. If one is indignant at a perceived injustice, what tells one that the object of one's indignation is an evil is not that one apprehends one's flushed face or racing pulses in association with one's thought (or 'image') of the unjust act. On the contrary, one feels indignant at the malefactor's action because it is unjust – not because one flushes in indignation when one hears about it. Indeed, the flush is a flush of indignation (and not of shame or guilt, for example) only because the object of one's feeling *is* an injustice of another (as opposed, for example, to an injustice one committed oneself). And, to be sure, one will feel indignant thus only because, and in so far as, one *cares* about the protection of the rights of others. The matter of *caring*, wholly disregarded by Damasio, brings us to our final point.

(9) Damasio associates the capacity for effective practical reasoning and for pursuit of goals with the ability to feel emotions (hence the title of his book, *Descartes's Error*). According to his somatic marker hypothesis, this is because the emotions are partly inherited and partly conditioned somatic responses to the beneficial and the harmful, and to good and evil – and, as such, they are efficient guides to action. It does indeed appear to be the case that damage to the ventromedial prefrontal cortex or even the amygdala in humans is accompanied by changes in the capacity to feel emotions, and by deterioration in the ability to pursue goals effectively. Since feeling an emotion is not a way of informing oneself of the state of one's body, since the emotions are misconstrued as somatic markers of good and evil, and since one's somatic responses to circumstances are not a litmus test for right and wrong, it is implausible to suppose that what is wrong with patients suffering from such lesions is that their somatic responses are awry or uninformative for them. A more plausible hypothesis, which would perhaps be worth investigating, is whether such brain damage affects their capacity to care or persist in caring about such circumstances as provide objects of standing emotional attitudes, on the one hand, and about goals, on the other. One feels no emotions concerning things about which one is indifferent, and one does not pursue goals efficiently unless one cares about achieving one's objective. Such deficiency in the ability to care would affect both the patients' emotions and their ability to pursue goals over time. This would indeed provide an integrative neuroscientific explanation linking emotion, motivation and action.

6

Motor Action and Cortical–Spinal Cord Function: Galen to Broca and Sherrington

6.1 The Ventricular Doctrine, from Galen to Descartes

6.1.1 Galen: motor and sensory centres

The archaic Greek (Homeric) conception of the soul or *psuchē* was of 'life breath', which was thought to be what differentiates a living human being from a dead one. Hence the *psuchē* was conceived to be 'expired' at the moment of death. It was philosophers who detached the conception of *psuchē* from these common associations with breath. They conceived of the *psuchē* as an entity distinct from the body, and capable of surviving the death of the body. This conception is patent in the writings of Plato. It was Aristotle who broke with this dualist tradition. He did not conceive of the *psuchē* as an immaterial entity distinct from the body. On his view, the *psuchē* is the 'principle' of life – it is what distinguishes living things from inanimate nature. Accordingly, he differentiated between the vegetative (or nutritive) *psuchē* that characterizes all forms of life, the sensitive *psuchē* that further characterizes animal self-moving sentient (non-human) life, and the rational *psuchē* that is the mark of human beings. The constitutive features of the vegetal *psuchē* are the functions of growth, nutrition and reproduction. Plants possess only a vegetal *psuchē*, and their organs are correctly understood as enabling them to exercise those functions definitive of plant life. Animals possess, in addition to a vegetal *psuchē*, a sensitive *psuchē* constituted by the powers of perception, desire and locomotion. Human beings possess not only a vegetal and sensitive *psuchē*, but also a rational *psuchē*, constituted by the powers of will (rational volition) and of intellect. Although it is customary to translate Aristotle's use of '*psuchē*' by 'soul', this is misleading. For his concept is a biological, not a theological, one. The *psuchē*, in his view, is neither a substance, nor a part of a substance. It is constituted by the essential powers of kinds of living beings. A living being, according to Aristotle, retains its *psuchē* as long as it is capable of exercising its characteristic functions. If these powers are lost, if a living being loses the ability to engage in its essential activities, it is effectively destroyed, even though its constitutive matter may survive. Unlike the Platonist, and later Christian, dualist conception of the body and soul, according to Aristotle, the body and *psuchē* make up an animal 'just as the pupil and sight make up the eye' (*De Anima* 413^{a}1–2). Consequently, as he wrote, 'we can dismiss as unnecessary the question of whether the soul and body are one: it is as though we were to ask whether the wax and its shape are one, or generally the matter of a living thing and that of which it is the matter' (*De anima* 412^{b}6–7).

Aristotle, like Empedocles before him, believed that there were four sublunary elements: earth, water, air and fire. To this list he added a further supra-lunary element, the 'first element', subsequently called 'the aether', from which, he thought, heavenly bodies are constituted. Aristotle conceived of this 'divine' element as making up the 'natural principle' in the breath (*pneuma*). The *pneuma*, he conjectured, is passed from the bronchioles of the lungs via the intrapulmonary veins to the pulmonary vein and thence to the heart, where it is converted to '*vital pneuma*'. The *vital pneuma* can then be conducted in blood vessels to muscles, in order to effect their contraction.

Aristotle's ideas had to modified with the discovery by Hierophilus (third century BC) of nerves, and by the observations by Galen and his students (second and third century AD) that the nerves arise from the brain and spinal cord and are necessary for the initiation of muscle contraction. Accordingly, Galen held that the *vital pneuma* is delivered by the blood vessels to the brain, where it is converted to *psychic pneuma*. The composition of *psychic pneuma* was unclear, but it was held to be conducted from the brain along nerves, conceived as conduits, to the muscles (Galen, 1854a, p. 323). This supposedly allowed the muscles to contract, presumably as a consequence of their ballooning as they filled with *psychic pneuma* (see Bennett, 1999).

On the basis of dissections, Galen discovered that all the motor nerves for the voluntarily moved parts of an animal's body below its neck originate in the spinal cord. The nerves that move the thorax arise from the cervical cord. Transverse incisions that sever the cord deprive all parts of the body below the incision of both sensation and movement, since the cord receives the powers of sensation and voluntary movement from the brain (Galen, 1859). Elsewhere, he noted that the degree of damage to respiration and vocalization depended on the extent of lesions to the nerves that subserve the muscles responsible for these functions (Galen, 1962, pp. 22–6).

As a consequence of his observations on injured chariot drivers, Galen was also able to distinguish sensory from motor nerves. He did so in terms of their relative hardness, motor nerves being hard and sensory nerves soft (Galen, 1854a, pp. 597f). He associated the hard motor nerves with their origins in the spinal cord or its marrow, and the soft sensory nerves with the brain. Very soft nerves he linked with the middle of the anterior parts of the brain, and he thought that there were mixed motor and sensory nerves originating at some intermediate position between the caudal part of the spinal cord, which gives rise to the hardest nerves, and the brain (Galen 1821a, p. 25; 1854a, pp. 592f).

Using the term 'soul' in an Aristotelian sense, Galen distinguished the motor soul from the sensory soul, these being not two entities but two principles of activity. He assigned five functions – namely, the five perceptual faculties – to the sensory soul, and considered the motor soul as having one function – namely, movement. The rational soul possessed three functions: imagination, reason and memory.

6.1.2   Galen: the functional localization of the rational soul in the anterior ventricles

This association of the pure sensory nerves with the brain, and the fact that these nerves were taken as very soft, carried important implications for brain function. Galen asserted that the brain is similar in substance to the nerves that arise from it. Unlike Aristotle, he conceived of the brain, rather than the heart, as the locus of sensation, perception, imagination and thought. Since the front of the brain is the source of the soft nerves of perception, and the anterior parts of the brain are the source of the hard nerves distributed to the entire body, and since contact between hard and soft parts would be dangerous, they are, he held, separated by the *dura mater* [*tentorium cerebelli*] (Galen, 1854c, pp. 541–3). It is noteworthy that Galen associated the whole brain with the psychological powers of human beings. But he did not ascribe any special function in mental life to the cortex. For he observed that donkeys have a highly convoluted brain, from which he inferred that cerebral convolutions could not be associated with intelligence. But although he associated the whole brain with psychological faculties in general, he linked the higher mental functions, such as reasoning, with the ventricles (Galen, 1859, p. 590).

Galen enjoyed absolute authority for more than a millennium. It is therefore no surprise that the association of the ventricles with the higher mental functions was elaborated in the following centuries.

6.1.3   Nemesius: the attribution of all mental functions to the ventricles

It was Nemesius (*c.* 390 AD), bishop of Emesa (now Homs) in Syria, who developed the doctrine of the ventricular localization of all mental functions, rather than just the intellectual ones. Unlike Galen, he allocated perception and imagination to the two lateral (anterior) ventricles, intellectual abilities to the middle ventricle, and memory to the posterior ventricles (fig. 6.1). His evidence for these hypotheses consisted in observations of the effects of lesions. He claimed that damage to the front ventricles impairs the senses, but not the intellect. Damage to the middle of the brain causes mental derangement, but does not affect the function of the senses. Damage to the cerebellum, he thought, causes loss of memory, but does not affect either thought or perception (Nemesius, 1955, pp. 341f). This localization of mental functions in the ventricles became known as the ventricular doctrine.

Nemesius believed that sensibility involves the frontal lobes and the psychic *pneuma* that they contain, the nerves that proceed from them and function as conduits for the psychic *pneuma*, and the sense-organs. He explained why there are two anterior ventricles by reference to the supposition that sensory nerves run from the ventricles to the paired sense-organs. The organs of sense, he remarked, are five, but their input is unified, as Aristotle had claimed, by the *sensus communis*, for we perceive the colour, taste, smell, texture and sound of a thing as unified qualities of a single object (a proposed solution to what is currently referred to as 'the binding problem'). So the function of perception, Nemesius held, is exercised by the soul, which apprehends the results of the synthesis effected by the *sensus communis*.

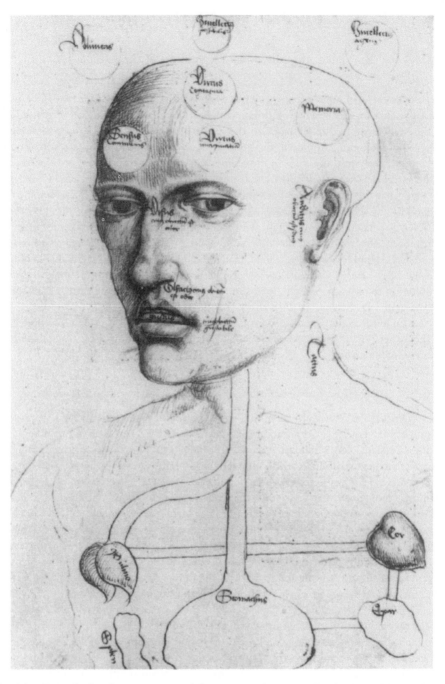

Fig. 6.1. From the fourth century AD until the seventeenth century, the 'faculties of the mind' were taken as housed in the four ventricles of the brain. Shown is a fifteenth-century illustration, with indistinct lettering, designed to illustrate the 1491 edition of Aristotle's *De Anima*. Four regions of the brain are labelled: *sensus communis, virtus cogitativa, virtus imaginativa* and *memoria*. (Courtesy of the Incunabula Collection at the National Library of Medicine, Bethesda.)

It is noteworthy that Nemesius conceived of the soul in very different terms from Aristotle and his followers. Nemesius was a Christian, more influenced by Neoplatonism than by Aristotelian philosophy (he was attracted by the doctrine of the pre-existence of the soul, and also by metempsychosis). He did not conceive of the soul (*psuchē*) as something that 'informs' the organism, constituting its essential powers, as Aristotle had done, but rather as a separate, indestructible, spiritual substance, linked to the material substance constituted by the body in a 'union without confusion' in which the identity of each substance is fully preserved. Consequently, he attributed perception and cognition not to the human being (i.e. to the animal as a whole), but to the soul. The attribution of psychological attributes to a constituent *part* of a living creature deviates importantly from the Aristotelian conception. The misguided tendency to explain how a living creature perceives, thinks, feels emotions, etc. by reference to a subordinate part of that creature's perceiving, thinking, feeling emotions, etc. runs like a canker through the history of neuroscience to this day.

6.1.4   One thousand years of the ventricular doctrine

The ventricular doctrine for the localization of psychological functions, established in the early centuries of the first millennium, was still accepted by scholars at the beginning of the second millennium. The great physician Avicenna (Abu Ali al-Husain ibn Abdullah ibn Sina (980–1037)) held that the *sensus communis* is located in the forepart of the front ventricle of the brain. He believed that the synthesis of the sensory input is effected in the rear part of the front ventricle. The 'sensitive imagination' he thought to be located in the middle ventricle, and the recollective and retentive faculties in the rear ventricle (Rahman, 1952, p. 31).

Ventricular localization still held sway in quattrocento Italy. Physicians – for example, Antonio Guainerio (d. 1440) – ascribed mnemonic deficiencies in patients to excessive accumulation of phlegm in the posterior ventricle, thus impairing the organ of memory (Benton and Joynt, 1960). The doctrine was still being taught at the best teaching centres at the beginning of the sixteenth century, as is shown by the illustrations produced in the 1494 edition of Aristotle's *De Anima*. Leonardo da Vinci (1452–1519; fig. 6.2a) went to great lengths to determine the first accurate description of the ventricles, given their presumed importance in the mental life of human beings. To achieve this, he poured molten wax into the cavities in the brains of cattle. His drawings provide detail of a kind unmatched in accuracy, although they still localize the mental faculties in the different ventricles (fig. 6.3a). In these drawings, Leonardo's only deviation from the doctrine laid down by Nemesius 1,100 years earlier was to localize perception and sensation in the middle ventricle rather than the lateral ventricles, on the ground that most sensory nerves converge on the midbrain.

Andreas Vesalius (1514–64; fig. 6.2b) described the dominance of the ventricular doctrine when he was at the University of Louvain in 1503:

> I have not yet forgotten how, when I was following the philosophical course in the Castle School, easily the most distinguished school of the University of Louvain, in such commentaries

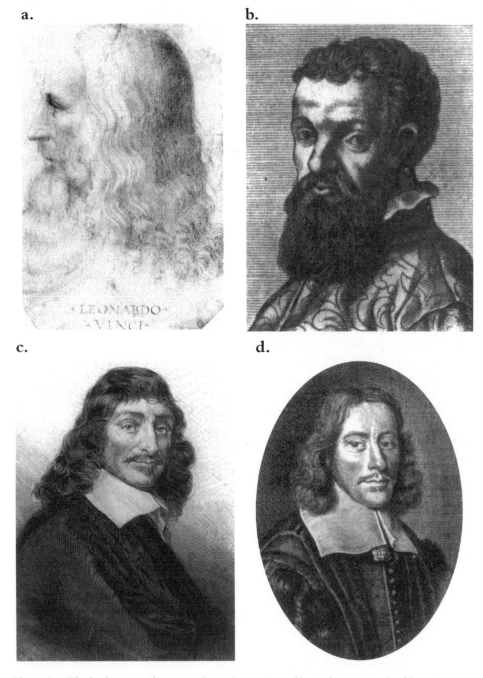

Fig. 6.2. The leading contributors to the understanding of brain function in the fifteenth to seventeenth centuries. **a:** Leonardo da Vinci (1472–1519). (Drawing from the collection of Her Majesty Queen Elizabeth II, Windsor Castle Royal Library.) **b:** Andreas Vesalius (1514–64), a professor of anatomy at Padua, whose dissections and observations rekindled the study of anatomy during the Renaissance (Archives, Washington University Medical School, St Louis, Mo.). **c:** René Descartes (1596–1650), the philosophical theorist of the new science of the seventeenth century, who singled out the pineal gland as the locus of the interaction between mind and body. (By Franc Hals, 1650. Museé de Louvre.) **d:** Thomas Willis (1621–75), author of *Cerebri anatome* (1664). (By G. Vertue, 1742. Archiv für Kuust and Geschiclite, Berlin.)

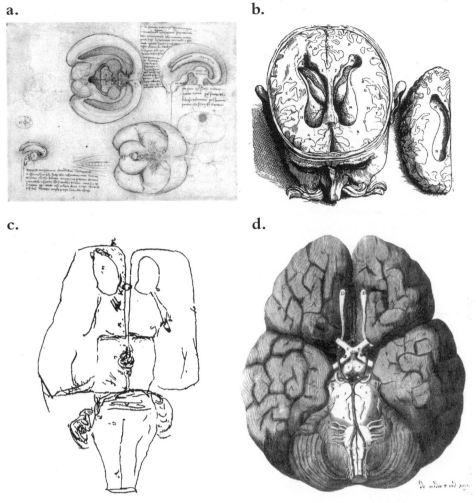

Fig. 6.3. Structure of the brain as determined in the fifteenth to seventeenth centuries.

a: Leonardo da Vinci's determination of the correct structure of the ventricles. (Finges, 1994, fig. 2.5.) **b:** a view of the brain from Vesalius's *De humani coporis fabrica* (1543) showing the ventricles. (Archives, Washington University Medical School, St Louis, Mo.) **c:** Descartes's incorrect drawing of the relationship between the pineal gland and the ventricles. (From *L'Homme*, 1664.) **d:** Illustration of the base of the brain by Christopher Wren from Thomas Willis's book *Cerebri anatome*. (Tercentenary edn, 1664–1964, pub. 1965, ed. William Feindel, Montreal: McGill University Press.)

on Aristotle's treatise *De Anima* as were read to us by our teacher, a theologian by profession and therefore, like the other instructors at the school, ready to introduce his own pious views into those of the philosophers, the brain was said to have three ventricles. The first of these was anterior, the second, middle, and the third, posterior, thus taking their names from their sites; they also had names according to their function. Indeed, those men believed that the first or anterior, which was said to look forwards towards the forehead, was called the ventricle of the *sensus communis* because the five senses, odours, colours, tastes, sounds and tactile qualities are brought into this ventricle by the aid of the five nerves which subserve them. Therefore, the chief use of this ventricle, which use we usually call 'the common sense', was considered to be that of receiving the objects of the five senses and transmitting them to the second ventricle, joined by a passage to the first so that the second might be able to imagine and reason, and cogitate about those objects; hence cogitation or reasoning was assigned to the latter ventricle. The third ventricle was consecrated to memory, into which the second desired that all things sufficiently reasoned about those objects be sent and suitably deposited. (Vesalius, 1543, p. 623)

Vesalius gave detailed and accurate drawings of the human ventricles in 1543 and accompanied these in his *Fabrica* with descriptions of how *psychic pneuma* is generated in the ventricles and then distributed to the nerves (fig. 6.3b). His descriptions are similar to those given by Galen 1,300 years previously. He held the ventricles to be cavities in which inhaled air is mixed with *vital pneuma* from the heart, and then transformed by the brain into *psychic pneuma*. The *psychic pneuma*, he held, is transmitted by the nerves to the organs of sensation and motion to enable them to function. He thought that some of the psychic *pneuma* is distributed from the fourth ventricle into the spinal cord and thence into the nerves arising from it. The lateral and third ventricles dispense *psychic pneuma* to the nerves originating in their vicinity, which transmit it to organs of sensation and movement. He remained agnostic on the question of whether the *psychic pneuma* was transmitted through a conduit in the nerves, or along the sides of the nerves like light along a column, or through the substance of the nerves (Vesalius, 1543, p. 632).

Although Vesalius accepted the hypothesis that the ventricles are the source of *psychic pneuma*, he was, like Galen, sceptical about the idea that the psychological functions originate in the ventricles. This anticipated Thomas Willis (see below, pp. 213–16), who, in search of the physical basis of psychological functions, shifted attention away from the ventricles to the substance of the brain itself (see §6.2.1 below). Vesalius observed that the shape of the ventricles in many mammals is much the same as in humans, so it is difficult to associate the uniquely human intellectual functions with the ventricles (Singer, 1952, p. 40).

6.1.5   Fernel: the origins of neurophysiology

Although some writers hold Aristotle, in his biological writings, to have dealt with physiological subjects, and conceive of Galen's *On the Use of Parts* as the earliest separate surviving treatise dealing with human physiology, it is the sixteenth-century physician and scholar Jean Fernel (1495–1558) who should be credited with the first formal treatment of physiology. Fernel's *De naturali parte Medicinae*, published in Paris in 1542, contains the term 'physiology' for the first time. 'Physiology', he explained, 'tells us the causes of the actions of the body' (Fernel, 1542; Physiol. Ii, praefatro). He distinguished anatomy, which indicates only *where* processes take place, from physiology, which studies *what* the processes and functions of the various organs are. The book was renamed *Physiology* in the 1554 edition, and was soon regarded as the major treatise on the subject.

Fernel's empirical observations, as well as his general reflections, were accommodated within the framework of late medieval Aristotelian thought as modified by Christian thinkers (in particular, Aquinas's great synthesis). Like Aristotle, Fernel held that plants and animals have a soul (*psuchē*) or principle of life. Possession of a rational soul (i.e. the powers of intellect and will) is distinctive of man. Fernel conceived of the rational soul of man, as distinct from his vegetative (or nutritive) and sensitive soul, as separable from the body and as immortal. It is far from clear whether the Aristotelian conception of the *psuchē* as an array of powers and capacities (second-order powers) informing living things can coherently be married with Christian doctrines concerning the immortality of the soul. But that was precisely what Aquinas had endeavoured to do. Other scholastic philosophers also contributed to this synthesis of Christianity and Aristotelian thought. Fernel was heir to this confused tradition.

Fernel conceived of perception as produced by the transmission of images from the sense-organs to the *sensus communis* (or common sensorium) in the brain. The function of the *sensus communis* was to present the soul with the unified or synthesized inputs from the several senses. Memory and imagination, he held, are two subordinate faculties of the sentient soul, enabling the sentient animal to apprehend what is pleasant or unpleasant, beneficial or harmful. Appetite causes a movement towards a pleasing or beneficial object, or a movement away from a displeasing or harmful one. This is effected by the contraction of the brain, forcing the *psychic pneuma* from the front ventricle into the fourth (rear) ventricle, and thence down the spinal cord and out along the nerves into the muscles.

All this was received doctrine. What is pertinent to our present concerns is that Fernel noted that some of our acts occur non-voluntarily: for example, certain movements of eyes and eyelids, of the head and hands during sleep, as well as movements involved in breathing. These muscular movements, he held, do not involve an act of will, and can therefore be regarded as *reflexes*, motor acts in which the will or thought play no role (Fernel, 1542, vol. 9, 109a; ch. 8 of the original edition). This insight marks the beginning of an investigation that was completed only with the work of Sherrington in the twentieth century.

Physiology went through several editions and had an influence that extended for a century. However, it could not continue as the definitive text in physiology beyond the middle of the seventeenth century, since the Aristotelian concepts and conceptions on which it was based ceased to be viable. What, above all, made them obsolete was the rise of Keplerian astronomy and Galilean mechanistic physics. The spectacular success of the new physics led to the rapid demise of Aristotelian physics – that is, to the replacement of teleological explanations of natural phenomena by mechanistic explanations. This was no less evident in the advances in the biological sciences than in those of the physical sciences. Descartes argued persuasively that the activities of the body, the subject matter of physiology, should be considered in purely mechanical terms.

6.1.6   Descartes

Descartes (1596–1650; fig. 6.2c) marks a profound upheaval in European thought. Although aspects of his philosophy are still rooted in scholastic Aristotelian thought, the novelty of his philosophical reflections are the starting point of modern philosophy. Although much of his neuroscientific research proved wrong, it provided a crucial impetus and shift of direction for neuroscience. Descartes agreed with the Aristotelian scholastics that the intellect can operate independently of the body, that the soul or mind is incorporeal, and can exist independently of the body, and that it is immortal. However, he broke with them radically over the following four matters.

First, he held that the mind, as he conceived it, is the *whole* soul. The scholastics, by contrast, conceived of the mind (understood as the intellect and the will) as merely a part of the soul (the immortal part that is separable from the body). The other parts of the soul – namely, the nutritive and sensitive functions – are to be conceived, according to the scholastics, in Aristotelian fashion, as the form of the body. Descartes disagreed radically. Unlike Aristotle, he conceived of the soul not as the principle of *life*, but as the principle of *thought* or *consciousness*. The functions of the Aristotelian vegetative or nutritive soul (nutrition, growth, reproduction) and of the sensitive soul (perception *physiologically conceived*, and locomotion) are essential functions *not* of the Cartesian mind, but of the body. All the essential functions of animal life, he argued, are to be conceived in purely mechanistic terms. This was to have profound effects for the further development of neurophysiology.

Secondly, Descartes redrew the boundaries of the mental. The essence of the Cartesian mind is not that of the scholastic-Aristotelian rational soul, i.e. intellect and will, but rather *thought* or *consciousness*. A person is essentially a *res cogitans*, a thinking thing – and Descartes extended the concepts of thought and thinking far beyond anything that Aristotle or the scholastics would have ascribed to the rational soul. The functions of the rational soul, according to the scholastics, included the ratiocinative functions of the intellect and the deliberative-volitional functions of the will (rational desire), but excluded sensation and perception, imagination and animal appetite. By contrast, Descartes understood *thought* as including 'everything which we are aware of as happening within us, in so far as we have awareness of it' (Descartes (1644), *Principia Philosophiae*, CSM (1985) I, p. 195). Hence *thinking* is to be identified here not merely with understanding, willing, imagining, but also with sensory awareness. Thought, therefore, was, in a revolutionary way, defined in terms of consciousness – that is as that of which we are immediately aware within us. And consciousness was thereby assimilated to self-consciousness, inasmuch as it was held to be impossible to think and have experiences (to feel pain, seem to perceive, feel passions, will, imagine, cogitate) without knowing or being aware that one does. The identification of the mental with consciousness remains with us to this day and casts a long shadow over cognitive neuroscientific reflection.

Thirdly, he held that the union of the mind with the body, though 'intimate', is a union of two distinct substances. Contrary to scholastic thought, according to which a human being is a unitary substance (an *ens per se*), Descartes intimated that a human being is *not* an individual substance, but a composite entity. The person (the *ego*), on the other hand, is an individual substance and is identical with the mind. To be sure, *because* the human mind is united with the body, it has perceptions (*psychologically understood*). But perceptions are conceived of as modes of thought or consciousness, produced by the union of the mind with the body. Indeed, it is precisely by reference to the intimate union of mind and body that Descartes explained the non-mechanical perceptual qualities (i.e. colours, sounds, tastes, smells, warmth, etc.) as being produced in the mind in the form of ideas consequent upon psycho-physical interaction. Similarly, the mind, *because* it is united with the body, can bring about movements of the body through acts of will. Hence neuroscience must investigate the forms of interaction between the mind and the brain that produce sensation, perception and imagination (which are 'confused' forms of thought), on the one hand, and voluntary movement on the other.

Fourthly, just as he conceived of the mind as having a single essential property – namely, thought – so too he conceived of matter as having a single essential property – namely, extension. He conceived of the principles of explanation in the physical and biological sciences alike as purely mechanical, save in the case of the neuropsychology of human beings, who are unique in nature in possessing a mind.

Descartes contributed substantially to advances in neurophysiology and visual theory (Descartes (1985), *Optics*, CSM, pp. 130–7). Although his neurophysiological theories proved to be largely wrong, they were essential steps on the path to a correct understanding. Moreover, his conviction that fundamental biological explanation at the neurophysiological level will be in terms of efficient causation has been triumphantly vindicated by the development of neurophysiology since the seventeenth century (Bennett, 1999). He rejected the Aristotelian and Galenian conception of *psychic pneuma*, arguing instead that the body consists of a set of corpuscularly constituted, mechanically interacting parts, so that the ultimate level of analysis concerns only corpuscular motion. Each part of the body can be activated by the transfer to it of motion that is ultimately derived from heat, which itself is just the agitation of particles engaged in fermentation. Descartes thought that this took place in the heart and therefore involved blood particles. This description has a modern ring about it, except, of course, for the placing of heat generation in the heart.

In Descartes's scheme, large blood particles, when they reach the brain, are used to nourish it, whereas fine blood particles are transformed in the ventricles into a different kind of particle that can be used by the brain for the purposes of conduction along the nerves leaving the brain and spinal cord. These particles he referred to as *animal spirits* (Descartes (1985), *Treatise on Man*, CSM, p. 129). The name reminds one of the *psychic pneuma*, but according to Descartes, the animal spirits are material corpuscles accessible to physiological inquiry. He states:

what I am calling 'spirits' here are merely bodies; they have no property other than that of being extremely small bodies which move very quickly, like the jets of flame that come from a torch. They never stop in any place, and as some of them enter the brain's cavities, others leave it through the pores in its substance. These pores conduct them into the nerves, and then to the muscles. In this way the animal spirits move the body in all the various ways it can be moved. (Descartes (1985), *Passions of the Soul*, CSM I, p. 10)

Descartes's own dissections of the nervous system in his early twenties led him to describe nerves as hollow tubules with a sleeve-like double outer sheath, the inner and outer membrane of the sheath being continuous with the inner and outer meninges of the brain. Each nerve tubule contained a central marrow of longitudinal fibrils, surrounded by animal spirits moving outward from the brain, the animal spirits being composed of highly volatile material particles derived from the blood. Conduction in the nerves involves the passage of small particles derived from the heart. Transmission is due to these particles leaving the ends of the nerves and entering the muscle (Bennett, 1999).

Descartes retained the Galenic idea that the heart is the source of the material used to allow conduction by the nerves, after its transformation in the brain. According to Galen and his students, that material passed from the heart as *vital pneuma*, was transformed in the brain into *psychic pneuma*, whence it was used by the nerves that leave the brain and spinal cord for conduction. According to Descartes, coarse and fine particles in the blood leave the heart and are sorted by the brain in such a way that the coarse particles are used to nourish it, whereas the small particles, ceasing to have the form of blood, become *animal spirits*. These are able to enter the pores and conduits of the brain, from which they are guided eventually into appropriate nerves to generate a particular motor action. He argued that, in the case of motor action, the flow of *animal spirits* from the ventricles involved the opening of particular valves in the walls of the ventricles, with a consequent flow of spirits into the appropriate motor nerve, leading to the contraction of muscle. In the case of involuntary behaviour associated, for example, with a pinprick, this would lead to a tension on just those filaments which open the appropriate valves in the walls of the ventricles to release the animal spirits into the motor nerves that contract the muscles for moving the limb away from the point of the indentation.

Descartes used the word 'reflex' only once in developing his conception of non-human animals as automata, although it is implied throughout his descriptions of animal behaviour and human non-volitional reactions. Although he did not quote Fernel's *Physiology* in his *Treatise on Man*, it is clear that his development of the doctrine of mindless motor acts in humans and animals has for its foundations the concept of the reflex first enunciated by Fernel (see Sherrington, 1951, p. 152). *Treatise on Man* argues that such motor acts require not only an excitatory process, but also an inhibitory one, a speculation that was later to be confirmed experimentally by Sherrington and analysed at the cellular level by his student John Eccles. Descartes then argued that the excitatory and inhibitory processes, when acting together, allow animals and the bodies of human beings (when functioning independently of the intervention of the mind) to be described as automatons.

These hypotheses about the mechanism of reflex and involuntary movement raised the question of the mechanism of *voluntary* movement. Here Descartes departed fundamentally from the ventricular doctrine. He denied that the ventricles are the seat of the sensitive and rational (including volitional) powers of human beings. He also denied that non-human animals have any sensitive powers *in the sense in which human beings do*, inasmuch as they lack consciousness. And he held that the human mind interacts with the body in the pineal gland, which he incorrectly placed inside the ventricle (fig. 6.3c). In his words:

> We need to recognize also that although the soul is joined to the whole body, nevertheless there is a certain part of the body where it exercises its functions more particularly than in all the others. It is commonly held that this part is the brain, or perhaps the heart – the brain because the sense organs are related to it, and the heart because we feel the passions as if they were in it. But on carefully examining the matter, I think I have clearly established that the part of the body in which the soul directly exercises its functions is not the heart at all, or the whole of the brain. It is rather the innermost part of the brain, which is a certain very small gland situated in the middle of the brain's substance and suspended above the passage through which the spirits in the brain's anterior cavities communicate with those in the posterior cavities. The slightest movements on the part of this gland may alter very greatly the course of these spirits, and conversely any change, however slight, taking place in the course of the spirits may do much to change the movements of the gland. (Descartes (1649) *Les Passions de l'Ame*, CSM (1985) I, p. 31; fig. 6.4a)

It is interesting to note the reasoning whereby Descartes concluded that the pineal gland is the locus of the *sensus communis* and of interaction between the body and soul. It was because it is located *between* the two hemispheres of the brain and is not itself bifurcated. Consequently, he argued, it must be in the pineal gland that 'the two images coming from a single object through the two eyes, or the two impressions coming from a single object through the double organs of any other sense [e.g. hands or ears] can come together in a single image or impression before reaching the soul, *so that they do not present it with two objects instead of one*' (Descartes (1649), *Les Passions de l'Ame*, CSM (1985), I, p. 340; AT XI, p. 353; our italics). These images or figures 'which are traced in the spirits on the surface of the gland' are 'the forms of images which the rational soul, united to this machine [i.e. the body], will consider directly when it imagines some object or perceives it by the senses' (Descartes (1664) *L'Homme de René Descartes*, CSM (1985) I, p. 106; AT XI, p. 119).

It is noteworthy that Descartes warned that although the image generated on the pineal gland does bear some resemblance to its cause (immediately, the retinal image; mediately, the object perceived), the resultant sensory perception is not caused by the resemblance. For, as he observed, that would require 'yet other eyes within our brain with which we could perceive it' (Descartes (1637) *La Dioptrique*, CSM (1985) I, p. 167; AT VI, p. 130). Rather, it is the movements composing the image on the pineal gland which, by acting directly on the soul, cause it to have the corresponding perception. The warning was apt, but the caution insufficient. Descartes was wrong to identify the pineal gland as the locus of a *sensus communis*. He was wrong to think that an image corresponding to the retinal image (and hence to what is seen) is reconstituted in the brain. These are factual errors, and it is noteworthy that they still have analogues in current neuroscientific thought, in particular in the common characterization of the so-called binding problem (see above, pp. 32–8). He was right to caution that whatever occurs in the brain that enables us to see whatever we see, our seeing cannot be explained by reference to *observation* of such brain events or configurations. For, as he observed, that would require 'yet other eyes within our brain'. Nevertheless, he was confused, *conceptually* confused, to suggest

(i)   that images or impressions coming from double organs of sense must be united in the brain to form a single representation *in order that the soul should not be presented with two objects instead of one*;

(ii)   that the soul 'considers directly' the forms or images in the brain when it perceives an object;

(iii) that it is the *soul*, rather than the living animal (human being) that perceives.

The first error presupposes precisely what he had warned against. For only if the images or impressions are actually *perceived* by the soul (or mind) would there be any reason to suppose that the 'two images' would result in double vision or double hearing. The second error is the incoherence of supposing that in the course of perceiving, the soul (or mind) 'considers' anything whatsoever *in the brain*. And the third is the error of supposing that it is the *soul* (or *mind*) rather than the living animal that perceives. The latter commits a *mereological fallacy*. For it consists in ascribing to a part of a an entity attributes which logically can be ascribed only to the entity as a whole. The particular form which this fallacy took in Descartes consisted in ascribing to the soul or mind attributes which can be ascribed only to the animal as a whole.

Descartes explained his theory as follows:

> Let us now take it that the soul has its principal seat in the small gland located in the middle of the brain. From there it radiates through the rest of the body by means of the animal spirits, the nerves, and even the blood, which can take on the impressions of the spirits and carry them through the arteries to all the limbs. Let us recall what we said previously about the mechanism of the body. The nerve-fibres are so distributed in all the parts of the body that when the objects of the senses produce various different movements in these parts, the fibres are occasioned to open the pores of the brain in various different ways [fig. 6.4a]. This, in turn, causes the animal spirits contained in these cavities to enter the muscles in various different ways [fig. 6.4b]. In this manner the spirits can move the limbs in all the different ways they are capable of being moved. And all the other causes that can move the spirits in different ways are sufficient to direct them into different muscles. To this we may now add that the small gland which is the principal seat of the soul is suspended within the cavities containing these spirits, so that it can be moved by them in as many different ways as there are perceptible differences in the objects. But it can also be moved in various different ways by the soul, whose

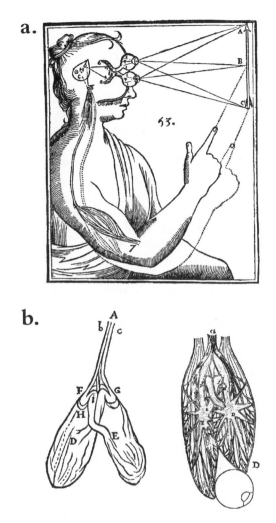

Fig. 6.4. Descartes's conception of the role of motor nerves in initiating muscle contraction.

    a: drawing from *De homine* (1662) by Descartes showing how light enters the eye and forms images on the retina. Hollow nerves from the retina project to the ventricles; the motion of the pineal gland (H) then releases the animal spirits into the motor nerves to produce motion. **b:** *left* shows Descartes's sketch of reciprocal muscles of the eye (*De homine*, Latin translation by Schuyl); *right* is a redrawing showing closure of valves on relaxation, opening on contraction to allow animal spirits to flow in and swell the muscle (*L'homme*, French edition of 1677, p. 16).

nature is such that it receives as many different impressions – that is, it has as many different perceptions as there occur different movements in the gland. And conversely, the mechanism of our body is so constructed that simply by this gland's being moved in any way by the soul or by any other cause, it drives the surrounding spirits towards the pores of the brain, which direct them through the nerves to the muscles; and in this way the gland makes the spirits move the limbs. (Descartes (1985), *The Passions of the Soul*, CSM I, P. 34)

By the middle of the seventeenth century, Descartes had replaced the ventricular doctrine localizing psychological functions in the ventricles of the brain with his idiosyncratic *inter-actionist* doctrine localizing all psychological functions in the pineal gland, which he conceived to be the point of interaction between mind and brain. This is how he met the objection of Vesalius that it is difficult to reconcile the idea that the different ventricles are associated with different psychological attributes with the fact that the ventricles of humans are so similar to those of other mammals. However, his contemporaries were soon to point out that the pineal gland was not inside the ventricles, and furthermore, as other mammals possessed this gland, Descartes's response to Vesalius was inadequate.

Nevertheless, Descartes had made the fundamental contribution of opening up all animal activity to mechanical analysis, i.e. to what became physiology and neuroscience. The shift of attention away from the ventricles to the substance of the brain, which Descartes's theory initiated, was to reach its conclusion in the hands of a young man, Thomas Willis, who was 29 years old when Descartes died.

6.2   The Cortical Doctrine: from Willis to du Petit

6.2.1   Thomas Willis: the origins of psychological functions in the cortex

As a consequence of his observations on the passage of blood through the animal cortex and on patients with neurological problems who could be examined post-mortem, the Professor of Medicine at Oxford, Thomas Willis (1621–75; fig. 6.2d), reached the conclusion that the psychological attributes of human beings are functionally dependent on the cortex, and not on the ventricles (fig. 6.3d). This he argued with great force in his classic work *De anima brutorum* (1672) and in his *Cerebri anatome, cui accessit nervorum descriptio et usus* (1664), the power of which was greatly assisted by the magnificent drawings made from Willis's sketches by the young Christopher Wren. Willis gave the first cortical theory of the control of the musculature and of reflex control. This is of such importance in the history of the integrative action of the nervous system that it warrants a full description.

Willis assigned to man and to all other animals a system of particles found throughout their bodies which he called 'the corporeal soul'. The corporeal soul depends wholly upon the body, is born and dies with it, actuates its parts and is extended through them, and, although imperceptible, is plainly 'of a material nature'. It arises out of matter and is known by inference from its manifest effects. The corporeal soul is the material basis (or vehicle) of certain distinctive vital functions of living organisms (Willis, 1683, pp. 1, 6f).

Willis described in detail the role of *Animal Spirits* that circulate in the brain and nerves. They are derived from the *Vital Spirits* of the blood:

The life and flame of the blood, the vital flame, is not visible and is not destructive like normal flames . . . so that it does not destroy the blood. . . . but rather dissolves the blood in such a way that of the particles which arise, some are burnt and others are let go. Amongst these latter particles, the most subtle, which like beams of light sent from a flame, are distilled into the brain and cerebellum. These most subtle particles are called the *Animal Spirits*. (Willis, 1683, pp. 22f)

The animals spirits are generated in the cortex and cerebellum, and stored in the brain for use by the corporeal soul. From the brain, the animal spirits flow down the spinal cord into the nerves, whence they are distilled from the ends of the nerves into the muscles, membranes and viscera, thereby activating them, the sense-organs and the organs of motion.

How is this flow of animal spirits initiated? Willis first described what occurs in the brain when an organ of perception is excited. The images of external objects, impressed upon the organs of sense, are transmitted inwards by the animal spirits, to the 'common sensory' (or *sensus communis*). If the sense impression is weak, it terminates in the common sensory, and the perception of the object quickly ceases without any further consequence. But

if (which more often happens) the impulse of the object be stronger, the sense excited from thence, like the vehement waving of water in a whirlpool, both partly passes through the streaked bodies, and going forward to the callous body, it often raises up two other internal senses, to wit, the imagination and memory, either one or both of them; and also is partly reflected from them, and from thence, by a declining of the spirits, leaping into the nerves, local motions are made. (Willis, 1683, p. 59)

This description places the cortex in a reflex arc from sensation to motor act, and it is clear that Willis thought – in a thoroughly Cartesian fashion – that in all animals other than man, all motor acts are reflex, for he comments that 'because brutes or men, whilst they as yet know not things, want spontaneous appetite. So long, therefore, they, being destitute of the internal principle of motion, move themselves or members, only as they are excited from the impulse of the external object, and so sensation preceding motion, is in some manner the cause of it' (ibid.). He also noted that some animals, despite decapitation, continue to move and leap about. He explained this by reference to the supposition that animal spirits are intermingled with the blood and so still bring about motion and sense (purely physiologically conceived).

So, animal sensation and perception are, Willis held, purely bio-mechanical phenomena. But human perception is different. His explanation of perception, conceived as a psychological phenomenon associated with consciousness, followed Cartesian lines. Sense impressions are conveyed to the common sensory, whence the animal spirits transmit minute pictures or representations of perceived objects along the little pipes of the nerves.

it is possible to conceive of a middle part of the brain, a kind of interior chamber of the soul equipped with dioptric lenses; in the innermost part of which images or representations of all sensible things, sent in through the passages of the nerves, like tubes or narrow openings, first pass through the corpora striata as through a lens; then they are revealed upon the corpus callosum as if on a white wall, and so induce perception. (Willis, 1672, pp. 43f)

It is striking that Willis should invoke the model of the most recent optical technology of the day – namely, the *camera obscura* – to explain conscious perception, as opposed to the merely bio-mechanical perception characteristic of 'mere brutes'. His conception of an *internal representation* upon the corpus callosum is a direct heir of Descartes's idea that an image of what is seen must be produced on the surface of the pineal gland, where it is 'presented to the soul'. Willis's supposition that the Rational Soul 'beholds the image of the thing there painted' commits precisely the error against which Descartes warned (and then committed) – the error of trying to explain how human beings can see an object by appealing to the soul's perceiving a representation of the object in the brain. But if we are puzzled as to how an animal can see an object before it, it is no explanation to say that this is made possible by reference to some part of the animal (its soul) seeing a picture of that object in its brain. For now we are just as puzzled how the soul can see a picture of an object (without any eyes either!).

The rational soul not only perceives representations of things on the internal screen of the corpus callosum, it also initiates acts of volition there. Willis linked the functions of conscious perception, memory and volition with the cerebral cortex. In particular, he associated them with the gyri of the cortex. He argued that

> for the various acts of imagination and memory, the animal spirits must be moved back and forth repeatedly within certain distinct limits and through the same tracts or pathways, therefore numerous folds and convolutions of the brain are required for these various arrangements of the animal spirits; that is, the appearances of perceptible things are stored in them, just as in various storerooms and warehouses, and at given times can be called forth from them. Hence these folds or convolutions are far more numerous and larger in man than in any other animal because of the variety and number of acts of the higher faculties, but they are varied by a disordered almost haphazard arrangement so that the operations of the animal function might be free, changeable and not limited to one. (Willis, 1664, pp. 65f)

He held that the brain consists of two different substances, cortical and medullary (i.e. white and grey matter). This, he conjectured, was because the animal spirits are generated in the cortical substance, whereas the medullary substance serves for the operation and distribution of the animal spirits.

Willis's acceptance of the conception of the rational soul (the mind) as an immaterial, immortal entity, that interacts with the body via the cortex, and that perceives and initiates intentional action, left him with the insurmountable problem of explaining the interaction between the immaterial mind and the material corporeal soul in the corpus callosum. To this problem he had no answer.

6.2.2   The cortex 100 years after Willis

The cortical revolution due to Willis led in the following century to a focus on the relationship between the cortex and those nerve trunks that seemed to be intimately related to it. But there was no advance in functional localization. At the end of the eighteenth century attempts were still being made to locate the *sensus communis* and mental processes

a.

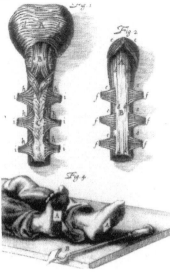

b.

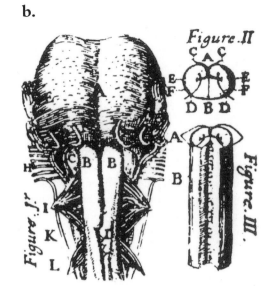

c.

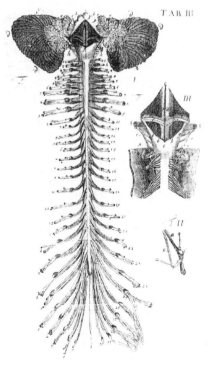

d.

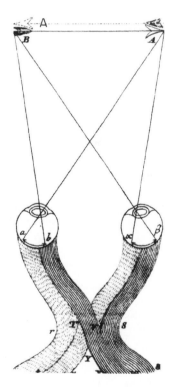

in the brain. However, there was a remarkable contribution during this period by Domenico Mistichelli (1675–1715) and Francois Pourfour du Petit (1664–1741). They both described the decussation of the pyramids: that is, the crossing over of nerves from left to right and right to left at the spino-medullary junction called 'the pyramid'. Mistichelli, in 1709, made this clear in his drawing of the decussation (fig. 6.5a) and his comments on it:

> what I have recently observed, that is, that the medulla oblongata externally is interwoven with fibres that have the closest resemblance to a women's plaited tresses. Whence it occurs that many nerves that spread out on one side have their roots on the other; so, for example, those that extend to the right arm, through such plaiting, can readily have their roots in the left fibres of the meninges. The same may be understood of those on the left proceeding from the right; and so one may go on describing many, if not all the other nerves, that have their origin immediately from the spinal cord. (Mistichelli, 1709, pp. 282f)

Petit went even further than this in 1727, tracing the origins of the fibres that decussate back to the cortex:

> All the cortical substance of the cerebral hemispheres supplies the medullary part, which is itself but a mass of an infinite number of tubes, some of which constitute the corpus callosum, while others collect together to form the middle-fluted bodies. The inferior part of the cerebral peduncles [i.e. the midbrain, pons and medulla oblongata] which can be seen between the optic nerve [optic tract] and the pons, is a continuation of the middle-fluted bodies. The medullary fibres of which it is composed pass through the pons, separated from each other by the pontine fibres with which they are intertwined. They collect together again at the inferior part of the pons in order to form exclusively the pyramidal bodies. (Pourfour du Petit, 1727 [see fig. 6.5 b])

Each pyramidal body divides at its inferior part into two large bundles of fibres. But more often there are three, and sometimes four. Those on the right pass to the left, and those on the left pass to the right, binding themselves together. Du Petit's remarkable work placing the origins of the pyramidal fibres in the cortex, was further elaborated by his identifying the function of the fibres as motor. Du Petit was a military surgeon, and he observed that wounds to the cerebral cortex caused contra-lateral motor paralysis. He inferred that move-

Fig. 6.5. Conceptions in the eighteenth century of the origins of motor and sensory nerves. **a:** Domencio Mistichelli's (1709) figure showing the decussation of the pyramids and the outward rotation of a paralysed limb. (From *Trattato dell' Apoplessia*, Roma: A. de Rossi alla Piazza di Ceri. In Clarke and O'Malley, 1968, p. 282.) **b:** The crossing of the pyramids as described and experimentally demonstrated on injury to the brain in dogs by a pupil of Duverney. His drawings are from his *Lettres d'un medicin* (1727). (From the copy in the Bibliothèque Nationale; reproduction by courtesy of Dr Auguste Tournay.) **c:** Procháska's illustration of the spinal roots and their ganglia. (Prochàska, 1984.) **d:** John Taylor's (1750) diagram showing the partial crossing of the optic nerves at the chiasma. (Finger, 1994, p. 184).

ment was generated by the passage of animal spirits from the cortex, through the striatum and basal ganglia, and then across the pyramids to muscle. He gave the first explicit description of the motor cortex's controlling movement through the pyramidal tract. This prescient work of Du Petit has a remarkably modern ring about it.

6.3   The Spinal Soul, the Spinal Sensorium Commune, and the Idea of a Reflex

6.3.1   The spinal cord can operate independently of the enkephalon

It had been noted since time immemorial that cutting off the head of a snake did not stop its movements in response to touch for some days. However, a thorough study of the ability of the spinal cord to mediate the contraction of muscle and movement in the absence of the enkephalon was not made until the investigations of Alexander Stuart (1637–1742). In his Croonian Lecture to the Royal Society in 1739, Stuart described experiments in which he first cut off the head of a frog and then gently inserted a small blunt instrument to bring pressure on the medulla, resulting in the movement of limbs (fig. 6.7a). The same instrument, pushed through the hole of the occiput of the skull on the medulla oblongata resulted in the movement of eyes and mouth (Stuart, 1739, p. 36; fig. 6.7a). He explained these phenomena along traditional lines. The pressure exerted forced a quantity of animal spirits to pass through the spinal cord into the slender canals of the nerves, and thence into the muscles. The experiments were thought to confirm the received account of voluntary movement: namely, that (putting aside Cartesian qualms about non-human animals) an impulse of the mind or will causes the motion of animal spirits though the nerves into the muscles, thus causing them to contract.

The problem of how decorticate animals can still move and display a degree of sensitivity to being touched was taken up by Robert Whytt (1714–66); fig. 6.6a) in his books *Essays on the Vital and Involuntary Motions of Animals* (1751 a, b) and *Observations on the Sensibility and Irritability of the Parts of Man and Other Animals*, written *c.* 1751 in Edinburgh. Assuming that the motions of insects and reptiles after decollation are biological in origin, Whytt argued, in explicit opposition to Descartes's mechanism, that they must be attributed to the same 'sentient principle' or 'soul' as moves the whole animal. For the movements of the decollated animal are similar to those of the whole animal, although of shorter duration (Whytt, 1751, p. 115). So the sentient principle or soul cannot be confined to the brain alone. Indeed, given the behaviour of decorticate animals, there must be a 'spinal soul' too. Whytt, unlike Descartes and Willis, rejected the mechanical conception of a reflex, that requires no conscious intervention to be initiated. On the contrary, he argued:

> *The motions performed by us in consequence of irritation*, are owing to the original constitution of our frame, whence the soul or *sentient principle*, immediately, and *without any previous ratiocination*, endeavours by all means, and in the most effectual manner, to avoid or *get rid of every disagreeable sensation* conveyed to it by *whatever hurts or annoys the body*. (Whytt, 1751, p. 113)

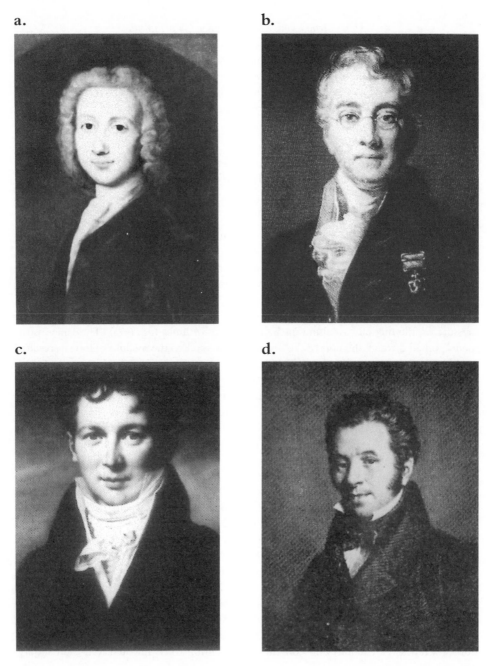

Fig. 6.6. Pioneers in our understanding of the functions of the spinal cord in the eighteenth and nineteenth centuries. **a:** Robert Whytt (1714–66), whose experiments demonstrated reflex action in decapitated animals as well as the effects of spinal shock (From the portrait in the Royal College of Physicians, Edinburgh, by courtesy of Mr G. R. Pendrill.) **b:** Sir Charles Bell (1774–1842), who investigated the functions of the spinal roots and published his findings in a privately printed pamphlet in 1811. (Archives, Washington University Medical School, St Louis, Mo.) **c:** François Magendie (1783–1855), French scientist who made many contributions to anatomy and physiology including a clear description of the difference between the dorsal and ventral roots of the spinal cord. (Courtesy of the Collège de France.) **d:** Marshall Hall, F.R.S. (1790–1857), who gave the first description of the relation between the nerves and spinal cord involved in a reflex act. From a pastel portrait James Lumley, 1856. (By courtesy of the Wellcome Trustees.)

Although he anticipated Sherrington on the stretch reflex, he was unable to grasp the essentially mechanical nature of a reflex.

The idea of a 'soul' or sentient principle operating throughout the nervous system after decollation was advanced by Jiri Procháska (1749–1820) too. He resurrected the notion of the *common sensorium*, but detached it from its ancient role of synthesizing sensory input to generate unified perception (the ancient solution proposed to what is currently called 'the binding problem'). In the heyday of the ventricular doctrine, the *sensus communis* was associated with the lateral ventricles. Prochaska associated it with the brain and spinal cord (fig. 6.5c). He conceived of its function as being not to process sensory input and transform it into perceptual experience, but rather to reflect and transmit sensory impressions from the sensorial nerves to the motor nerves, where they allegedly become motor impressions. This process, he held, takes place irrespective of whether the animal be conscious or not. The cerebrum and cerebellum, he argued, are the locus of mind–body interaction in perception and voluntary action. But, he conjectured, the locus of the *sensorium commune* (as he called it) extends to the medulla oblongata, the crura cerebri and cerebelli, part of the thalami optici, and the whole spinal marrow (Procháska, 1784, part II, p. 123). That it must extend to the spinal marrow, he averred, is demonstrated by the movements and reactions of decorticate animals. It is not unconscious behaviour alone that is determined by the *sensorium*

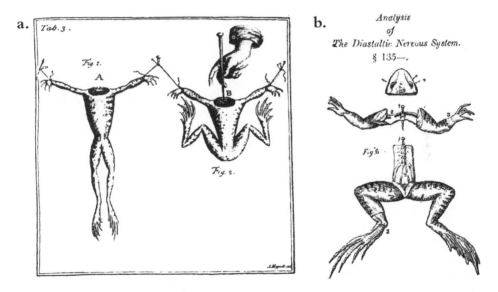

Fig. 6.7. Experiments in the eighteenth century showing that the isolated spinal cord mediates reflex actions. **a:** Alexander Stuart's experiment confirming the observations of Stephen Hales that a decapitated frog convulses on being pithed and then becomes immobile. (Stuart, 1739.) **b:** One of Hall's experiments to demonstrate the three parts of the reflex arc; the arc was broken by either of the following procedures: (i) skinning the extremity (at 3; the 'esodic' nerves); (ii) sectioning of the Òbrachial or the lumbar or femoral nerve (Hall, 1850).

commune, but all manner of conscious involuntary actions too, such as sneezing, coughing, vomiting and so forth. Voluntary actions are also mediated by processes in the *sensorium commune*, but they are directed and moderated by the mind, and so are to be deemed animal rather than automatic (ibid., p. 129).

The production of animal spirits was a function assigned to the brain. But the reflex behaviour of decorticate animals made their operation puzzling. For to explain that behaviour, one was forced to hypothesize a residuum of animal spirits remaining in the spinal cord after decollation. The solution, which rendered the whole idea of animal spirits obsolete, was given by Luigi Galvani (1737–98). He showed that nerves can conduct electricity just as metal wires can, and that the nerves themselves can generate the necessary electrical current to explain decorticate behaviour (see Bennett, 1999). His key experiment to show that nerves conduct electricity involved suspending a frog's spinal cord/leg preparation in a sealed jar by means of a wire passed through the spinal cord and then through the seal at the top of the jar. Lead shot was present at the bottom of the jar. A wire was then strung across the ceiling to pick up the charge from a frictional machine and to convey it by induction to the wire from which the frog's remains were suspended. This enabled Galvani to demonstrate that when the frictional machine sparked, the legs twitched – from which he concluded that the spinal cord and nerves conduct electricity (Galvani, 1791). This made altogether redundant the hypothesis of the brain's storing animal spirits derived from *psychic pneuma*, which are transmitted along the spinal cord and through the nerves.

6.3.2   Bell and Magendie: the identification of sensory and motor spinal nerves

A clearer grasp of reflex action could not emerge until the sensory and motor nerves were differentiated. This was done by Charles Bell (1774–1842; fig. 6.6b), who identified the anterior roots of the spinal cord as motor, and by François Magendie (1783–1855; fig. 6.6c), who discovered that the posterior roots are sensory. (Much controversy attended the attribution of these discoveries.)

In a letter to his brother in 1810, Bell described his experiments. He opened the spine of a dog and destroyed the posterior part of the spinal marrow. No convulsive movement followed. But when he injured the anterior part, the animal was convulsed. He therefore concluded that the posterior nerves are sensory.

Bell confirmed his hypothesis that the anterior nerves are motor by further ingenious experiments on animals. In one of these, using an ass, he cut the 'portio dura of the seventh nerve', which he describes as 'a respiratory nerve of the face', and noted that movement of the nostrils on the same side ceased instantly (Bell, 1821, p. 398). In another experiment, he cut the respiratory nerve on one side of a monkey's face and observed that 'the very peculiar activities of his features on that side ceased altogether. The timid motion of his eyelids and eyebrows were lost, and he could not wink on that side, like a paralytic drunkard, whenever he showed his teeth in rage' (Bell, 1821, p. 80). These experiments established Bell's claim to have discovered the motor function of the anterior roots.

It is striking that the arguments developed for the claim that the anterior roots are motor in function did not involve reference either to the spinal soul postulated in the seventeenth century or to the *sensorium commune* in the spine postulated by Procháska. The reason is clear. Bell's and Magendie's experiments did not involve disruption of the spinal cord or removal of the head, so questions as to how reflexes can be elicited without the brain did not arise. Their research was focused on the effects of cutting nerves that lead from the brain and spinal cord to the peripheral parts of the body. Bell had satisfied himself by dissection that the anterior and posterior roots were continuous with particular columns of the spinal cord connected with the brain. So there was no conflict between the idea that the soul ('the principle of life') or mind (consciousness) resides only in (or interacts only with) the brain and the fact that severing the roots produced the effects observed.

In a remarkably incisive passage, Bell seems to have understood correctly the integrative power of the spinal cord in decapitated animals:

> the spinal marrow has much resemblance to the brain, in the composition of its cineritious and medullary matter. In short, its structure declares it to be no more than a nerve, that is, to possess properties independently of the brain. Another consideration presses upon us. Where are the many relations existing between the different parts of the frame, and necessary to their combined operations, established? There must be a relation between the four quarters of an animal. That these combined motions and relations are not established in the brain, the phenomena exhibited on stimulating the nervous system of the decapitated animal sufficiently evince. They must therefore depend on an arrangement of fibres somewhere in the spinal marrow. Comparative anatomy countenances this idea, since the motions of the lower animals are concatenated independently of the anterior ganglion. Such arguments induce me to believe that the brain does not operate directly on the frame of the body, but through the intervention of a system of nerves whose proper roots are in the spinal marrow. (Bell, 1834, p. 48)

In this passage, the requirement of a 'soul' (or principle of life) in the spinal cord is abandoned, even though decorticate animals are being considered.

Bell does not seem to have made any reference to the posterior roots possessing a sensory function. This may be explicable by reference to the fact that most of his work was carried out on stunned rabbits. It was Bell's contemporary, Magendie, who first made the distinction between motor and sensory nerves in relation to the anterior and posterior roots. It was in 1822 that the French Academy of Science reported that Magendie had discovered that with the severing of the posterior roots of the spinal nerves, only sensation is lost, whereas severing the anterior roots causes loss of motor function (Magendie, 1822, pp. 88–95). The experiments of Bell and Magendie provided the grounds for what became known as the Bell–Magendie hypothesis of spinal roots.

6.3.3   Marshall Hall: isolating sensation from sense-reaction in the spinal cord

Bell and Magendie avoided becoming caught up in the controversies concerning the existence of a spinal soul responsive to touch and capable of initiating motion independently of the cerebrum. Nevertheless, the question still remained of how sensation could be associated with the spinal cord independently of the brain. This was largely answered by Marshall Hall (1790–1857; fig. 6.6d) in the 1830s, through his careful distinction between sensation and reflex action. The animals on which Hall experimented were salamanders, frogs and turtles. He noted that a salamander's tail, entirely removed from the body, will still move as in the living animal on being excited by the point of a needle being lightly passed over its surface. However, all motion ceased on destroying the spinal marrow within the caudal vertebrae. Hall gave a full communication to the Royal Society in 1833 entitled 'On the reflex function of the medulla oblongata and medulla spinalis'. In it he declared that the excited motions of decapitated animals are dependent upon a principle different from sensation and volition.

By 1837, Hall had given an account of the spinal cord as containing a reflex centre that operated in a non-sentient and non-volitional manner, by contrast with the operations of the nerves of sensation that pass up to the brain and the motor nerves of volition that pass down from the brain. The results of his work are summarized by his statements (Hall, 1832, 1837a, b, 1843):

1. That reflexes do not involve sensation and therefore do not involve the brain.
2. That the excito-motor property or power mediated by the true spinal marrow is independent of the nerves which connect the spinal cord to the brain. So the true spinal marrow is not to be thought of as a group of nerve fibres.
3. The true spinal marrow does not possess sensation, volition or consciousness.
4. The true spinal marrow possesses its own excito- or sensory-nerves which are separate from the nerves of sensation, and therefore not sentient.
5. The true spinal marrow possesses its own motor nerves that are not voluntary and are therefore distinct from the nerves of volition.
6. Generally, the spinal and cerebral nerves lie side by side in the same fasciculi.
7. Experiments in which the nerves of one lower limb are stimulated to generate movements of the upper limbs, as well as of the opposite lower limb, show that the excito-motor system is positioned next to the voluntary system of the cerebrum. However, the two systems are not independent, as the excito-motor system can be modified during a volitional act. The true spinal system is susceptible to modification by volition.

These conclusions were revolutionary. They clearly stated that there are sensory nerves that do not produce sensations, and that there are motor nerves that do not merely mediate volitional acts. So reflex acts do not require a nervous arc from muscle to brain, and then from brain to muscle, as Charles Bell had thought. Rather, the reflex arc required a nerve leading from the point irritated into the spinal cord marrow, the spinal marrow itself, and nerves passing out of the spinal cord marrow (Hall, 1850; fig. 6.7b). Hall gave an example of how the true spinal marrow operates in his analysis of the stepping reflex, which lay the foundations for, and in some respects anticipated the work of, Charles Sherrington later in the nineteenth century.

In the influential textbook by Johannes Müller (1801–58), *Elements of Physiology* (1838), the full significance of Marshall Hall's work was recognized. Müller stated explicitly that the spinal cord is a reflector, and that the phenomena of reflection are independent of any *senso-*

rium commune in the spine. The *sensorium commune* is indeed still invoked, but only to explain *experienced sensation* (and perception). It is conceived to be located only in the brain.

6.3.4 Elaboration of the conception of the 'true spinal marrow'

Although Marshall Hall, with his conception of 'the true spinal marrow', had arrived at the correct view of the relationship between the brain and the spinal cord, there was still much resistance to the abandonment of the idea of the spinal soul. Eduard Pfluger (1829–1910), for example, still argued that the spinal cord was sentient and even possessed consciousness (Pfluger, 1853). Similarly, Friedrich Goltz, as late as 1869, subscribed to the view that a spinal soul must exist in order to explain how a decerebrate frog could still possess 'soul-faculties' of movement and sensation. However, he was not consistent, suggesting elsewhere in his book *Beiträge zur Lehre den Funktionen der Nervenzentrendes des Frosches* that the decerebrate frog has only simple reflex mechanisms, and does not feel any sensations. And Michael Foster, ten years later, was still reluctant to dismiss the idea that the spinal cord of a frog may nevertheless be conscious and feel sensation (Foster, 1879). Others took a different view. Claude Bernard, in his *Leçons sur la physiologie et la pathologie du système nerveux* (1858) argued against Pfluger and in support of Hall that spinal reflexes initiated by excitation of sensory nerves need not involve consciousness, but merely a reflex arc in the spinal cord (fig. 6.8b; see also fig. 6.8d). So too, Alfred Vulpian in his *Leçons sur la physiologie . . . du système nerveux* (1866), ridiculed the idea that explanation of reflex action in decapitated salamanders and frogs required postulating the intervention of a spinal soul.

Ivan Sechenov (1829–1905), having experimented on the reflexes of frogs, elaborated in detail what he took to be the relationship between 'the true spinal marrow' and the brain (see fig. 6.8c). The true spinal marrow mediates the reflex pathway a–d in fig. 6.8c, whereas the brain at N exerts its influence on this pathway through Nc.

In 1879 Michael Foster (1836–1907) published the third edition of his great work *A Textbook of Physiology*. Here he gave a succinct account of the relationship between spinal reflexes and the brain, which is worth quoting in full:

> The phenomena of reflex action have shown us that the cord contains a number of more or less complicated mechanisms capable of producing, as reflex results, co-ordinated movements altogether similar to those which are called forth by the will. Now it must be an economy to the body, that the will should make use of these mechanisms already present, by acting on their centres, rather than that it should have recourse to a special apparatus of its own of a similar kind. And from an anatomical point of view, it is clear that the white matter of the upper cervical cord does not contain a sufficient number of fibres, even of attenuated dimensions, to connect the brain, by afferent or efferent ties, with every sensory and motor nerve-ending of the trunk and limbs. (Foster, 1879, quoted in Liddell, 1960)

It is interesting that although clarity regarding reflex action was being achieved, the conceptual confusions regarding voluntary action were as great as ever. Foster's conception of the will as an agent acting on the brain merely perpetuated ancient conceptual confusions. The puzzling question of how *the will* can *act on* parts of the cerebral cortex was not confronted, just as Descartes three centuries earlier had failed to confront the

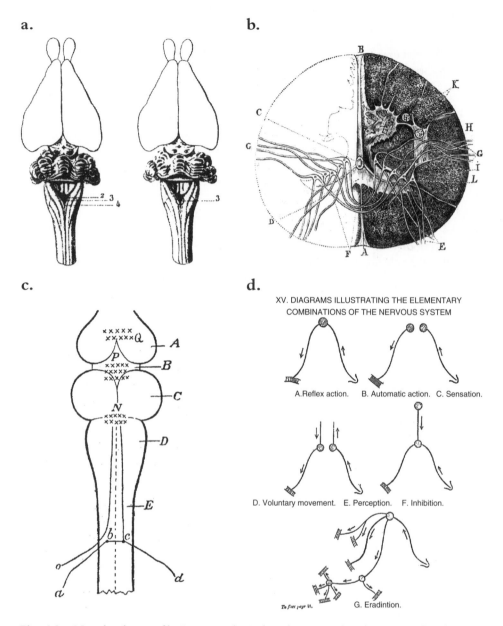

a.

b.

c.

d.

XV. DIAGRAMS ILLUSTRATING THE ELEMENTARY
COMBINATIONS OF THE NERVOUS SYSTEM

A.Reflex action.   B. Automatic action.   C. Sensation.

D. Voluntary movement.   E. Perception.   F. Inhibition.

G. Eradintion.

Fig. 6.8. Neural pathways of brain stem and spinal cord ascertained in the nineteenth century. **a:** location of the respiratory centre in the medulla of young rabbits; this drawing was made by Alfred Vulpian and accompanied a memoir written in 1858 by Marie-Jean-Pierre Flourens, with whom he was working (see Olmstead, 1944). **b:** schema of the connections between the posterior and anterior roots of the spinal cord as taught to students in the days before the neuron doctrine and the theory of the synapse. (Bernard, 1858.) **c:** Ivan Michailovich Sechenov's (1863, p. 42) diagram illustrating reflex arcs in the spinal cord and brain of the frog. Letters a–b–c–d represent a spinal reflex arc with sensory (a–b), central (b–c) and motor (c–d) components. The reflex arc of the brain consists of the sensory nerve (0), the central component (N–c) and the motor efferent (c–d). P is the region in the brain-stem which Sechenov concluded was the location of the inhibitory apparatus. **d:** connections in the nervous system as taught to students in 1885. (Pye-Smith, 1885.)

question of how the will can act on the pineal gland. It is a problem that calls out for conceptual disentangling by philosophical methods, rather than for scientific investigation and experimentation.

6.3.5   Implications of the conception of a reflex for the function of the cortex

Sechenov, by contrast with Foster, went down the road already pioneered in the eighteenth century by philosophers such as Diderot, D'Holbach and La Mettrie (author of *L'Homme Machine* (1747)). He in effect opted for a synthesis of physicalism and behaviourism. Since Marshall Hall had shown the redundancy of the notion of a spinal soul to explain reflex action and the behaviour of decorticate animals, and since the spinal cord could be viewed as operating purely bio-mechanically, Sechenov saw no reason not to treat the brain itself and all animal behaviour in the same way. He pointed out that the psychological attributes of humans, such as pleasure, fear, anger, etc., were all identified by reference to what human beings say and do. They all involve muscle contractions, whether of the larynx or of the limbs, that are part of a particular reflex. He conceived of a reflex pathway as consisting essentially in afferent nerves bringing in sensory information, together with a central pro-cessing unit, either in the spinal cord or in the brain, leading to an efferent nerve responsible for the contraction of muscles. In 'willed movement' (voluntary and intentional action that is not a response to an immediate sensory stimulus), the role of the afferent nerves is fulfilled by that of memory traces in the brain left by previous events that did involve afferent sensory flow. In rational behaviour, an inhibition emanating from the brain itself exerted control on the reflexes, preventing or permitting them to proceed. Self-consciousness, Sechenov argued, is a delusion. What appear to be rational cognitive acts are in effect no more than psychical reflexes (Sechenov, 1863). In this way Sechenov anticipated the work of Pavlov fifty years later.

6.4   The Localization of Function in the Cortex

6.4.1   Broca: the cortical area for language

Although the first experiments indicating a specialized area of the cortex for motor control were reported by Fritsch and Hitzig in 1870 (see below, §6.4.2), it could be claimed that the first evidence for cortical specialization was discovered by Paul Broca (1824–80; fig. 6.9a) in 1861. Broca reported the results of an autopsy on the cortex of one of his patients, a Monsieur Leborgne, who had suffered from loss of speech (aphasia). Broca found a lesion in the left anterior (frontal) lobe. This, he suggested, was the language area of the cortex. It subsequently became known as 'Broca's area' (Broca, 1861; see figs. 6.10a and b).

6.4.2   Fritsch and Hitzig: the motor cortex

There was little progress in understanding the functions of the cortex for nearly 200 years between the death of Thomas Willis in 1675 and the experiments of Fritsch and Hitzig

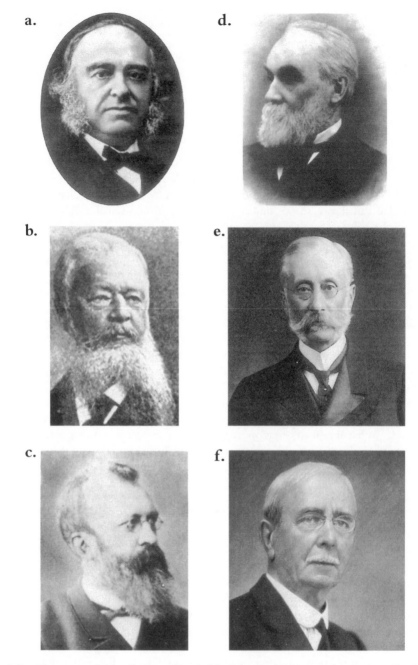

Fig. 6.9. Pioneers on the localization of cortical functions in the nineteenth century. **a:** Paul Broca (1824–80), whose association between aphasia and damage to the frontal cortex in M. Leborgne ('Tan'), in 1861, became the first cortical localization that was widely accepted (courtesy of the Académie de Médécin, Paris). **b:** Gustav Fritsch (1838–1927). **c:** Edouard Hitzig (1838–1907) (both **b** and **c** reproduced by kind permission of Dr A. E. Walker, from whom Professor Stender of Berlin obtained the picture of Hitzig). **d:** John Hughlings Jackson (1835–1911), who inferred the presence of a somatotopically organized motor cortex on the basis of epileptic seizures and other clinical evidence. (Finger, 1994, fig. 14.2.) **e:** David Ferrier (1843–1928), one of the leaders of the localizationist movement in the last quarter of the nineteenth century (courtesy of Yale Medical Historical Library, New Haven). **f:** Charles Scott Sherrington (1857–1952). (Sherrington, 1947.)

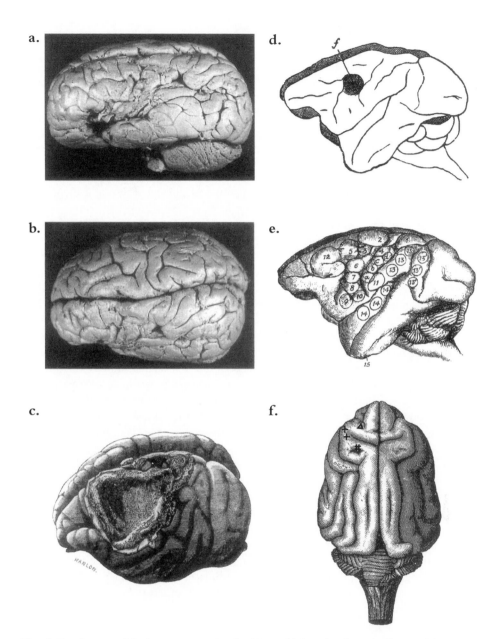

Fig. 6.10. Images of the human cortex involved in establishing localization of cortical functions. **a** and **b:** two photographs of the brain of Leborgne ('Tan'), Paul Broca's celebrated case, 1861. (Musée Dupuytren; courtesy of Assistance Publique, Hôpitaux de Paris). **c:** drawing showing the lesion of a monkey who became hemiplegic after cortical surgery; the monkey was presented at the International Medical Congress in London in 1881 by David Ferrier. **d:** David Ferrier's (1886) diagram of the left hemisphere of the monkey brain showing the locus of the ablation that resulted in a paralysis of the biceps on the right side. (Ferrier, 1876b, fig. 113.) **e:** David Ferrier's (1886) diagram of the left hemisphere of the monkey brain showing the regions that gave rise to movements (circles with numbers) when electrically stimulated. (Ferrier, 1886, fig. 70) **f:** drawing of the brain of a dog from Fritsch and Hitzig, 1870; this figure shows the areas (triangle, cross, hatch marks) from which movements of the opposite side of the body were evoked with electrical stimulation. (von Bonin, 1960, p. 73.)

c. 1870. For example, the leading French physiologist in the first half of the nineteenth century, Marie-Jean-Pierre Flourens (1794–1867), claimed, as a consequence of his research on pigeons, that the cortex was concerned only with perception, intellectual abilities and the will, not with motor action (Flourens, 1823). Furthermore, according to Flourens, the functions which the cortex does perform cannot be ascribed to different areas, for the cortex acts as a whole: 'All sensations, all perceptions, and all volition occupy concurrently the same seat in these organs. The faculty of sensation, perception and volition is then essentially one faculty' (Flourens, 1824, p. 57). Later, in 1858, he was to argue that the motor action involved in respiration is limited to the medulla, and does not involve the brain (fig. 6.8a).

It was not until the second half of the nineteenth century that progress was made in understanding the role of the cortex in motor control. In 1870, Gustav Fritsch (1838–1927; fig. 6.9b) and Edouard Hitzig (1838–1907; fig. 6.9c) published their monumental work 'Über die elektrische Erregbarkeit des Grosshirns', in which they described the results of their experiments on stimulating the brains of dogs with galvanic currents that led them to the idea of a 'motor cortex' (fig. 6.10f). In these experiments, the exposed cortex of the dogs was excited at different sites with levels of electrical stimulation just detectable when applied to the human tongue. They found areas on the surface of the cortex that gave muscular contractions to a dog's face and neck on the opposite side to the hemisphere being stimulated, as well as forepaw extension and flexion. On unilateral ablation of the forepaw area of the cortex, they observed that sensation was unaffected, but that the dog's powers of movement and posture were impaired. This led them to the hypothesis that a discrete area of the cortex has a motor function. They generalized this idea, suggesting that psychological powers too require circumscribed areas of the cortex. This conception of cortical localization was a major advance in our understanding of cortical functions.

Following this work of Fritsch and Hitzig on dogs, John Hughlings Jackson (1835–1911; fig. 6.9d) reached similar conclusions, based on observations of epileptic patients. He noted that in many cases, especially of syphilitic epilepsy, convulsions were limited to one side of the body. Autopsies confirmed that such patients suffered from degenerative disease on the opposite side of the cortex, often on the surface of the hemisphere (Jackson, 1863). The temporal pattern of contraction across muscle groups during seizures in progressive epilepsy attracted Hughlings Jackson's attention. He conjectured that the motor cortex must be organized along somatotopic lines, so that the hands, face, tongue and feet, which possess the greatest capacity for specialized movement, were correlated with larger areas of the motor cortex than other movable parts of the body.

These brilliant suggestions of Hughlings Jackson were confirmed by the work on primates by David Ferrier (1843–1928; fig. 6.9e) in 1874. Using alternating current stimulation of discrete sites on the cortex, he was able to delineate clearly the area of the cortex that produces the twitching of muscles as well as movements that in some cases resembled attempts at walking (fig. 6.10e). On introducing small lesions into the motor area of the cortex which he had mapped, Ferrier showed that in some cases these resulted in a paralysis of the opposite hand and forearm, and in another case to the paralysis of the biceps muscle (fig. 6.10d; see also fig. 6.10c). By contrast, these animals showed normal sensitivity to touch and noxious stimuli. Such observations clearly pointed to a somatotopic organization of the motor cortex (Ferrier, 1873–4, 1876a, b). This work on primates was subsequently confirmed and extended by Victor Horsley (1857–1916), who in 1887 showed that the precentral gyrus was predominantly motor and the postcentral predominantly sensory, so that the motor cortex was to be found exclusively anterior to the Rolandic fissure (Beevor and Horsley, 1887, 1890, 1894).

6.4.3 Electrical phenomena in the cortex support the idea of a motor cortex

In 1875, Richard Caton (1842–1926) discovered that electrical oscillations could be recorded through two electrodes placed on the surface of the cortex of a monkey and that these oscillations were altered by various forms of sensory stimulation as well as by anoxia and anaesthesia. Caton noted that a galvanometer recorded electrical currents in all areas of the brain he had examined. Of particular interest was his discovery that a negative current was generated by these areas of cortex previously identified by Ferrier as involved in motor acts, such as rotation of the head or mastication, or areas of cortex involving sensory elicited activity such as movement of the eyelids in response to stimulation of the opposite retina by light. The electrical changes due to stimulation of the retina with light were later confirmed by Adolf Beck (1863–1942), adding credence to Caton's observations on the localization of electrical activity during movement of the kind predicted by Ferrier's work (Beck, 1890).

6.5 Charles Scott Sherrington: the Integrative Action of Synapses in the Spinal Cord and Cortex

6.5.1 Integrative action in the spinal cord

It is to Charles Sherrington (1857–1952; fig. 6.9f) that one must turn to find the experimental plan for elucidating the mechanism of the 'true spinal marrow'. The thoroughness and methodical nature of Sherrington's researches on the subject are at a new level. These were dependent not so much on technical advances at the time as on the brilliance and clarity of his thinking, coupled with formidable and indefatigable capacity for experiment. Sherrington first tackled the problem of the spinal origin of the efferent nerves innervating a particular muscle (Sherrington, 1892). He went on to show that the positions of the motoneurons supplying a muscle are scattered throughout the length of the spinal cord segments supplying nerves to the muscle. In 1910, he published his great paper, 121 pages long, which established the flexion-reflex of the limb, the crossed-extensor-reflex, as well as the process of reflex stepping and standing (Sherrington, 1910). In this work, he shows that application of a noxious stimulus to a limb evokes a flexion-reflex which is naturally protective. The crossed extensor-reflex is revealed here in experiments in which Sherrington showed that stimuli that evoke flexion in one limb result in extension of the opposite limb, a discovery which then led him to research that established the role of the spinal cord in reflex processes involved in stepping and standing. Sherrington's description of inhibition in the spinal cord is particularly beautiful:

a.

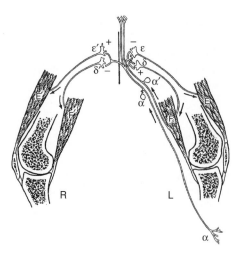

b.

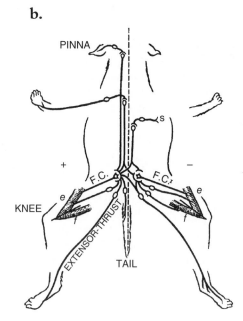

c.

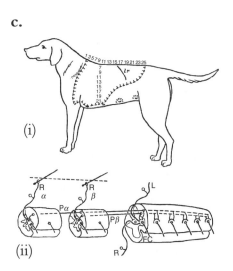

(i)

(ii)

d.

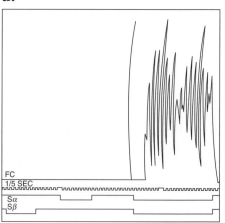

Fig. 6.11. Sherrington's elucidation of the principles of operation of the spinal cord. **a:** 'diagram indicating connexions and actions of two afferent spinal root-cells, α and α', in regard to their reflex influence on the extensor and flexor muscles of the two knees. The α root-cell afferent from skin below knee; α', root-cell afferent from flexor muscle of knee, i.e. in hamstring nerve; ε and εI, efferent neurones to the extensor muscles of the knee, left and right; δ and δ', efferent neurones to the flexor muscles; E and EI, extensor muscles; F and FI, flexor muscles. The 'schalt-zellen' (v. Manokow) probable between the afferent and efferent root-cells are for simplicity omitted. The sign +ve indicates that at the synapse which it marks the afferent fibre α (and α') excites the motor neurone to discharging activity, whereas the sign −ve indicates that at the synapse which it marks the afferent fibre α (and α') inhibits the discharging activity of the motor neurones. The effect of strychnine and of tetanus toxin is to convert the minus sign into plus sign.' (Sherrington, 1947, fig. 37.)

b: 'The final common path is therefore an instrument passive in the hands of certain groups of reflex-paths. I have attempted to depict this very simply in the figure. There certain type-reflexes are indicated by lines representing their paths. The final common path (F.C.) selected is the motor neurone of the vasto-crureus of the dog or cat. Reflexes that act as 'allied reflexes' on F.C. are represented as having their terminals joined together next to the final common path. Reflexes with excitatory effect (+ sign) are brought together on the left, those with inhibitory (− sign) on the right. Of the reflex pairs formed by the two reflexes which two symmetrical receptive points, one right and one left, yield in regard to the final common path, one of the pair only is represented, in order to simplify the diagram. To have a further indication of the reflexes playing upon F.C., all that is required is to add to the reflexes indicated in the diagram for FC, a set of reflexes similar to those given in the diagram for FC', for they must be added if the remaining members of the right and left reflex pairs from various parts of the body be taken into account. It is noteworthy that in many instances the end-effect of a spinal reflex initiated from a surface point on one side is bilateral and takes effect at symmetrical parts, but is opposite in kind at those two parts, e.g. is inhibition at one of them, excitation at the other. Hence reflexes initiated from points corresponding one with the other in the two halves of the body are commonly antagonistic. S stands for scratch-receptor, e and f are extensor and flexor muscles of knee respectively.' (Sherrington, 1947, fig. 44.)

c: Sherrington's classic picture of the areas for the scratch-reflex in the dog. (i) shows the 'receptive field', as revealed after low cervical transection, a saddle-shaped area of dorsal skin, whence the scratch-reflex of the left hind-limb can be evoked. lr marks the position of the last rib, (ii) shows a diagram of the spinal arcs involved; L, receptive or afferent nerve-path from the left foot; R, receptive nerve-path from the opposite foot; $R\alpha$, $R\beta$, receptive nerve-paths from hairs in the dorsal skin of the left side; F.C., the final common path, in this case the motor neurone to a flexor muscle of the hip; $P\alpha$, $P\beta$, proprio-spinal neurones. (Sherrington, 1947, fig. 39.)

d: 'Records from above downwards (read from left to right): F.C., myograph curve of flexor muscle of hip (scratch-reflex). The vertical arc (preceding the response) coincides with the descent of the signal lines ($S\alpha$, $S\beta$). Time in 1/5 sec. Signal line $S\alpha$: each descent of the line marks the period of stimulation of the skin belonging to arc $R\alpha$ [fig. 6.11c] of the shoulder skin. The strength of stimulus is arranged to be subliminal, so that a reflex-response in F.C. is not obtained. Signal line $S\beta$: each descent of the line marks the period of stimulation, also subliminal of a point of shoulder skin 8 cm. from $R\alpha$. Though the two stimuli applied separately are each unable to evoke the reflex, when applied contemporaneously they quickly evoke the reflex. The two arcs $R\alpha$ and $R\beta$, therefore, reinforce each other in their action on the final common path F.C. (summation effect, immediate spinal induction).' (Sherrington, 1947, fig. 38.)

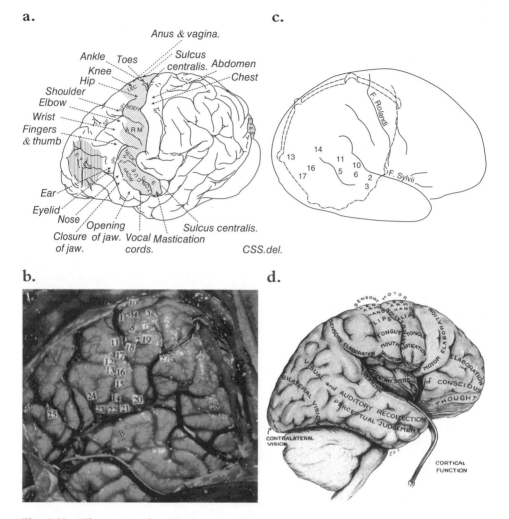

Fig. 6.12. The motor and somatosensory cortex in humans and other primates. **a:** brain of a chimpanzee (*Troglodytes niger*); left hemisphere viewed from side and above so as to obtain as far as possible the configuration of the sulcus centralis area. The figure involves, nevertheless, considerable foreshortening about the top and bottom of sulcus centralis. The extent of the 'motor' area on the free surface of the hemisphere is indicated by the black stippling, which extends back to the sulcus centralis. Much of the 'motor' area is hidden in sulci; for instance, the area extends into the sulcus centralis and the sulcus precentrales, also into occasional sulci which cross the precentral gyrus. The names printed large, in enhanced black, on the stippled area indicate the main regions of the 'motor' area; the names printed small, outside the brain, indicate broadly by their pointing lines the relative topography of some of the chief subdivisions of the main regions of the 'motor' cortex. But there exists much overlapping of the areas and of their subdivisions, which the diagram does not attempt to indicate. The shaded regions, marked 'Eyes', indicate in the frontal and occipital regions respectively the portions

The striking correspondence observed between the reflex inhibition and the reflex contraction, when examined in one and the same type-reflex, allows the inference that the nerve fibres from the receptive field of the reflex each divide in the spinal cord into end-branches (e.g. collaterals), one set of which, when the nerve fibre is active, produces excitation, while another set, when the nerve fibre is active, produces inhibition. (Sherrington, 1900, 1905a, b) The single afferent nerve-fibre would therefore, in regard of one set of its terminal branches, be specifically

---

Fig. 6.12. (*Continued*)
of cortex which, under faradization, yield conjugate movements of the eyeballs. But it is questionable whether these reactions resemble those of the 'motor' area sufficiently to be included with them. They are therefore marked in vertical shading instead of stippling as is the 'motor' area. S.F. = superior frontal sulcus. S.Pr. = superior precentral sulcus. I.Pr. = inferior precentral sulcus. (Sherrington and Grünbaum, 1902, plate 4.)

b: Brain of a human. Here, and in c, are shown the responses to electrical stimulation of the surface of the cortex of patient prior to undergoing surgery for epilepsy. The dura has been turned back to expose the cortex. The left temporal lobe is seen below the fissure of Sylvius. The numbered tickets dropped on the surface of the cortex indicate points of positive response to electrical stimulation. A few of the patients' responses during the operation are as follows (Penfield and Roberts, 1959, fig. VII-3):

Postcentral Gyrus

1. Tingling right thumb and slight movement
2. Sensation in lower lip outside
3. Sensation right upper lip inside
4. Tingling in right side of tongue at the tip
5. Sensation in the 'joint of the jaw and in the lower lip inside'

Precentral Gyrus

11. Feeling in my throat which stopped my speech
12. Quivering of jaw in a 'sidewise manner'
13. Pulling of jaw to right

c: brain of a human. 'Broken line indicates craniotomy exposure. The responses to stimulation (thyratron stimulator) were as follows:

Points 13 and 17: Contralateral coloured stars (points lie on visual (occipital) cortex.

Points 14 and 16: Complicated visual hallucinations, like the aura of her attack. At points near to 14 and 16, stimulation had the following effect. She stared suddenly and then cried: 'Oh, I can see something come at me! Don't let them come at me!' She remained staring and fearful for 30 secs, although the stimulation was of much shorter duration.

Points 11, 5, 10, 6, 2, and 3: Auditory hallucinations that she heard the voices of her mother and brothers 'yelling at her in an accusing manner, producing terror and tears'. (From Penfield and Rasmussen, 1968, fig. 87.)

d: functions of the human cortex. 'This illustration serves as a summary restatement of conclusions, some hypothetical (e.g. The elaboration zones), others firmly established. The suggestion that the anterior portion of the occipital cortex is related to both fields of vision rather than to one alone is derived from the results of stimulation.' (Penfield and Rasmussen, 1968, fig. 110.)

excitor, and in regard to another set of its central endings, be specifically inhibitory. It would, in this respect, be duplex centrally. (fig. 6.11a; Sherrington, 1947, p. 107)

Sherrington (1947, pp. 121–151) goes on to show how the action of excitatory and inhibitory nerves works within the spinal cord to determine the activity in a set of motoneurons to a muscle (the 'final common pathway'). He cites as an example the effects of simultaneous stimulation of the skin at different points exciting a scratch reflex which cannot be evoked by stimulation of either point alone (fig. 6.11d). This he interprets as due to the connections from the two points to the motoneurons (Ra and Rb in fig. 6.11c) as reinforcing each other through excitatory connections to the motoneurons. However in the case of stimulation of the skin at corresponding points on opposite sides of the body, the motoneurons are affected by both inhibitory and excitatory influences (see fig. 6.11b).

Sherrington, in his great papers at the beginning of the last century (1887, 1907, 1910), laid down the general scheme for the analysis of the integrative functions of the spinal cord. In so doing, he not only laid the foundations for twentieth-century research on the spinal cord, but also completed the research program initiated eighty years earlier by Marshall Hall. As a result, the notion of a 'spinal soul' was finally eliminated from further consideration.

6.5.2   The motor cortex

The twentieth-century study of motor cortical function is also founded on Sherrington's ideas. Although Ferrier in 1886 had first located the motor cortex in primates (fig. 6.10d), it was Sherrington and Grünbaum in 1902 who first gave a detailed description of the spatial extent of this area of the cortex of primates. They noted that it does not extend behind the sulcus centralis, and thus clearly distinguished it from the area that we now know as somatosensory (fig. 6.12a). In the same work, they also identified what we now call 'the frontal eye fields', noting that they are wholly separated spatially from the motor area of the Rolandic region. Their method of unipolar faradization (alternating current) stimulation of the cortex allowed for much finer localization than had been possible with the double-point electrodes used up to this time. In addition to numerous actions of limbs, they determined the cortical localization of movements of the ear, nostril, palate, sucking, mastication, the vocal chords, chest wall, abdominal wall, pelvic floor, anal orifice and vaginal orifice. This led them to the discovery of the somatotopic organization of the motor cortex. Their classic paper (1902), established unequivocally the conception of a motor cortex, and hence too that different parts of the cortex are specialized for different functions. Their method of experimentation was later followed by Penfield and his colleagues on human cortex (figs. 6.12b–d).

Sherrington conceived of long reflexes involving the motor cortex as attached to the direct reflex pathways of the spinal cord. In this way, the motor cortex is able to coordinate such reflex pathways even though they may involve sites that are widely separated (Sherrington, 1947, p. 148). He provided the basis for twentieth-century investigations of the motor cortex and the spinal cord through his structural and functional studies and the remarkable use of his observations to generate prescient hypotheses for further investigation.

7

Conceptual Presuppositions of Cognitive Neuroscience

7.1 Conceptual Elucidation

In *Philosophical Foundations of Neuroscience* (Bennett and Hacker, 2003),[1] we aimed to contribute to neuroscientific research in the only way in which philosophy can assist science – not by offering scientists empirical theories in place of their own, but by clarifying the conceptual structures they invoke. The systematic elucidations we gave of sensation, perception, knowledge, memory, thought, imagination, emotion, consciousness and self-consciousness are not theories.[2] Their purpose was to clarify the psychological concepts that cognitive neuroscientists use in *their* empirical theories. The conceptual clarifications we gave demonstrated numerous incoherences in current neuroscientific theorizing. They showed why these mistakes are committed and how to avoid them.

Criticisms of our work, from three of the leading philosophers who concern themselves with cognitive neuroscience and its philosophical implications, Professors Churchland, Dennett and Searle, are the subject of this chapter. Responding to them will serve three purposes. First, it will defend and clarify further the fundamental philosophical principles that inform our work. Secondly, it will rectify a variety of misunderstandings and

---

[1] Page references to this book will be flagged '*PFN*'. The main critics of our book that we here address are Paul Churchland, in his critical notice 'Cleansing Science' (2005), John Searle and Daniel Dennett, both of whom responded to us at an 'authors and critics' session at the meeting of the American Philosophical Association (Eastern Division) in New York, December 2005, and whose papers, together with a version of the current chapter, were published in Bennett et al., 2007. All page references to their critical essays are to this publication.

[2] Searle, in his APA paper, objected to our insistence that our observations are not a theory. He asserted that a conceptual result is significant only as a part of a general theory (p. 122). If by 'a general theory' he means an overall account of a conceptual network, rather than mere piecemeal results, we agree. Our denial that our general accounts are theoretical is a denial that they are logically on the same level as scientific theories. They are descriptions, not hypotheses; they are not confirmable or refutable by experiment; they are not hypothetico-deductive, and their purpose is neither to predict nor to offer causal explanations; they do not involve idealizations in the sense in which the sciences do (e.g. the notion of a point-mass in Newtonian mechanics), and they do not approximate to empirical facts within agreed margins of error; there is no discovery of new entities and no hypothesizing entities for explanatory purposes.

misinterpretations. Thirdly, it will advance further criticisms of views that we hold to be mistaken.

Cognitive neuroscience is an experimental investigation that aims to discover empirical truths concerning the neural foundations of human faculties and the neural processes that accompany their exercise. A precondition of truth is sense. If a form of words makes no sense, then it won't express a truth. If it does not express a truth, then it can't explain anything. Philosophical investigation into the conceptual foundations of neuroscience aims to disclose and clarify conceptual truths that are presupposed by, and are conditions of the sense of, cogent descriptions of cognitive neuroscientific discoveries and theories.[3] If conducted correctly, it will illuminate neuroscientific experiments and their description, and the inferences that can be drawn from them. In *Philosophical Foundations of Neuroscience* we delineated the conceptual network formed by families of psychological concepts. These concepts are presupposed by cognitive neuroscientific research into the neural basis of human cognitive, cogitative, affective and volitional powers. If the logical relations of implication, exclusion, compatibility and presupposition that characterize the use of these concepts are not respected, invalid inferences are likely to be drawn, valid inferences are likely to be overlooked, and nonsensical combinations of words are likely to be treated as making sense.

In this book, *History of Cognitive Neuroscience*, we have delineated some of the major experimental investigations into cognitive neuroscience over the past century or so. We have outlined what the neuroscientists in question thought they had discovered and what conclusions they drew from their work. We have subjected their descriptions of the results of their experiments to critical analytic scrutiny. For, we have argued, it is common for experiments and consequences taken to follow from them to be flawed by conceptual confusions and unclarities. Our criticisms have been wholly analytic, concerned not with errors of fact or experimental infelicity, but only with conceptual error.

Some philosophers, especially in the USA, have been much influenced by Quine's philosophy of logic and language, according to which there is no significant difference

---

[3] Dennett, in his reply to our book at the APA, seemed to have difficulties with this thought. In his criticisms (p. 79), he quoted selectively from our book: 'Conceptual questions antecede matters of truth and falsehood' (*PFN* 2); 'What truth and falsity is to science, sense and nonsense is to philosophy' (*PFN* 6). From this he drew the conclusion that in our view philosophy is not concerned with truth at all. However, he omitted the sequel to the first sentence:

> They are questions concerning our forms of representation, not questions concerning the truth or falsehood *of empirical statements*. These forms are presupposed by true (and false) scientific statements, and by correct (and incorrect) scientific theories. They determine not what is empirically true or false, but rather what does and does not make sense. (*PFN* 2, emphasis added)

He likewise omitted the observation on the facing page that neuroscience is discovering much concerning the neural foundations of human powers, 'but its discoveries in no way affect *the conceptual truth* that these powers and their exercise . . . are attributes of human beings, not of their parts' (*PFN* 3, emphasis added). As is patent, it is our view that philosophy is concerned with conceptual truths, and that conceptual truths determine what does and does not make sense.

between empirical and conceptual truths.[4] According to Quine, the sentences of a theory face experience as a totality, and are confirmed holistically. So, from a theoretical point of view, a Quinean will hold that there is no essential difference between the sentence 'Memory is knowledge retained' and the sentence 'Memory is dependent upon the normal functioning of the hippocampus and neo-cortex'. But this is wrong. The former is a conceptual truth, the latter a scientific discovery. 'Memory is knowledge retained' is an expression of a rule of description (or norm of representation) in the *guise* of a statement of fact, whereas 'Memory is dependent upon the normal functioning of the hippocampus' *is* a statement of fact. To confuse and conflate the two is akin to confusing or conflating the rules of chess with moves in chess, or a measure with a measurement. Note that the distinction between conceptual and empirical truth is *not* an epistemological, but a logical, one. A conceptual proposition ascribes internal properties or relations, whereas an empirical proposition ascribes external ones. A conceptual truth is partly constitutive of the meanings of its constituent expressions, whereas an empirical proposition is a description of how things stand. Precisely because such statements are partly constitutive of the meanings of their constituent expressions, failure to acknowledge a conceptual truth (e.g. that red is darker than pink) is a *criterion* of lack of understanding of one or another of its constituent expressions. But that does not make the distinction epistemological.

It would be similarly mistaken to suppose that the theorems of the differential calculus, which are non-empirical truths, were confirmed holistically by the predictive success of Newtonian mechanics (as is implied by the Quinean doctrine). They were confirmed by mathematical proofs. It would be equally erroneous to suppose that 'vixens are female' is confirmed by the success of zoological theory or that 'bachelors are unmarried' is confirmed by the sociology of marital habits. So too, that red is darker than pink is not verified by confirmation of the theory of colour, but rather is presupposed by it. Non-empirical propositions, whether they are propositions of logic or mathematics or straightforward conceptual truths can be neither confirmed nor infirmed by empirical discoveries or theories.[5] Conceptual truths delineate the logical space within which facts are located. They determine what makes sense. Consequently, facts can neither confirm nor conflict with them.[6]

---

[4] Paul Churchland proposes, as a consideration against our view, that 'Since Quine, the bulk of the philosophical profession has been inclined to say "no"' to the suggestion that there are 'necessary truths, constitutive of meanings, that are forever beyond empirical or factual refutation' 2005, p. 474). We doubt whether he has done a social survey (do most philosophers really think that truths of arithmetic are subject to empirical refutation together with any empirical theory in which they are embedded?); and we are surprised that a philosopher should think that a head-count is a criterion of truth.

[5] For canonical criticism of Quine on analyticity, see Grice and Strawson, 1956. For more recent, meticulous criticism of Quine's general position, see Glock, 2003. For a contrast between Quine and Wittgenstein, see Hacker, 1996, ch. 7. Williamson (2006), construes conceptual truths as epistemological and argues that there are no such truths. His criticisms of *that* notion of conceptual truth, whether valid or not, are therefore irrelevant to the conception that we advance.

[6] It is mistaken to suppose, as Churchland does (2005, pp. 467f), that the Cartesian claim that the non-physical mind can affect events in the physical world via its action on the pineal gland is refuted by the fact that it would

A final point of clarification: it has been suggested by critics that we are committed to something called 'Ordinary Language Philosophy' (Churchland, 2005, p. 465). The suggestion is misplaced. We are concerned with ordinary language only when the problematic concepts we are dealing with are non-technical concepts of natural language. But we have no qualms or hesitations about discussing technical concepts in neuroscience (in other sciences or in mathematics) and pointing out when they are misused. Nor, as is patent in *Philosophical Foundations of Neuroscience*, do we have qualms about identifying conceptual incoherences that stem from the misuse of technical concepts. That they are misused is not, in our view, shown by whether their application does or does not accord with that of non-technical concepts. It has also been suggested that we possess and deploy something called 'a theory of meaning' (Churchland, 2005, p. 476). If a theory of meaning is a set of axioms, formation and transformation rules that will allow the derivation of the truth conditions of any well-formed sentence of a language, then we certainly have no theory of meaning. Our observations about the meanings of words and about the boundaries between sense and nonsense are not a part of any *theory*, but clarifications of the concepts of word-meaning, sense and nonsense. Churchland supposes that our claim that a word is used according to standards of correct use (rules of use) is a theoretical claim. It is no more theoretical than the claim that law-abiding citizens act in accordance with the law.

7.2   Two Paradigms: Aristotle and Descartes

Philosophical reflection on human nature, on the body and soul, goes back to the dawn of philosophy. The polarities between which it fluctuates were set out by Plato and Aristotle. According to Plato, and the Platonic-Christian tradition of Augustine, the human being is not a unified substance, but a combination of two distinct substances, a mortal body and an immortal soul. According to Aristotle, a human being *is* a unified substance, the soul (*psuchē*) being the form of the body. To describe that form is to describe the characteristic powers of human beings: in particular, the distinctive powers of intellect and will that characterize the rational *psuchē*. Modern debate on this theme commences with the heir to the Platonic-Augustinian tradition: namely, the Cartesian conception of human beings as two

violate the law of Conservation of Momentum. The Cartesian claim could be empirically refuted only if it made sense. For it to make sense, it would have to provide criteria of identity for immaterial substances – but that is just what it does not do. We would have to know what counts as an immaterial substance, how to distinguish the same immaterial substance again on a subsequent occasion, and how to distinguish one such substance from two or twenty or 200 (each of which may be thinking the very same Cartesian thoughts). But we do not. We would have to understand what it would be for an immaterial substance to possess causal powers to act on a material substance. Then we might find out that immaterial substances do not in fact possess such powers. But we do not understand what it would be, for the idea is incoherent. If one thinks that the supposition that an immaterial substance causes movements of a human being's limbs when he moves voluntarily is subject to empirical disconfirmation, then we must also think that it is, in principle, subject to empirical confirmation – that something conceivable could confirm it, even if nothing in fact does. But what experimental result could conceivably confirm that the movement of one's arm, when one moves one's arm voluntarily, is caused by an immaterial substance?

one-sided things, a mind and a body. Their two-way causal interaction was invoked to explain human experience and behaviour.

The greatest figures of the first two generations of twentieth-century neuroscientists, e.g. Sherrington, Eccles and Penfield, were avowed Cartesian dualists. The third generation retained the basic Cartesian structure, but transformed it into brain–body dualism: substance dualism was abandoned, but structural dualism retained. For neuroscientists now ascribe much the same array of mental predicates to the brain as Descartes ascribed to the mind, and conceive of the relationship between thought and action, and experience and its objects, in much the same way as Descartes – essentially merely replacing the mind by the brain. The central theme of our book was to demonstrate the incoherence of brain–body dualism, and to disclose its misguided crypto-Cartesian character. Our constructive aim was to show that an Aristotelian account, with due emphasis on first- and second-order active and passive abilities and their modes of behavioural manifestation, supplemented by Wittgensteinian insights that complement Aristotle's, is necessary to do justice to the structure of our conceptual scheme and to provide coherent descriptions of the great discoveries of post-Sherringtonian cognitive neuroscience.[7]

7.3   Aristotle's Principle and the Mereological Fallacy

In *Philosophical Foundations of Neuroscience* we identified a pervasive error that we called 'the mereological fallacy in neuroscience'.[8] Correcting this error is a leitmotiv (but *only* a leitmotiv) of our book. We called the mistake 'mereological', because it involves ascribing to parts attributes that can be ascribed intelligibly only to the wholes of which they are parts. A form of this error was pointed out *c.* 350 BC by Aristotle, who remarked that 'to say that the soul [the *psuchē*] is angry is as if one were to say that the soul weaves or builds. For it is surely better not to say that the soul pities, learns or thinks, but that a man does these with his soul' (*De anima* 408^{b}12–15) – doing something with one's soul being like doing something with one's talents. It is mistaken to ascribe to the soul of an animal attributes that are properly ascribable only to the animal as a whole. We might call this 'Aristotle's principle'.

Our primary concern was with the neuroscientific cousin of this: namely, the error of ascribing to the *brain* – a part of an animal – attributes that can be ascribed literally only to the animal as a whole. We were not the first to have noted this – it was pointed out by Anthony Kenny in his brilliant paper 'The Homunculus Fallacy' of 1971.[9] This error is more properly *mereological* than its Aristotelian ancestor, since the brain is literally a part of

---

[7] The Aristotelian, anti-Cartesian, points that we emphasize are (i) Aristotle's principle, which we discuss below; (ii) Aristotle's identification of the *psuchē* with a range of capacities; (iii) that capacities are identified by what they are capacities to do; (iv) that whether a creature possesses a capacity is to be seen from its activities; (v) Aristotle's realization that whether the *psuchē* and the body are one thing or two is an incoherent question.

[8] It is, of course, not strictly a fallacy, but it leads to fallacies – invalid inferences and mistaken arguments.

[9] We preferred the less picturesque but descriptively more accurate name 'mereological fallacy' (and, correlatively, 'the mereological principle'). We found that neuroscientists were prone to dismiss as childish the fallacy of sup-

the sentient animal, whereas, contrary to the claims of Plato and Descartes, the soul or mind is not. In Aristotelian spirit we now observe that to say that the brain is angry is as if one were to say that the brain weaves or builds. For it is surely better to say not that the brain pities, learns or thinks, but that a man does these.[10] Accordingly, we deny that it makes sense to say that the brain is conscious, feels sensations, perceives, thinks, knows or wants anything – for these are attributes of animals, not of their brains.

We were a little surprised at the APA meeting to find that Dennett thinks that his distinction in *Content and Consciousness* of 1969 between personal and sub-personal levels of explanations is what *we* had in mind. He there wrote, correctly, that being in pain is not a property of the brain. But his reason was that pains are 'mental phenomena' that are 'non-mechanical', whereas cerebral processes are 'essentially mechanical' (p. 91). The contrast *we* drew between properties of wholes and properties of parts is not between what is non-mechanical and what is mechanical. It is the bracket clock as a whole that keeps time, not its *fusée* or great wheel – although the process of keeping time is wholly mechanical. It is the aeroplane that flies, not its engines – although the process of flying is wholly mechanical. Moreover, verbs of sensation, such as 'hurts', 'itches', 'tickles', *do* apply to the parts of an animal, whose leg may hurt, whose head may itch, and whose flanks may tickle (*PFN* 73). These attributes are, as Dennett puts it, 'non-mechanical'; nevertheless, they *are* ascribable to parts of an animal. So the mereological point we made is quite different from Dennett's distinction between personal and sub-personal levels of explanation, and, applied to animals, is quite different from his distinction between what is 'mechanical' and what is not.[11]

The mereological principle that we advance was rejected by Barry Dainton (2007) in his review of *Neuroscience and Philosophy*. Dainton appears to think that the brain is a limiting case of a mutilated human being. He writes that he is able to think, and that 'it seems very plausible to think that I would continue to have this ability if I were reduced to the condition of a healthy living brain (maintained by life-support machinery, say). If I am essentially a human being, as Bennett and Hacker suggest, then I am still a human being in my diminished condition. . . . If there's nothing to distinguish me from my brain, won't my brain be able to do everything I can do?'

posing that there is a homunculus in the brain, and to proceed in the next breath to ascribe psychological attributes to the brain.

[10] Not, of course, *with* his brain, in the sense in which one does things *with* one's hands or eyes, nor in the sense in which one does things with one's talents. Of course, he would not be able to do any of these things but for the normal functioning of his brain.

[11] We were more than a little surprised to find Dennett declaring that his 'main points of disagreement' are that he does not believe that 'the personal level of explanation is the *only* level of explanation when the subject matter is human minds and actions', and that he believes that the task of relating these two levels of explanation is 'not outside the philosopher's province' (p. 79). There is no disagreement at all over *this*. Anyone who has ever taken an aspirin to alleviate a headache or imbibed excessive alcohol to become jocose, bellicose or morose, and wants an explanation of the sequence of events, must surely share Dennett's first commitment. Anyone who has concerned himself, as we have done throughout the 452 pages of *Philosophical Foundations of Neuroscience*, with clarifying the relationships between psychological and neuroscientific concepts and the phenomena they signify, share his second one.

One needs to exercise one's ability to think a little more strenuously than this in order to see the error of this reasoning. That something seems plausible is no reason for thinking it to be true. (The argument from design seemed plausible for many centuries, as did the invariability of species – until both were shown to be mistaken by Darwin.) It all depends on the grounds advanced for the alleged plausibility. To suppose that I might be 'reduced' to the condition of a healthy living brain is precisely to beg the question at issue, not an argument for the ascription of psychological predicates to the brain.

Human brains are not kinds of human beings, and dead brains are not the corpses of human beings. When a brain is removed from a cadaver and put into a jar of formalin, what the jar contains is not a human corpse or the mutilated remains of a human being. Human beings have brains, but human brains do not have brains – they *are* brains. Human beings have bodies, but a human brain does not have a body, it is a part of a human body. Human beings have minds. But brains don't have minds (there is no such thing as the brain making up its mind, having a dirty mind, or having a thought cross its mind). The fact that human beings have the distinctive capacities constitutive of having a mind is dependent upon the normal functioning of their brain. That no more shows the brain to be a human being, or a limiting case of a mutilated human being, than the fact that an aeroplane's capacity for flight depends upon the normal functioning of its engines shows that the engines fly, let alone that an engine is an aeroplane or a limiting case of a damaged aeroplane.

To be sure, one may fantasize about brains being removed from bodies, inserted into complex gadgetry that will support its continued existence, and perhaps hooked up to prosthetic eyes and ears, maybe even limbs and a computerized voice box. And then, so the science fiction runs, the voice and limbs may exhibit thought and volition. Does this not show that it is the brain that thinks? No! It shows that this imaginary being, which we may dub 'a cerebroid' (partly organic and partly metallic and electronic), thinks. Brains do not think, and they are neither thoughtful nor thoughtless. Only beings the behavioural reperloire of which includes thoughtful behaviour can be said, truly or falsely, to think, be thoughtful or thoughtless. A condition for the literal, intelligible application of cogitative predicates to a being is that the being could, logically, satisfy the behavioural criteria for the ascription of such attributes. But there is nothing a brain could do that would satisfy the complex criteria for thinking, reasoning, being thoughtful or thoughtless, reflective or ruminative, attentive or considerate.

Magritte might have painted a brain on a pedestal, with a 'bubble' coming out of it with 'cogito ergo sum' inscribed in the bubble. This painting could have been named 'Professor Dainton thinking'. But it would be a joke, not the illustration of a truth.

7.4 Is the Mereological Fallacy Really Mereological?

Searle objected that what we characterize as a paradigm of a mereological fallacy – i.e. the ascription of psychological attributes to the brain – is no such thing, for the brain is not a part of a person, but rather a part of a person's body (p. 107). This, we think, is a red-herring. The dictum of Wittgenstein that we quoted was 'Only of a *human being* and of what resembles (behaves like) a living human being can one say: it has sensations; it sees, is blind;

hears, is deaf; is conscious or unconscious' (Wittgenstein, 1953, §281; our emphases). The brain *is* a part of the human being.

Searle suggests that if ascribing psychological attributes to the brain really were a mereo-logical error, then it would vanish if one ascribed them to what he calls 'the rest of the system' to which the brain belongs. He thinks that the 'rest of the system' is the body that a human being *has*. He observes that we do not ascribe psychological predicates to the body one has. With the striking exception of verbs of sensation (e.g. 'My body aches all over'), the latter point is correct. We do not say 'My body perceives, thinks, or knows'. However, 'the system' to which the human brain can be said to belong is *the human being*. The human brain is a part of the human being, just as the canine brain is a part of a dog. My brain, the brain I have, is as much a part of me – of the living human being that I am – as my legs and arms are parts of me. But it is true that my brain can also be said to be a part of my body.

How is this to be explained? Our talk of our mind is largely *non-agential, idiomatic* talk of our rational powers of intellect and will, and of their exercise. Our talk of our body is talk of our corporeal properties. To speak of *my body* is to speak of corporeal features *of the human being that I am* – features pertaining to appearance (an attractive or ungainly body), to the superficies of the human being (his body was covered with mosquito bites, was lacer-ated all over, was painted blue), to aspects of health and fitness (a diseased or healthy body), and, very strikingly, to sensation (my body may ache all over, just as my leg may hurt and my back may itch).[12] But knowing, perceiving, thinking, imagining, etc. are not corporeal features of human beings and are not ascribable to the body a human being has, any more than they are ascribable to the brain that a human being has. Human beings are not *their bodies*. Nevertheless, they *are* bodies, in the quite different sense of being a particular kind of sentient spatio-temporal continuant – *homo sapiens*; and the brain is a part of the living human being, as are the limbs.[13] It is not, however, a conscious, thinking, perceiving part – and nor is any other part of a human being. For these are attributes of the human being as a whole.

Nevertheless, Searle has noted an interesting feature of our corporeal idiom. Human beings are persons – that is, they are intelligent, language-using animals, are self-conscious, possess knowledge of good and evil, are responsible for their deeds, and are bearers of rights and duties. To be a person is, roughly speaking, to possess such abilities as qualify one for the status of a moral agent. We would probably not say that the brain is part of

[12] It is important to note that the Cartesian conception of the body is quite mistaken. Descartes conceived of his body as an insensate machine – a material substance without sensation. But our actual conception of our body ascribes verbs of sensation to the body we have – it is our body that aches all over or that itches intolerably.

[13] The human brain is part of the human being. It can also be said to be part of the body a human being is said to have. It is, however, striking that one would, we suspect, hesitate to say of a living person, as opposed to a corpse, that their body *has* two legs or, of an amputee, that their body *has* only one leg. The misleading possessive is applied to the human being and to a human corpse, but not, or only hesitantly, to the body the living human being is said to have. Although the brain is a part of the human body, we surely would not say 'My body *has* a brain' or 'My body's brain has meningitis'. That is no coincidence.

the person, but rather that it is part of the person's body, whereas we would not hesitate to say that Jack's brain is a part of Jack, part of *this* ☞ human being, just as his legs and arms are parts of Jack. Why? Perhaps because 'person' is, as Locke stressed, 'a forensic term', but not a substance-name. So, if we use the term 'person' in contexts such as this, we indicate thereby that we are concerned primarily with human beings *qua* possessors of those characteristics that render them persons, in relative disregard of corporeal characteristics. Perhaps the following analogy will help: London is a part of the UK; the UK belongs to the European Union, but London does not. That does not prevent London from being part of the UK. So too Jack's being a person does not prevent his brain being part of him.

7.5 The Rationale of the Mereological Principle

Why should one accept Aristotle's principle and its neuroscientific heir? Why should we discourage neuroscientists from ascribing *consciousness, knowledge, perception*, etc. to the brain?

7.5.1 Consciousness

It is animals that are conscious or unconscious, and that may become conscious of something that catches their attention. It is the student, not his brain, who awakes and becomes conscious of what the lecturer is talking about, and it is the lecturer, not his brain, who is conscious of his students' boredom as they surreptitiously yawn. The brain is not an organ of consciousness. One sees with one's eyes and hears with one's ears, but one is not conscious with one's brain any more than one walks with one's brain.

An animal may be conscious without showing it. That is the *only* sense in which one can say, with Searle, that 'the very existence of consciousness has nothing to do with behaviour' (p. 104). But, *the concept* of consciousness is bound up with the behavioural grounds for ascribing consciousness to the animal. An animal does not have to exhibit such behaviour in order for it *to be* conscious. But only an animal to which such behaviour *can intelligibly be ascribed* can also be said, *either truly or falsely*, to be conscious. It makes no sense to ascribe consciousness or thought to a chair or an oyster, because there is no such thing as a chair or an oyster falling asleep and later waking up, or losing consciousness and then regaining it; and there is no such thing as a chair or an oyster behaving thoughtfully or thoughtlessly.[14] The 'ontological question' (as Searle put it) – the question of truth (as we should prefer to

---

[14] We agree with Searle that the question of which of the lower animals are conscious cannot be settled by 'linguistic analysis' (p. 104). But whereas he supposes that it can be settled by investigating their nervous system, we suggest that it can be settled by investigating the behaviour the animal displays in the circumstances of its life. Just as we find out whether an animal can see by reference to its responsiveness to visibilia, so too we find out whether an animal is capable of consciousness by investigating its behavioural repertoire and responsiveness to its environment. (That does not imply that being conscious is behaving in a certain way, only that the criteria for being conscious are behavioural.)

put it) – presupposes the antecedent determination of the question of sense. Agreement on the behavioural grounds for ascription of consciousness, i.e. on what *counts* as a manifestation of consciousness, is a precondition for scientific investigation into the neural conditions for being conscious. Otherwise one could not even identify what one wants to investigate. To distinguish the question of sense from the question of truth is not to confuse 'the rules for using words with the ontology', as Searle suggested (p. 105) – on the contrary, it is to distinguish them.[15]

Searle insisted that consciousness is a property of the brain. Sherrington, Eccles and Penfield, being Cartesians, thought it to be a property of the mind. What recent neuroscientific experiment can Searle cite to show that it is *actually* a property of the brain? After all, the only thing neuroscientists *could* discover is that certain neural states are inductively well correlated with, and causal conditions of, an *animal's* being conscious. But *that* discovery cannot show that it is *the brain* that is conscious. Is Searle's claim, then, a conceptual insight? No – for that is not the way the concept of *being conscious* is deployed. It is human beings (and other animals), not their brains (or their minds), that fall asleep and later awaken, that are knocked unconscious and later regain consciousness. So is it a linguistic recommendation: namely, that when a human being's brain is in a state that is inductively well correlated with the human being's being conscious, we should describe his brain as being conscious too? This is a convention we could adopt. We could introduce this derivative use of 'to be conscious'. It is necessarily parasitic on the primary use that applies to the human being as a whole. It is difficult, however, to see anything that recommends it. It is certainly not needed for the sake of clarity of neuroscientific description, and it adds nothing but an empty form to existing neuroscientific explanation.

7.5.2   Knowledge

Knowledge comprises abilities of complex kinds. The identity of an ability is determined by what it is an ability to do. The simplest grounds for ascribing an ability to an animal is that it engages in corporeal activities that manifest its abilities. The more complex the ability, the more diverse and diffuse the grounds. If an animal knows something, it can act and respond to its environment in ways that it cannot if it is ignorant; if it does so, it manifests its knowledge. The brain can be said to be the *vehicle* of these abilities, but what this means

---

[15] The warrant for applying psychological predicates to others consists of evidential grounds. These may be inductive or constitutive (criterial). Inductive grounds, in these cases, presuppose non-inductive, criterial grounds. The criteria for the application of a psychological predicate consist of behaviour (not mere bodily movements) in appropriate circumstances. The criteria are defeasible. That such-and-such grounds warrant the ascription of a psychological predicate to another is partly constitutive of the meaning of the predicate, but does not exhaust its meaning. Criteria for the application of such a predicate are distinct from its truth conditions – an animal may be in pain and not show it, or exhibit pain-behaviour without being in pain. (We are no behaviourists.) The truth conditions of a proposition ascribing a psychological predicate to a being are distinct from its truth. Both the criteria and the truth conditions are distinct from the general conditions under which the activities of applying *and* of denying the predicate of creatures can significantly be engaged in. But it is a mistake to suppose that a condition of 'the language-game's being played' (as Searle put it), is the *occurrence* of publicly observable behaviour. For the language-game with a psychological predicate is played with its denial no less than with its affirmation.

is that in the absence of the appropriate neural structures the animal would not be able to do what it can do. The neural structures in the brain are distinct from the abilities *the animal* has, and the operations of these structures are distinct from the exercise of the abilities *by the animal*. In short, the knower is also the doer, and his knowing is exhibited in what he does.

We pointed out that J. Z. Young, like so many neuroscientists, held that the brain contains knowledge and information 'just as knowledge and information can be recorded in books or computers' (1978, p. 192).[16] Dennett averred that we did nothing to establish that there is no concept of knowledge or information such that it cannot be said to be encoded in both books and brains (p. 91). In fact, we did discuss this (*PFN* 152f). But we shall explain again.

A code is a system of encrypting and/or information-transmission conventions parasitic on language. A code is not a language. It has neither a grammar nor a lexicon (cf. Morse code). Knowledge is not *encoded* in books, unless they are written in code. One can encode a message only if there is a code in which to do so. There is a code only if encoders and intended decoders agree on encoding conventions. In this sense there isn't, and couldn't be, a neural code. In the sense in which a book contains information, the brain contains none. In the sense in which a human being possesses information, the brain possesses none. That information can be derived from features of the brain (as dendrochronological information can be derived from a tree trunk) does not show that information is encoded in the brain (any more than it is in the tree trunk).

So, in the ordinary sense of 'knowledge', there can be no knowledge recorded, contained in, or possessed by the brain. Dennett then changed tack, and recommended that we attend to the cognitive scientific literature on *extensions* of the term 'knowledge' that might allow knowledge, in an extended sense, to be ascribed to the brain. And he recommended to our attention Chomsky's attempt to explain an extended concept of knowledge – namely, 'cognizing' – according to which human beings, and even neonates, cognize the principles of universal grammar (Chomsky, 1980).[17] According to Chomsky, someone who cognizes cannot tell one what he cognizes, cannot display the object of his cognizing, does not recognize what he cognizes when told, never forgets what he cognizes (but never remembers it either), has never learnt it and could not teach it. Apart from that, cognizing is just like knowing! Does *this* commend itself as a model for an intelligible extension of a term?

7.5.3   Perception

The perceptual faculties are powers to acquire knowledge by the use of one's sense-organs. An animal uses its eyes in glancing at, watching, peering at and looking at things. It is

---

[16] Dennett suggested (p. 91) that we misrepresented Crick in holding that because he wrote that our brain believes things, and makes interpretations on the basis of its previous experience or information (Crick, 1995, pp. 28–33, 57), therefore Crick really thought that the brain believes things and makes interpretations on the basis of its previous experience or information.

[17] Far from being oblivious to this, as Dennett asserted (p. 91), the matter was critically discussed in Baker and Hacker, 1984, pp. 340–5.

thus able to discriminate things that are coloured, that have distinctive shapes and move-ments. It exhibits its visual acumen in what it does in response to what it sees. It would not have these perceptual powers or be able to exercise them but for the proper func-tioning of appropriate parts of its brain. However, it is not the cerebral cortex that sees, but the animal. It is not the brain that moves closer to see better, looks through the bushes and under the hedges. It is not the brain that leaps to avoid a predator seen or charges the prey it sees – it is the perceiving animal. In short, the perceiver is also the actor.

In *Consciousness Explained*, Dennett ascribed psychological attributes to the brain. He asserted that it is conscious, gathers information, makes simplifying assumptions, makes use of supporting information, and arrives at conclusions (Dennett, 1993, pp. 142–4). This is to commit the very fallacy that both Aristotle and Wittgenstein warned against – the mereo-logical fallacy, as we called it. In his APA paper, Dennett conceded that it would be a fallacy to attribute *fully fledged* psychological predicates to parts of the brain (p. 87). Nevertheless, he holds, it is theoretically fruitful, and consistent with accepting the erroneous character of attributing predicates of wholes to their parts, to extend the psychological vocabulary, *duly attenuated*, from human beings and other animals to (a) computers and (b) parts of the brain. Indeed, he apparently holds that there is no difference of moment between these two extensions. But there *is* a difference. Attributing psychological properties (attenuated or otherwise) to computers is mistaken, but does not involve a mereological fallacy. Attributing such psychological properties to the brain or its parts is mistaken and does involve a mereo-logical fallacy. Taking the brain to be a computer and ascribing such psychological properties to it or its parts is doubly mistaken. We shall explain.

It is true that we do, in casual parlance, say that computers remember, that they search their memory, that they calculate, and sometimes, when they take a long time, we jocularly say that they are thinking things over. But this is merely a *façon de parler*. It is not a literal application of the terms 'remember', 'calculate' and 'think'. Computers are devices designed to fulfil certain functions for us. We can store information in a computer, as we can in a filing cabinet. But filing cabinets cannot remember anything, and neither can computers. We use computers to produce the results of a calculation – just as we used to use a slide-rule or a cylindrical mechanical calculator. Those results are produced without anyone or anything literally calculating – as is evident in the case of a slide-rule or a mechanical cal-culator. In order literally to calculate, one must have a grasp of a wide range of concepts, follow a multitude of rules that one must know, and understand a variety of operations. Computers do not and cannot.

Dennett suggests that 'it is an empirical fact . . . that *parts* of our brains engage in processes that are *strikingly like* guessing, deciding, believing, jumping to conclusions, etc. and it is *enough* like these personal level behaviors to warrant stretching ordinary usage to cover it' (p. 86). He agrees that it would be mistaken to 'attribute *fully-fledged* belief', decision, desire or pain to the brain. Rather, 'Just as a young child can *sort of* believe that her daddy is a doctor . . . , so . . . some part of a person's brain can *sort of* believe that there is an open door a few feet ahead' (p. 87).

This is part of what Dennett characterizes as 'the intentional stance' – a research meth-odology that supposedly helps neuroscientists to explain the neural foundations of human powers. He claims that adoption of the intentional stance has accomplished 'excellent scientific work . . . generating hypotheses to test, articulating theories, analysing distressingly complex phenomena into their more comprehensible parts' (p. 87). It seems committed to the idea that some parts of the brain 'sort of believe', that others *sort of decide*, and yet others *sort of oversee* these activities. All this, presumably, is supposed to *sort of explain* what neuroscientists want to explain. But if the explananda are uniformly sorts of believings, pseudo-expectings, proto-wantings and demi-decidings (as Dennett suggests), they at best only *sort of make sense*, and presumably are only *sort of true*. And how one can make valid inferences from such premises is more than just sort of obscure. How precisely such premises are supposed to *explain* the phenomena is equally obscure. For the logic of such putative explanations is altogether unclear. Does sort of believing, pseudo-believing, proto-believing or demi-believing (p. 89) something furnish a part of the brain with a reason for acting? Or only a sort of reason? – for a sort of action? When asked whether parts of the brain are, as Dennett puts it, 'real intentional systems', his reply is 'Don't ask' (p. 89).[18]

Cognitive neuroscientists ask *real* questions – they ask *how* the prefrontal cortices are involved in human thinking, *why* re-entrant pathways exist, *what* precisely are the roles of the hippocampus and neocortex in a human being's remembering. Being told that the hippocampus sort of remembers for a short while and that the neocortex has a better sort of long-term memory provides no explanation whatsoever. No well-confirmed empirical theory in neuroscience has emerged from Dennett's explanations, for ascribing 'sort of psychological properties' to parts of the brain does not *explain* anything. We shall revert to this when we discuss Sperry and Gazzaniga's account of commissurotomy. Not only does it not explain; it generates further incoherence.[19]

---

[18] See his autobiographical entry in Guttenplan, 1994, p. 240.

[19] Of course, we are not denying that analogical extension of concepts and conceptual structures is often fruitful in science. The hydrodynamical model generated a fruitful, testable, and mathematicized, theory of electricity. Nothing comparable to this is evident in the poetic licence of Dennett's intentional stance. It is evident that poetic licence allows Dennett to describe thermostats as *sort of believing* that it is getting too hot, and so switching off the central heating. But this adds nothing to engineering science or to the explanation of homeostatic mechanisms.

Dennett asserted (p. 87) that we did not address his attempts to use what he calls 'the intentional stance' in explaining cortical processes. In fact, we discussed his idea of the intentional stance at some length (*PFN* 427–31), giving seven reasons for doubting its intelligibility. Since Dennett has not replied to these objections, we have, for the moment, nothing further to add on the matter.

In the debate at the APA, Dennett proclaimed that there are 'hundreds, maybe thousands, of experiments' to show that a part of the brain has information which it contributes to 'an on-going interpretation process in another part of the brain'. This, he insisted, is a 'sort of asserting – a sort of telling "Yes, there is colour here", "Yes, there is motion here"'. This, he said, 'is just obvious'. But the fact that cells in the visual striate cortex fire in response to impulses transmitted from the retina does not mean that they have *information* or *sort of information* about objects in the visual field, and the fact that they respond to impulses does not mean that they *interpret* or *sort of interpret* anything. Or should we also argue that an infarct shows that the heart has sort of information about the lack of oxygen in the bloodstream and sort of interprets this as a sign of coronary obstruction? Or that my failing torch has information about the amount of electric current reaching its bulb and interprets this as a sign of the depletion of its batteries?

We agree with Dennett that many of a child's beliefs are beliefs in an attenuated sense. A little girl's grasp of the concept of a doctor may be defective, but she will rightly say 'Daddy is a doctor', and reply to the question 'Where is the doctor?' by saying 'In there ☞ (pointing to Daddy's office)'. So she can be said to believe, in an attenuated sense, that her father is a doctor. She satisfies, in her verbal and deictic behaviour, *some* of the normal criteria for believing that her father is a doctor (but also satisfies some of the criteria for lacking this belief). But there is no such thing as a part of a brain asserting things, as the child does, answering questions, as the child does, or pointing at things, as the child does. So in the sense in which, in her verbal and deictic behaviour, the child can manifest *rudimentary* belief, a part of a brain can no more do so than the whole brain can manifest fully-fledged belief. Or can Dennett suggest an *experimentum crucis* that will demonstrate that her prefrontal cortex sort of believes that the cat is under the sofa?

The child can also exhibit rudimentary belief in her non-verbal behaviour. If she sees the cat run under the sofa and toddles over to look for it, then she can be said to think that the cat is under the sofa. But brains and their parts cannot *behave*, cannot toddle over to the sofa, cannot look under it, and cannot look nonplussed when there is no cat there. Brain parts can neither voluntarily act nor take action. Unlike the child, brain parts cannot satisfy *any* of the criteria for believing something, even in a rudimentary sense. Brains (and their parts) can only 'sort of believe' in the sense in which they are 'sort of oceans' (since there are brainwaves), and are 'sort of weather-systems' (since there are brainstorms). The similarity between a brain and an ocean is at least as great as the similarity of brain processes to human beings' believings, decidings or guessings. After all, both brains and oceans are grey, have wrinkles on their surface, and have currents running through them.

7.6   The Location of Psychological Attributes

The question of whether the brain is a possible subject of psychological attributes is distinct from the question of whether the brain is the locus of those psychological attributes to which a corporeal location can intelligibly be assigned (*PFN* 122f, 179f). Our reasons for denying that the brain can be the subject of psychological attributes do not show that the brain is not the locus of such attributes to which it makes sense to assign a corporeal location. Nor were they meant to. Our view is that sensations such as pains and itches *can* be assigned a location. The location of a pain is where the sufferer points, in the limb that he assuages, in the part of his body he describes as hurting – for it is these forms of pain-behaviour that provide criteria for the location of pain. By contrast, thinking, believing, deciding and wanting, for example, cannot be assigned a *somatic* location. The answer to the questions 'Where did you think of that?', 'Where did he acquire that strange belief?', 'Where did she decide to get married?', is *never* 'In the prefrontal lobes, of course'. The criteria for where a human being thought of something, acquired a belief, made a decision, got angry or was astonished involve behaviour, to be sure, but not somatic-location-indicative behaviour. The location of a human being's thinking, recollecting, seeing, deciding, getting angry or being astonished is *where the human being is when he thinks*, etc.[20] Which part of his brain is involved in his doing so is a further, important question about which neuroscientists are gradually learning more. But they are not learning where thinking, recollecting or deciding occur – they are discovering which parts of the cortex are causally implicated in a human being's thinking, recollecting, deciding.

Of course, thinking about something, deciding to do something, seeing something, are, as Searle rightly said (p. 110), real events – they really happen somewhere, somewhen, in the world. I thought up that argument in the library and decided how to phrase it in my study; I saw Jack when I was in the street, and I listened to Jill's recital in the concert hall. Searle suggested that the question 'Where do mental events occur?' is no more philosophically puzzling than the question 'Where do digestive processes occur?' So, he argued, digestive processes occur in the stomach, and consciousness occurs in the brain. This is mistaken. Being conscious, as opposed to unconscious, being conscious of something, as opposed to not noticing it or not attending to it, do not occur *in* the brain at all. Of course, they occur *because of certain events in the brain*, without which a human being would not have regained consciousness or had his attention caught. 'Where did you become conscious of the sound of the clock?' is to be answered by specifying where I was when it caught my attention, just as 'Where did you regain consciousness?' is to be answered by specifying where I was when I came round.

Both digesting and thinking are predicated of animals. But it does not follow that there are no logical differences between them. The stomach can be said to be digesting food, but the brain cannot be said to be thinking. The stomach is the digestive organ, but the brain is no more an organ of thought than it is an organ of locomotion.[21] If one opens the stomach, one can see the digestion of the food going on there. But if one wants to see thinking going on, one should look at *le penseur* (or the surgeon operating, or the chess-player playing or the debater debating), not at his brain. All his brain can show is what goes on there *while he is thinking*; all that fMRI scanners can show is which parts of his brain are metabolizing more oxygen than others when the patient in the scanner is thinking.[22] (We

---

[20] Thinking does not occur *in* the human being, but rather is done *by* the human being. The *event* of my thinking that you were going to V is located wherever I was located when I thought this; the *event* of my seeing you V-ing is located wherever I was when I saw you V. That is the only sense in which thinking, perceiving, etc. have a location. To ask, as Searle does (p. 109), where *exactly* did the thinking occur, in any *other* sense, is like asking where exactly did a person weigh 160 pounds, in some sense other than that specified by the answer 'When he was in New York last year'. Sensations, by contrast, have a somatic location – if my leg hurts, then I have a pain in my leg. To be sure, my state (if state it be) of having a pain in my leg obtained wherever I was when my leg hurt.

[21] One needs a normally functioning brain to think or to walk, but one does not walk *with* one's brain. Nor does one think *with* it, any more than one hears or sees with it.

[22] Searle contended that because we repudiate qualia as understood by philosophers, therefore we can give no answer to the question of what *going through a mental process* consists in (p. 110). If *reciting the alphabet in one's imagination* (Searle's example) counts as a mental process, it consists in first saying to oneself 'a', then 'b', then 'c', etc. until one reaches 'x, y, z'. That mental process is not identified by its qualitative feel, but by its being the recitation of the alphabet. The criteria for its occurrence include the subject's say-so. Of course, it can be supposed to be accompanied by as yet unknown neural processes, the locus of which can be roughly identified by inductive correlation using fMRI.

ascribe length, strength and having cracks to steel girders. But it does not follow that *length* and *strength* have the same logical character; and one can ask where the crack is, but not where the strength is.)

So, sensations, such as pains, *are* located in our bodies. But Searle holds that they are all *in the brain*. It is, he admits, counterintuitive – after all, we complain of stomach-ache, of gout in our foot, or arthritis in our knees. Nevertheless, he claims, the brain creates a body image, and the pain that we describe as being in the foot, and which we assuage by rubbing the foot, is an awareness-of-the-pain-as-in-my-foot, which is in the body-image that is in one's brain. It is interesting that Descartes took a very similar view, remarking that 'pain in the hand is felt by the soul not because it is present in the hand but because it is present in the brain'. The advantage of his account, Searle suggests, is that it means that we can describe the phenomenon of phantom pain without the absurdity of suggesting that the pain is in physical space, in the bed or underneath the sheet. But that absurdity, he holds, is what we are committed to by claiming that pains are in the body. We agree on the absurdity, but deny that we are committed to it.

There are many locative uses of 'in', some spatial, some non-spatial ('in the story', 'in October', 'in committee'). Among spatial uses, there are many different kinds, depending on what is in what (*PFN* 123f). We agree with Searle that if there is a coin in my jacket pocket, and if my jacket is in the dresser, then there is a coin in the dresser. But not all spatial locative uses of 'in' are thus transitive. If there is a hole in my jacket and the jacket is in the wardrobe, it does not follow that there is a hole in the wardrobe. In the case of the jacket and the coin, we are concerned with spatial relations between two independent objects, but not in the case of the jacket and the hole. Similarly, if there is a crease in my shirt, and my shirt is in the suitcase, it does not follow that there is a crease in the suitcase. The coin may be taken out of the jacket pocket, and the shirt may be taken out of the suitcase, but the hole cannot be taken out of the pocket – it has to be sewn up, as the crease has to be ironed out, not taken out.

The use of 'in' with respect to the location of sensations is not like the coin, but more like the hole (though still different). A pain is not a substance. If I have a pain in my foot, I do not stand in any *relation* to a pain – rather, my foot hurts *there* ☞, and I can point to the place that hurts, which we call 'the location of the pain'. In the case of the phantom limb, it feels to the sufferer just as if he still has the limb that has been amputated, and he avows a pain in the illusory limb. It seems to him just as if his leg were hurting, although he has no leg. We agree with Searle that it is not the bed that hurts; nor is the pain that the amputee feels under the sheet. That he feels the pain where his leg would have been, and that his leg would have been under the sheet, do not imply that there is a pain under the sheet, any more than his having a pain in his unamputated leg and his leg being in his boot implies that he has a pain in his boot. Indeed, we agree with Searle about the phenomena, and disagree only over its description. That the amputee's pain is real, but its felt location is illusory (his leg does not hurt, as he has no leg), does not show that when a person who has *not* suffered an amputation feels a pain in his leg, its felt location is illusory too. It really is his leg that hurts! We do not think that there are body-images in the brain, and wonder what evidence there is for their existence – after all, one cannot find body-images if one opens up the brain of a human being. What Searle is apparently referring to is that physiological methods, beginning with those of Sherrington, have been used to establish that neurons in the somatosensory cortex can be excited in a topographical one-to-one relation with points stimulated on the surface of the body and with the spatial layout of the muscles of the limbs and trunk. But it is altogether unclear what Searle means by 'having a pain in a phenomenological phantom foot in a body image in the brain' (p. 119). One *can* have pains in one's *head* – they are commonly known as headaches. But one cannot have a backache or a stomach-ache in one's brain; or any other pain. And that is no coincidence, since there are no fibre-endings there save in the dura.

Finally, Searle claimed that when philosophers say that two people both have the same pain, what they mean is that they have the same type-pain, but different token-pains (p. 115). 'The token pain that they or I experience *exists only as it is perceived* by a particular conscious subject' (p. 116). This is mistaken. First of all, pains are not *perceived* by their sufferers. To *have* a pain is not to *perceive* a pain. 'I have a pain in my leg' no more describes a relation between me and an object called 'a pain' than does the equivalent sentence 'My leg hurts'. Secondly, Peirce's type/token distinction was applied to inscriptions and is dependent on orthographic conventions.[23] It no more applies to pains than it does to colours. If two armchairs are both maroon, then there are two chairs of the very same colour, and not two token-colours of the same type. For how is one to individuate the different tokens? Obviously not by location – since that merely distinguishes the two coloured chairs, not their colour. All one can say is that the first alleged token belongs to the first chair and the second to the second chair. But this is to individuate a property by reference to the pseudo-property of belonging to the substance that has it – as if properties were substances that are distinguished by means of Leibniz's law, and as if being the property of a given substance were a property that distinguishes, for example, the colour of *this* chair from the colour of *that* one. And that is absurd. The two chairs are both of the very same colour. Similarly, if two people have a splitting headache in their left temples, then they both have the very same pain. A's pain is not distinguishable from B's pain by virtue of the fact that it belongs to A, any more than the maroon colour of the first chair is distinguished from the maroon colour of the second chair by virtue of the fact that it belongs to the first. The distinction between qualitative and numerical identity does not apply to colours or to pains, and neither does the Peircean distinction between types and tokens.

7.7 Linguistic Anthropology, Auto-anthropology, Metaphor and Extending Usage

At the APA meeting, Professor Dennett suggested that to examine the use of words involves either a form of anthropology or a form of 'auto-anthropology'. For one has to discover the uses of words by doing appropriate social surveys, asking people to consult their intu-

---

[23] The American logician C. S. Peirce distinguished between type-words and token-words. In the sentence 'The cat sat on the mat' there are six token-words, but only five type-words, since there are two tokens of the same type-word 'the'. There are two tokens of the same type-word if and only if there are two distinct words inscribed, each containing the same letters in the same sequence. Peirce's distinction is adequate for his purposes, but not at all well defined. It should not be confused with the quite different distinctions between universal and particular, between a general concept and its instantiation, and between attribute and substance.

itions on correct word usage. Alternatively, one has to consult one's own intuitions; but then it might turn out that one's intuitions diverge from those of others. He averred that we did not consult the community of neuroscientists to discover their intuitions about their neuroscientific 'patois' of psychological predicates (p. 86), but only our own intuitions.

This is a misconception. A competent speaker of the language no more has to consult his intuitions (hunches, guesses) than a competent mathematician has to consult his intuitions concerning the multiplication tables or a competent chess-player has to consult his intuitions about the movements of chess pieces. It is an empirical fact, to be established by anthropologists, historical linguists, etc., that a given vocable or inscription is or was used in a certain way in a given linguistic community. It is not an empirical fact that a word, *meaning what it does*, has the conceptual connections, compatibilities and incompatibilities that it does. It is an empirical fact that the vocable 'black' is used by English speakers to mean what it does, but given that it means what it does, namely *this* ☞ ■ colour, it is not an empirical fact that the propositions 'Black is darker than white', 'Black is more like grey than like white', 'Nothing can be both black all over and white all over simultaneously' are true. These are conceptual truths specifying a part of the conceptual network of which *black* is a node. They are norms of representation, constitutive of the meaning of the word 'black'. They are, in effect, inference tickets. If A is black and B is white, such conceptual truths allow us to infer, independently of experience, that A is darker than B; and if C is grey, we may infer, without observation, that A is more like it (in respect of colour) than it is like B. Failure to acknowledge these truths and the validity of the corresponding inferences they license betokens a failure fully to have grasped the meaning of the word 'black'. A competent speaker is one who has mastered the usage of the common expressions of the language. It is not an intuition of his that black is *that* ☞ ■ colour, that a vixen is a female fox, or that to perambulate is to walk. It is not a hunch of his that a man is an adult male human being. And it is no guess of his that if it is ten o'clock, it is later than nine o'clock, or that if something is black all over, it is not also white all over.

Although competent speakers of a language agree in the language they use, deviations from common usage are not, *as such*, philosophically pernicious. Such deviations may betoken no more than a fragment of a personal idiolect or a special sociolect, a novel extension of a term or the appropriation of an existing term for a new technical use. That is why we wrote that if a competent speaker uses expressions contrary to usage, then it may well be that

> his words must not be taken to have their ordinary meaning. The problematic expressions were perhaps used in a special sense, and are really homonyms; or they were analogical *extensions* of the customary use, as is indeed common in science; or they were used in a metaphorical or figurative sense. If these escape routes are available, then the accusation that neuroscientists fall victim to the mereological fallacy is unwarranted. (*PFN* 74)

But that these escape routes are available is not a matter that can be taken for granted. Nor is the cogency of this application of the term a matter on which the speaker in question is the final authority. For even if he is introducing a new use, or employing his words figuratively, whether he does so coherently has to be seen. And whether he does so consistently, or rather moves unawares between a new use and an old one, drawing inferences from the former that are licensed only by the latter, has to be investigated. That is why we wrote:

> The final authority on the matter is *his own reasoning*. We must look at the consequences he draws from his own words – and it is his inferences that will show whether he was using the predicate in a new sense or misusing it. If he is to be condemned, it must be out of his own mouth. (*PFN* 74)

And we proceeded to demonstrate that numerous leading neuroscientists could indeed be condemned out of their own mouth, precisely because they draw inferences from their application of the psychological vocabulary to the brain that can only intelligibly be drawn from its customary application to the animal as a whole (*PFN* chs 3–8).

If a neuroscientist applies psychological expressions, or semantic expressions such as 'representations', or expressions like 'map', to the brain, then he is either using these in their customary sense or he is using them in a novel sense. The latter may be (i) a derivative sense, (ii) an analogical or other extension of the old term, (iii) a mere homonym, or (iv) a metaphorical or figurative sense. If psychological terms are applied to the brain in their customary sense, then what is said is not intelligible. We do not know what it means to say that the brain thinks, fears or is ashamed. The constitutive grounds upon which competent speakers of our language apply such expressions to animals and human beings – namely, what they say and do – cannot be satisfied by a brain or its parts – there is no such thing as a brain or part of a brain making thoughtful observations, running away in fear, or blushing in shame. We no more understand what it would be for a brain or its parts to think, reason, fear or decide something than we understand what it would be for a tree to do so. If such terms are being applied in a novel sense, then the user owes us an explanation of what that sense is. It may be a derivative sense, as when we apply the term 'healthy' to food or exercise – a use that needs a different explanation from the explanation appropriate for the primary use of 'health' in application to a living being. It may be an analogical use, as when we speak of the foot of a mountain or of a page – such analogies are typically evident, but obviously call out for a very different paraphrastic explanation than that demanded by their prototype. Or it may be a homonym, like 'mass' in Newtonian mechanics, which requires a quite different explanation from 'mass' in 'a mass of people' or 'a mass of poppies'.

Neuroscientists' use of 'representation' is, for the most part, intended as a mere homonym of 'representation' in its symbolic and semantic sense. This has turned out to be ill-advised, for eminent scientists and psychologists have succumbed to the confusion of using the word both to mean a causal correlate or a concomitance and also to mean a symbolic representation. For it is in the former sense alone that it makes sense to speak of representations in the brain. Hence our criticisms of David Marr (*PFN* 70, 76, 143–7). Neuroscientists' use of the term 'map' appears to have begun life as an extension of the idea of a mapping, but it rapidly became confused with that of a map. There is nothing wrong with calling the set of entities on to which members of another set can be mapped 'a map' of the latter – although it is neither necessary nor clear. But incoherence is afoot if one then suppose that this 'map' might be used by the brain in the manner in which readers of an atlas use maps. It is altogether obscure what is meant by the claim that the brain or its parts know, believe, think, infer and perceive things. The only coherent idea that might be lurking here is that these terms are applied to the brain to signify the neural activity that supposedly corresponds with the animal's knowing, believing, thinking, inferring and perceiving. But then one cannot intelligibly go on to assert (as Crick, Sperry and Gazzaniga do) that the part of the brain that is thinking communicates *what it thinks* to another part of the brain. For while human thinking has a content (given by the answer to the question 'What are you thinking?'), neural activity cannot be said to have any content whatsoever.

It might be suggested that neuroscientists' talk of *maps* or *symbolic descriptions* in the brain and of the brain's knowing, thinking, deciding, interpreting, etc. is metaphorical (as is asserted by Churchland, 2005, pp. 469f, 474). These terms, one might claim, are actually probing metaphors the aptness of which is already long established with regard to *electronic computers*, which are aptly described as 'following rules'. For computers were '*deliberately built* to engage in the rule-governed manipulation of complex symbols'. Indeed, one might think, such talk 'is not even metaphorical any longer, given the well developed theoretical and technological background against which such talk takes place' (Churchland, 2005, p. 470). Similarly, cognitive neuroscientists, in their use of the common psychological vocabulary, 'are indeed groping forward in the darkness; metaphors are indeed the rule rather than the exception'. But this is normal scientific progress, and in some cases, neuroscience has advanced beyond metaphor, e.g. in ascription of 'sentence-like representations' and 'map-like representations' to the brain.

This can be questioned. Computers cannot correctly be described as following rules any more than planets can correctly be described as complying with laws. The orbital motion of the planets is *described* by the Keplerian laws, but the planets do not *follow* the laws of nature. Computers were not built to 'engage in rule-governed manipulation of symbols', they were built to produce results that will *coincide* with rule-governed, *correct* manipulation of symbols. For computers can no more *follow* a rule than can a mechanical calculator. A machine can execute operations that accord with a rule, provided all the causal links built into it function as designed and assuming that the design ensures the generation of a regularity in accordance with the chosen rule or rules. But for something to constitute following a rule, the mere production of a regularity in accordance with a rule is not sufficient. A being can be said to be following a rule only in the context of a complex practice involving actual and potential activities of justifying, noticing mistakes and correcting them by reference to the rule, criticizing deviations from the rule, and, if called upon, explaining an action as being in accordance with the rule and teaching others what counts as following a rule. The determination of an act as being *correct*, in accordance with the rule, is not a causal determination but a logical one. Otherwise we should have to surrender to whatever results our computers produce. (For further discussion, see Hacker, 1993, pp. 72–81.)

To be sure, computer engineers use such language – harmlessly, until such time as they start to treat it literally and suppose that computers really think, better and faster than we do, that they truly remember, and unlike us never forget, that they interpret what we type in, and sometimes misinterpret it, taking what we wrote to mean something other than we meant. *Then* the engineers' otherwise harmless style of speech ceases to be an amusing shorthand and becomes a potentially pernicious conceptual confusion.

To say that computers or brains think, calculate, reason, infer and hypothesize *may* be intended metaphorically. Metaphors do not explain – they illustrate one thing in terms of another. A metaphor ceases to be a metaphor when it becomes a dead metaphor, like 'a broken heart' or 'at one fell swoop'. But it cannot cease to be a metaphor by becoming literal. What would it be for it to be *literally* true that the planets obey the laws of nature? A slide-rule, mechanical calculator or computer can be said to calculate – figuratively speaking. But what would it be for it to do so literally? If 'the computer remembers (calculates, infers, etc.)' makes perfect (non-figurative) sense to computer engineers, that is precisely because they treat these phrases as dead metaphors. 'The computer calculates' means no more than 'The computer goes through the electrico-mechanical processes necessary to produce the results of a calculation without any calculation', just as 'I love you with all my heart' means no more than 'I truly love you'.

It is noteworthy that neuroscientists' talk of there being maps in the brain, and of the brain using these maps as maps, is, in the cases that we criticized, anything but metaphorical. Colin Blakemore's remark that 'neuroanatomists have come to speak of the brain having *maps*, which are thought to play an essential part in the representation and interpretation of the world by the brain, *just as the maps of an atlas do for the reader of them*' (1990, p. 265; emphasis added) is obviously not metaphorical, since there is nothing metaphorical about 'Maps of an atlas play a role in the representation of the world for their readers'. Moreover, 'representation' here is patently used in the symbolic sense, not the causal correlate sense. Nor is J. Z. Young's assertion that the brain makes use of its maps in formulating its hypotheses about what is visible (1978, p. 112). For *to make use of a map in formulating a hypothesis* is to take a feature indicated by the map as a *reason* for the hypothesis. Dennett asserted that the brain '*does* make use of them *as* maps' (Bennett et al., 2007, n. 20 in Dennett's chapter, pp. 73–95), and in the debate at the APA he asserted that it is an empirical, not a philosophical, question whether 'retinotopical maps' are used by the brain *as* maps, 'whether any of the information-retrieval operations that are defined over them exploit features of maps that we exploit when we exploit maps in the regular world'. But it could be an empirical question only if it made sense for the brain to use a map as a map. However, to *use* a map as a map, there has to *be* a map – and there are none in the brain; one has to be able to read the map – but brains lack eyes and cannot read; one has to be familiar with the projective conventions of the map (e.g. cylindrical, conic, azimuthal) – but there are no projective *conventions* regarding the mappings of features of the visual field on to the neural firings in the 'visual' striate cortex; and one has to use the map to guide one's behaviour – one's perambulations or navigations – which are not activities that brains engage in. One must not confuse a map with the possibility of a mapping. That one can map the firing of retinal cells on to the firing of cells in the visual striate cortex does not show that there is a map of visibilia in the visual field in the visual striate cortex.

Churchland supposes that because the neurons in V1 are roughly spatially homologous to, and react to, the retinal cells stimulated by a light array, one can speak of there being *an image* of the external stimulus on the cortical surface. He seeks to persuade his readers of the truth of this claim by illustrating a computer-generated image of neural activity in V1 in response to a bull's-eye pattern placed before a monkey's eyes. But this is altogether deceptive. There is indeed an image on the electronic screen – a representation of the pattern of activated cells in the monkey's 'visual' striate cortex. But there is no *image* in the monkey's brain. (There is an image of the regional temperatures on the television weather forecast, but that does not imply that there is an image in the atmosphere.) Churchland further insists that populations of cortical neurons connected with the neurons of V1, for example, in V2, V4, MT, etc., 'are in a good position to exploit . . . the spatial information evidently contained in V1's cortical image of the original external stimulus' (2005, p. 466). But there is no *information* contained in the active cells of V1, and the further neurons can no more 'exploit information' than they can reflect on information, draw inferences and construct explanatory hypotheses. The fact that neuroscientists can *derive* information from their knowledge of the pattern of active neurons in an animal's 'visual' striate cortex does not show that the neurons possess information (as the animal may) or contain information (as books may). (That dendrochronologists can derive information about historical weather patterns from their knowledge of tree rings does not show that trees possess or contain information about past weather.)

Finally, we should like to rectify a misunderstanding. Some of our critics assume that we are trying to lay down a law prohibiting novel extensions of expressions in the language. Dennett asserted in the debate at the APA that we would outlaw talk of the genetic *code*, given that we insist that knowledge cannot be *encoded* in the brain. Churchland supposes that we would in principle exclude such conceptual innovations as Newton's talk of the moon constantly *falling* towards the earth as it moves upon its inertial path. This is a misunderstanding.

We are not prohibiting anything – only pointing out when conceptual incoherences occur in neuroscientific writings. We are not trying to stop anyone from extending usage in scientifically fruitful ways – only trying to ensure that such putative extensions do not transgress the bounds of sense through failure adequately to specify the novel use or through crossing the novel use with the old one. There is nothing wrong with talking about the *foot* of a mountain – as long as one does not wonder whether it has a shoe. There is nothing wrong with speaking of *unhealthy* food – as long as one does not wonder when it will regain its health. There is nothing wrong with talk of the *passing* of time – as long as one does not get confused (as Augustine famously did) about how to measure it. There was nothing wrong with Newton's talking about the moon's 'falling' towards the earth[24] – but

---

[24] Churchland parodies our criticism of neuroscientists by a mock criticism of Newton. But the fact that Newton was not confused in his extension of the term 'to fall' (or 'force' and 'mass') goes no way to show that contemporary neuroscientists are not confused in their application of the psychological vocabulary. Our criticisms should be compared not to Churchland's parody, but to Berkeley's criticisms of Newton's unclarities about infinitesimals in *The Analyst* and *A Defence of Free-Thinking in Mathematics*. These conceptual unclarities were not eradicated until the nineteenth-century work of Bolzano, Cauchy, Weierstrass and Dedekind. Of course, Berkeley's criticisms were not meant to undermine the calculus, and neither are our criticisms of cognitive neuroscience meant to undermine neuroscience. We aim only to eradicate conceptual confusions and incoherent explanations.

there would have been had he wondered what made the moon slip. There was nothing wrong with his speaking of forces acting on a body in space – but there would have been had he speculated whether the forces were infantry or cavalry. There is nothing wrong with geneticists speaking of the genetic code. But there would be if they drew inferences from the existence of the genetic code that can be drawn only from the existence of literal codes. For to be sure, the genetic code is not a code in the sense in which one uses a code to encrypt or transmit a sentence of a language. It is not even a code in 'an attenuated sense', as a sentence agreed between husband and wife to talk over the heads of the children might be deemed to be.

Our concern was with the use, by cognitive neuroscientists, of the common-or-garden psychological vocabulary (and other terms such as 'representation' and 'map') in specifying the explananda of their theories and in describing the explanans. For, as we made clear, neuroscientists commonly try to explain human beings' perceiving, knowing, believing, remembering, deciding by reference to parts of the brain perceiving, knowing, believing, remembering and deciding. So, we noted such remarks, made by leading neuroscientists, psychologists and cognitive scientists, as the following:

J. Z. Young (1978, p. 119): 'We can regard all seeing as a continual search for the answers to questions posed by the brain. The signals from the retina constitute "messages" conveying these answers. The brain then uses this information to construct a suitable hypothesis of what is there.'

C. Blakemore (1990, p. 265): 'the brain [has] maps, which are thought to play an essential part in the representation and interpretation of the world by the brain, just as the maps of an atlas do for the readers of them.'

G. Edelman (1994, p. 130): The brain 'recursively relates semantic to phonological sequences and then generates their syntactic correspondences . . . by treating rules developing in memory as objects for conceptual manipulation.'

J. Frisby (1980, p. 8): 'there must be a symbolic description in the brain of the outside world, a description cast in symbols which stand for various aspects of the world of which sight makes us aware.'

F. Crick (1995, p. 170): 'When the callosum is cut, the left hemisphere sees only the right half of the visual field . . . both hemispheres can hear what is being said . . . one half of the brain appears to be almost totally ignorant of what the other half saw.'

S. Zeki (1999, p. 2054): '. . . the brain's capacity to acquire knowledge, to abstract and to construct ideals . . .'

D. Marr (1982, pp. 20f): 'our brains must somehow be capable of representing . . . information . . . The study of vision must therefore include . . . an inquiry into the nature of the internal representations by which we capture this information and make it available as a basis for decisions . . .

. . . a representation is a formal scheme for describing . . . together with rules that specify how the scheme is to be applied. . . . [a formal scheme is] a set of symbols with rules for putting them together. . . . a representation, therefore, is not a foreign idea at all – we all use representations all the time.'

These are not metaphorical uses. They are not bold extensions of terms, introducing new meanings for theoretical purposes. They are simply misuses of the common psychological (and semantic) vocabulary – misuses that lead to incoherence and various forms of nonsense, which we pointed out from case to case. There is nothing surprising about this. It is no different, in principle, from the equally misguided applications of the same vocabulary *to the mind* – as if it were my mind that knows, believes, thinks, perceives, feels pain, wants and decides – but it is not; it is I, the living human being that I am, that does so. The former error is no less egregious than the (venerable) latter one, and is rife among cognitive neuroscientists – sometimes to the detriment of the experiments they devise, commonly to their theorizing about the results of their experiments, and often to their explaining animal and human cognitive functions by reference to the neural structures and operations that make them possible.

7.8   Qualia

In our discussion of consciousness (*PFN*, chs 9–12), we argued that characterizing the domain of the mental by reference to the 'qualitative feel' of experience is misconceived (*PFN*, ch 10). But *pace* Searle (p. 101), we did not deny the existence of qualia on the grounds that if they did exist, they would exist in brains. If, *per impossibile*, psychological attributes were all characterized by their 'qualitative feel', they would still be attributes of human beings, not of brains.

A quale is supposed to be 'the qualitative feel of an experience' (Chalmers, 1996, p. 4), or it is such a thing as 'the redness of red or the painfulness of pain' (Crick, 1995, pp. 9f). Qualia are 'the simple sensory qualities to be found in the blueness of the sky or the sound of a tone' (Damasio, 1999, p. 9); or 'ways it feels to see, hear and smell, the way it feels to have a pain' (Block, 1994, p. 514). According to Searle, conscious states are 'qualitative in the sense that for any conscious state . . . there is something that it qualitatively feels like to be in that state (1997, p. xiv). According to Nagel for every conscious experience, 'there is something it is like for the organism to have it' (1979, p. 170). These various explanations *do not amount to the same thing*, and it is questionable whether a coherent account emerges from them.

Searle remarks that there is a qualitative feel to a pain, a tickle and an itch. To this we agree – in the following sense: sensations, we remarked (*PFN* 124), have phenomenal qualities (e.g. burning, stinging, gnawing, piercing, throbbing); they are linked with felt inclinations to behave (to scratch, assuage, giggle or laugh); they have degrees of intensity which may wax or wane.

When it comes to perceiving, however, we noted that it is problematic to characterize what is meant by 'the qualitative character of experience'. Specifying what we see or smell, or, in the case of hallucinations, what it seems to us that we see or smell, requires specification of an object. Visual or olfactory experiences and their hallucinatory counterparts are individuated by what they are experiences or hallucinations of.

Seeing a lamp-post is distinct from seeing a postbox, smelling lilac is different from smelling roses, and so too are the corresponding hallucinatory experiences that are described in terms of their seeming to the subject to be like their veridical perceptual counterpart.[25]

To be sure, roses do not smell like lilac – what roses smell like is different from what lilac smells like. Smelling roses is quite different from smelling lilac. But the qualitative character of smelling roses does not smell of roses, any more than the qualitative character of smelling lilac smells of lilac. Smelling either may be equally pleasant – in which case the qualitative character of the smelling may be exactly the same, even though what is smelled is quite different. Searle, we suggest, confuses what the smells are like with what the smelling is like.

Seeing a lamp-post does not normally feel like anything. If asked 'What did it feel like to see it?', the only kind of answer is one such as 'It didn't feel like anything in particular – neither pleasant nor unpleasant, neither exciting nor dull'. *Such* epithets – 'pleasant', 'unpleasant', 'exciting', 'dull' – *are* correctly understood as describing the 'qualitative character of the experience'. In this sense, *many* perceptual experiences have no qualitative character at all. *None* is individuated by its qualitative feel – they are individuated by their object. And if we are dealing with a hallucination, then saying that the hallucinated lamp-post was black is still a description of the object of the experience – its 'intentional object' in Brentano's jargon (which Searle uses). The quality of the hallucinatory experience, on the other hand, is probably: *rather scary*.

Contrary to what Searle suggests, we did not argue that 'if you do not define qualia as a matter of pleasantness or unpleasantness then you will have to individuate the experience by its object' (p. 115). Our argument was that we *do* individuate experiences and hallucinations by their objects – which are specified by the answer to the question 'What was your experience (or hallucination) an experience (or hallucination) *of?*'[26] Of course, the object need not be the cause, as is evident in the case of hallucinations. But, we insisted, the qualitative character of the experience should not be confused with the qualities of the object of the experience. That what one sees when one sees a red apple is red and round does not imply that one enjoyed a red, round visual experience. That what one seems to see when one hallucinates a red apple is red and round does not imply that one enjoyed a red, round visual hallucination. 'What did you see (or hallucinate)?' is one question; 'What was it like to see what you saw (or hallucinate what you hallucinated)?' another. One does not individuate perceptual experiences by their qualitative character. These are simple truths; but they seem to have been overlooked.

---

[25] Searle (like Grice and Strawson) supposes that perceptual experiences are to be characterized in terms of their highest common factor with illusory and hallucinatory experiences. So all perceptual experience is, as it were, hallucination, but veridical perception is a hallucination with a special kind of cause. This, we think, is mistaken.

[26] Searle asserts that we deny the existence of qualitative experiences (p. 100). We certainly do not deny that people have visual experiences, i.e. that they see things. Nor do we deny that seeing things may have certain qualities. What we deny is that whenever someone sees something, there is something it is like for them to see that thing, let alone that there is something it feels like for them to see what they see. And we deny that 'the *qualitative* feel of the experience' is its 'defining essence' (p. 115). Seeing or hearing is not defined by reference to what it feels like, but by reference to what it enables us to detect.

7.9   Enskulled Brains

Searle suggests that human beings are 'embodied brains' (p. 121). According to his view, the reason why we can say both 'I weigh 160 lbs' and 'My body weighs 160 lbs' is that what makes it the case that I weigh 160 lbs is that my body does. But I, it seems, am strictly speaking no more than an embodied (enskulled) brain. I *have* a body, and I am *in* the skull *of* my body. This is a materialist version of Cartesianism. One major reason why we wrote our book was the firm belief that contemporary neuroscientists, and many philosophers too, still stand in the long, dark shadow of Descartes. For while rejecting the immaterial substance of the Cartesian mind, they transfer the attributes of the Cartesian mind to the human brain instead, leaving intact the whole misconceived structure of the Cartesian conception of the relationship between mind and body. What we were advocating was that neuroscientists, and even philosophers, leave the Cartesian shadow-lands and seek out the Aristotelian sunlight, where one can see so much better.

If I were, *per impossibile*, an embodied brain, then I would have a body – just as the Cartesian embodied mind has a body. But I would not *have* a brain, since brains do not have brains. And in truth my body would not weigh 160 lbs, but 160 lbs less 3 lbs – which is, strictly speaking, what *I* would weigh. And I would not be 6 foot tall, but only 7 inches tall. Doubtless Searle will assure me that I am my embodied brain – my brain *together* with my body. But that does not get us back on track. For my brain together with my brainless body, taken one way, is just my cadaver; taken another way, it is simply *my body*. But I am not my body, not the body *I have*. Of course, I am *a* body – the living human being that stands before you, a particular kind of sentient spatio-temporal continuant that possesses intellect and will and is therefore a person. But I am no more *my body* than I am *my mind*. And I am not an embodied brain either. It is mistaken to suppose that human beings are 'embodied' at all – that conception belongs to the Platonic, Augustinian and Cartesian tradition that should be repudiated. It would be far better to say, with Aristotle, that human beings are *ensouled* creatures (*empsuchos*) – animals endowed with such capacities as confer upon them, in the form of life that is natural to them, the status of persons.

7.10   Cognitive Neuroscience

Our critics suggested that our investigations are irrelevant to neuroscience, or – even worse – that our advice would be positively harmful if followed. Dennett averred that our refusal to ascribe psychological attributes (even in an attenuated sense) to anything less than an animal as a whole is retrograde and unscientific. This, he believes, stands in contrast to the scientific benefits of the 'intentional stance' that he advocates. In his view, 'the poetic license granted by the intentional stance eases the task' of explaining how the functioning of parts contributes to the behaviour of the animal (p. 89).

We note first that *poetic licence* is something granted to poets for purposes of poetry, not for purposes of empirical precision and explanatory power. Secondly, ascribing cognitive powers to parts of the brain provides only the semblance of an explanation where an explanation is still wanting. So it actually blocks scientific progress. Sperry and Gazzaniga claim that in cases of commissurotomy, the bizarre behaviour of subjects under experimental conditions of exposure to pictured objects is *explained* by the fact that one hemisphere of the brain is ignorant of what the other half can see. The hemispheres of the brain allegedly know things and can explain things, and, because of the severance of the corpus callosum, the right hemisphere allegedly cannot communicate to the left hemisphere what it sees. So the left hemisphere must generate its own interpretation of why the left hand is doing what it is doing (Wolford et al., 2000, p. 2). Far from explaining the phenomena, this masks the absence of any substantial explanation by redescribing them in misleading terms. The dissociation of functions normally associated is indeed partially explained by the severing of the corpus callosum and by the localization of function in the two hemispheres. *That* is now well known, but currently available explanation goes no further. It is an illusion to suppose that anything whatsoever is added by ascribing knowledge, perception and linguistic understanding ('sort of', or otherwise) to the hemispheres of the brain.

Searle claimed that central questions in neurobiological research would be rejected as meaningless if our account of the conceptual structures deployed were correct. So, he suggests, 'the central question in vision, how do neurobiological processes . . . cause conscious visual experiences, could not be investigated by anyone who accepted [our] conception' (p. 124). Our conception, he avers, 'can have potentially disastrous scientific consequences' (ibid.).

Research on the neurobiology of vision is research into the neural structures that are causally necessary for an animal to be able to see, and into the specific processes involved in its seeing. That we deny that visual experiences occur in the brain, or that they are characterized by qualia, affects this neuroscientific research program only in so far as it averts futile questions that could have no answer. We gave numerous examples, e.g. the binding problem (Crick, Kandel and Wurtz), the explanation of recognition by reference to the matching of templates with images (Marr), and the suggestion that perceptions are hypotheses of the brain that are conclusions of unconscious inferences it makes (Helmholtz, Gregory, and Blakemore). Our contention that it is the animal that sees or has visual experiences, not the brain, and Searle's contention that it is the brain, not the animal, are conceptual claims, not empirical ones. The issue is none the less important for all that; but it should be evident that what we said does not *hinder* empirical investigation into the neural processes that underpin vision. Rather, it guides the description of the results of such investigations down the highroads of sense.

In general, the conceptual criticisms in our work do no more than peel away layers of conceptual confusion from neuroscientific research and clarify the conceptual forms it presupposes. This cannot impede the progress of neuroscience. Indeed, it should facilitate it – by excluding nonsensical questions, preventing misconceived experiments, and reducing misunderstood experimental results. It is this that we have tried to do in this book by surveying the history of cognitive neuroscience of the last century.

References

Abel, T., Nguyen, P. V., Barad, M., Deuel, T. A. S., Kandel, E. R. and Bourtchouladze, R., 1997. Genetic demonstration of a role for PKA in the late phase of LTP and in hippocampus-based long-term memory. *Cell* 88, 615–26.

Albright, T. D., Jessel, T. M., Kandel, E. R. and Posner, M. I., 2000. Neural science: A century of progress and the mysteries that remain. *Cell* 100, S1–S55.

Altmann, G. T. M. (ed.), 2002. *Psycholinguistics: Critical Concepts in Psychology*. Routledge, New York.

Amaral, D., Price, J. L., Pitkanen, A. and Carhael, S. T., 1992. Anatomical organization of the primate amygdaloid complex. In J. P. Aggleton (ed.), *The Amygdala: A Functional Analysis*, pp. 1–66. Wiley-Liss, New York.

Andersen, P., Eccles, J. C. and Loyning, Y., 1963. Recurrent inhibition in the hippocampus with identification of the inhibitory cell and its synapses. *Nature* 198, 541–2.

Baker, G. P. and Hacker, P. M. S., 1984. *Language, Sense and Nonsense*. Blackwell, Oxford.

Bannerman, D. M., Good, M. A., Butcher, S. P., Ramsay, M. and Morris, R. G., 1995. Distinct components of spatial learning revealed by prior training and NMDA receptor blockade. *Nature* 378, 182–6.

Barlow, H. B., 1972. Single units and sensation: a neuron doctrine for perceptual psychology? *Perception* 1, 371–94.

Barlow, H. B., 1997. The neuron doctrine in perception. In M. S. Gazzaniga (ed.), *The New Cognitive Neurosciences*, ch. 26. MIT Press, Cambridge, Mass.

Bartsch, D., Ghirardi, M., Skehel, P. A., Karl, K. A., Herder, S. P., Chen, M., Bailey, C. H. and Kandel, E. R., 1995. *Aplysia* CREB2 represses long-term facilitation: relief of repression converts transient facilitation into long-term functional and structural change. *Cell* 83, 979–92.

Baynes, M. and Gazzaniga, M. S., 2000. Consciousness, introspection and the split brain. In Gazzaniga 2000, ch. 94.

Bechara, A., Damasio, H. and Damasio, A. R., 2000. Emotion, decision making and the orbitofrontal cortex. *Cereb. Cortex* 10, 295–307.

Bechara, A., Tranel, D., Damasio, H., Adolphs, R., Rockland, C. and Damasio, A. R., 1995. Double dissociation of conditioning and declarative knowledge relative to the amygdala and hippocampus in humans. *Science* 269, 115–18.

Bechara, A., Tranel, D., Damasio, H. and Damasio, A. R., 1996. Failure to respond autonomically to anticipated future outcomes following damage to prefrontal cortex. *Cereb. Cortex* 6, 215–25.

Beevor, C. E. and Horsley, V. A., 1887. A minute analysis (experimental) of the various movements produced by stimulating in the monkey different regions of the cortical centre for the upper limb, as defined by Professor Ferrier. *Phil. Trans. Roy. Soc. Lond.* 178, 153–67.

Beevor, C. E. and Horsley, V. A., 1890. A record of the results obtained by electrical excitation of the so-called motor cortex and internal capsule in an organg-outang (Simia satyrus). *Phil. Trans. Roy. Soc. Lond.* 181, 129–58.

Beevor, C. E. and Horsley, V. A., 1894. A further minute analysis by electrical stimulation of the so-called motor regions (facial area) of the cortex cerebri in the monkey, Macacus sinicus. *Phil. Trans. Roy. Lond.* 185, 39–81.

Bell, C., 1806. *Essay on the Anatomy and Physiology of Expression*. Longman, Reese, Hurst and Orme, London.

Bennett, M. R., 1993. Understanding the brain in the 21st century. *Proc. Roy. Soc. N.S.W.* 123/3–4, 167–90.

Bennett, M. R., 1997. *The Idea of Consciousness*. Gordon & Breach, London.

Bennett, M. R., 1999. The early history of the synapse: from Plato to Sherrington. *Brain Res. Bull.* 50, 95–118.

Bennett, M. R., 2001. *History of the Synapse*. Taylor & Francis, London.

Bennett, M. R. and Hacker, P. M. S., 2001. Perception and memory in neuroscience: a conceptual analysis. *Prog. Neurobiol.* 65, 499–543.

Bennett, M. R. and Hacker, P. M. S., 2003. *Philosophical Foundations of Neuroscience*. Blackwell, Oxford.

Bennett, M. R. and Hacker, P. M. S., 2005. Emotion and cortical-subcortical function: conceptual developments. *Proc. Neurobiol.* 75/1: 29–52.

Bennett, M. R., Dennett, D., Hacker, P. M. S. and Searle, J., 2007. *Neuroscience and Philosophy – Brain Mind and Language*. Columbia University Press, New York.

Bennett, M. R., Gibson, W. G. and Robinson, J., 1994. Dynamics of the CA3 pyramidal neuron autoassociative memory network in the hippocampus. *Phil. Trans. Roy. Soc. Lond.* B 343, 167–87.

Berger, H., 1930. Über das Elektrenkephalogramm des Menschen, II. *J. Psychol. Neurol.* 40, 160–79.

Bernard, C., 1858. *Leçons sur la Physiologie et la Pathologie du Système Nerveux*. Ballière, Paris.

Blair, R. J., Morris, J. S., Frith, C. D., Perrett, D. I. and Dolan, R. J., 1999. Dissociable neural responses to facial expressions of sadness and anger. *Brain* 122, 883–93.

Blakemore, C., 1973. The baffled brain. In R. L. Gregory and E. H. Gombrich (eds), *Illusion in Nature and Art*, Duckworth, London.

Blakemore, C., 1977. *Mechanics of the Mind*. Cambridge University Press, Cambridge.

Blakemore, C., 1990. Understanding images in the brain. In H. Barlow, C. Blakemore and M. Weston-Smith (eds), *Images and Understanding*, Cambridge University Press, Cambridge. pp. 257–83.

Bliss, T. V. and Gardner-Medwin, A. R., 1973. Long-lasting potentiation of synaptic transmission in the dentate area of the unanaesthetized rabbit following stimulation of the perforant path. *J. Physiol.* 232, 357–74.

Bliss, T. V. and Lomo, T., 1970. Plasticity in a monosynaptic cortical pathway. *J. Physiol.* (Lond.) 207, 61P.

Bliss, T. V. and Lomo, T., 1973. Long-lasting potentiation of synaptic transmission in the dentate area of the anaesthetised rabbit following stimulation of the perforant path. *J. Physiol. (Lond.)* 232, 331–56.

Block, N., 1994. Qualia. In Guttenplan, 1994, pp. 514–20.

Bolshakov, V. Y., Golan, H., Kandel, E. R. and Siegelbaum, S. A., 1997. Recruitment of new sites of synaptic transmission during the cAMP-dependent late phase of LTP at CA3–CA1 synapses in the hippocampus. *Neuron* 19, 635–51.

Braver, T. S., Cohen, J. D., Nystrom, L. E., Jonides, J., Smith, E. E. and Noll, D. C., 1997. A parametric study of prefrontal cortex involvement in human working memory. *Neuroimage* 5, 49–62.

Breiter, H. C., Ectoff, N. L., Whalen, P. J., Kennedy, D. N., Rauch, S. L., Buckner, R. L., Strauss, M. M., Hyman, S. E. and Rosen, B. X., 1996. Response and habituation of the human amygdala during visual processing of facial expression. *Neuron* 2, 875–87.

Brindley, G. S., 1967. The classification of modifiable synapses and their use in models for conditioning. *Proc. Roy. Soc. Lond.* B 168, 361–76.

Broadbent, D. E., 1958. *Perception and Communication*. Pergamon, New York.

Broadbent, D. E., 1970. Stimulus set and response set: two kinds of selective attention: In D. I. Mostofsky (ed.), *Attention: Contemporary Theory and Analysis*, pp. 51–60. Appleton-Century-Crofts, New York.

Broca, P., 1861. 'Remarques sur le siège de la faculté du language articulè, suivies d'une observation d'aphéme (perte de la parole)'. *Bulletins de la Societié Anatomique* (Paris), 6, 330–57, 398–407. Translated as 'Remarks on the seat of the faculty of articulate language, followed by an observation of aphemia', in von Bonin, 1960, pp. 49–72.

Brodmann, K., 1909. *Vergleichende Lokalisation-lehre der Grosshirnrinde: in ihren. Prinzipien dargestellt auf Grund des Zellengbaues*. J. A. Barth, Leipzig.

Bushnell, M. C., Goldberg, M. E. and Robinson, D. L., 1981. Behavioural enhancement of visual responses in monkey cerebral cortex. I. Modulation in posterior parietal cortex related to selective visual attention. *J. Neurophysiol.* 46, 755–72.

Butter, C. M. and Snyder, D. R., 1972. Alterations in aversive and aggressive behaviours following orbitofrontal lesions in rhesus monkeys. *Acta Neurobiol. Exp.* 32, 525–65.

Byrne, J. H. and Kandel, E. R., 1996. Presynaptic facilitation revisited: state and time dependence. *J. Neurosci.* 16, 425–35.

Cahill, L. and McGaugh, J. L., 1988. Mechanisms of emotional arousal and lasting declarative memory. *TINS* 21, 294–9.

Calder, A. L., Young, A. W., Rowland, D., Perrett, D. I., Hodges, J. R. and Etcoff, N. L., 1996. Facial emotion recognition after bilateral amygdala damage. Differentially severe impairment of fear. *Cogn. Neuropsychol.* 13, 699–745.

Caplan, D., 1994. Language and the brain. In M. A. Gernsbacher (ed.), *Handbook of Psycholinguistics*, ch. 31. Academic Press, San Diego.

Caramazza, A., 1996. The brain's dictionary. *Nature* 380, 485–6.

Carew, T. J. and Sahley, C. L., 1986. Invertebrate learning and memory: from behavior to molecules. *Annu. Rev. Neurosci.* 9, 435–87.

Carew, T. J., Hawkins, R. D. and Kandel, E. R., 1983. Differential classical conditioning of a defensive withdrawal reflex in *Aplysia californica*. *Science* 219, 397–400.

Carpenter, M., 1976. *Human Anatomy*. The Williams and Wilkins Company, Baltimore.

Carter, R. M., Hofstotter, C., Tsuchiya, N. and Koch, C., 2003. Working memory and fear conditioning. *Proc. Natl. Acad. Sci. USA* 100, 1399–1404.

Castellucci, V. F., Carew, T. J. and Kandel, E. R., 1978. Cellular analysis of long-term habituation of the gill-withdrawal reflex of *Aplysia californica*. *Science* 202, 1306–8.

Chalmers, D. J., 1996. *The Conscious Mind*. Oxford University Press, Oxford.

Chao, L. L., Haxby, J. V. and Martin, A., 1999. Attribute-based neural substrates in temporal cortex for perceiving and knowing about objects. *Nature Neurosci.* 2, 913–19.

Cherry, E. C., 1953. Some experiments on the recognition of speech, with one and two ears. *J. Acoust. Soc. Am.* 25, 975–9.

Chomsky, N., 1959. *Syntactic Structures*. Mouton, The Hague.

Chomsky, N., 1980. *Rules and Representations*. Blackwell, Oxford.

Christianson, S. A., 1989. Flashbulb memories: special, but not so special. *Mem. Cogn.* 17, 435–43.

Churchland, P., 2005. Cleansing science. *Inquiry* 48, 464–77.

Clarke, E. and O'Malley, C. D., 1968. *The Human Brain and Spinal Coral*. University of California Press, Berkeley.

Cohen, N. J. and Squire, L. R., 1980. Preserved learning and retention of pattern analyzing skill in amnesia: dissociation of knowing how and knowing that. *Science* 210, 207–9.

Collingridge, G. L., Kehl, S. J. and McLennan, H., 1983. Excitatory amino acids in synaptic transmission in the Schaffer collateral-commissural pathway of the rat hippocampus. *J. Physiol.* 334, 33–46.

Coltheart, M., Rastle, K., Perry, C., Langdon, R. and Ziegler J., 2001. DRC: A dual route cascaded model of visual word recognition and reading aloud. *Psychol. Rev.* 108, 204–56.

Corbetta, M., Miezin, F. M., Dobmeyers, S., Shulman, G. L. and Petersen, S. E., 1991. Selective and divided attention during visual discriminations of shape, color and speed: functional anatomy by positron emission tomography. *J. Neurosci.* 11, 2383–2402.

Crick, F., 1994. *The Astonishing Hypothesis*. Simon & Schuster, London.

Critchley, H. D. and Rolls, E. T., 1996. Hunger and satiety modify the responses of olfactory and visual neurons in the primate orbitofrontal cortex. *J. Neurophysiol.* 75, 1673–86.

Critchley, M., 1954. Parietal syndromes in ambidextrous and left-handed subjects. *Zentralbl. Neurochir.* 14, 4–16.

Dainton, B., 2007. Wittgenstein and the brain. *Science* 317, 901.

Damasio, A. R., 1983. The anatomic basis of pure alexia. *Neurology* 33: 1573–83.

Damasio, A. R., 1994. *Descartes' Error: Emotion, Reason and the Human Brain*. Grosset/Putnam Book, New York.

Damasio, A. R., 1999. *The Feeling of What Happens*. Heinemann, London.

Damasio, H., Grabowski, T. J., Tranel., D., Hichwa, R. D. and Damasio, A. R., 1996. A neural basis for lexical retrieval. *Nature* 380, 499–505.

Damasio, A. R., McKee, J. and Damasio, H., 1979. Determinants of performance in color anomia. *Brain Lang.* 7: 74–85.

Dapretto, M. and Bookheimer, S. Y., 1999. Form and content: dissociating syntax and semantics in sentence comprehension. *Neuron* 24, 427–432.

Darwin, C., 1965. *The Expression of the Emotions in Man and Animals*. University of Chicago Press, Chicago. (First pub. 1872.)

De Boysson-Bardies, B. and Vihman, M., 1991. Adaptation to language: evidence from babbling and first words in four languages. *Language* 67, 297–319.

Démonet. J-F., Thierry, G. and Cardebat, D., 2005. Renewal of the neurophysiology of language: functional neuroimaging. *Physiol. Rev.* 85: 49–95.

Dennett, D., 1969. *Content and Consciousness.* Routledge and Kegan Paul, London.

Dennett, D., 1993. *Consciousness Explained.* Penguin, Harmondsworth.

Descartes, R., 1662. *Renatus Des Cartes de homine,* ed. F. Schuyl, Leffen and Francis, Lyon.

Descartes, R., 1664. *L'Homme de René Descartes et un traitté sur la formation du foetus.*

Descartes, R., 1964–76. *Oeuvres de Descartes,* ed. Ch. Adam and P. Tannery, rev. ed. Vrin/C.N.R.S., Paris.

Descartes, R. – CSM. 1985. *The Philosophical Writings of Descartes,* 2 vols, trans. J. Cottingham, R. Stoothoof and D. Murdoch. (References to this translation are abbreviated 'CSM', 1985) Cambridge University Press, Cambridge.

Desimone, R., Moran, J. and Spitzer, H., 1988. Neural mechanisms of attention in extrastriate cortex of monkeys. In Michael Arbib and Dhun-ichi Amari (eds), *Dynamic Interactions in Neural Networks: Models and Data,* Research Notes in Neural Computing, vol. 1, pp. 169–82.

Duchenne de Bologne, G. B., 1862. *The Mechanism of Human Facial Expressions,* trans. and ed. R. A. Cuthbertson 1990. Cambridge University Press, Cambridge.

Duffy, C., Teyler, T. J. and Shashoua, V. E., 1981. Long-term potentiation in the hippocampal slice: evidence for stimulated secretion of newly synthesized proteins. *Science* 212, 1148–51.

Eason, R., Harter, M. and White, C., 1969. Effects of attention and arousal on visually evoked cortical potentials and reaction time in man. *Physiol. Behav.* 4: 283–9.

Edelman, G. M., 1993. Neural Darwinism: selection and reentrant signaling in higher brain function. *Neuron* 10, 115–25.

Edelman, G. M., 1992. *Bright Air, Brilliant Fire.* Penguin Books, London.

Ekman, P., 1971. Universals and cultural differences in facial expressions of emotion. In J. K. Cole (ed.), *Nebraska Symposium on Motivation,* vol. 19, pp. 207–84. University of Nebraska Press, Lincoln.

Ekman, P. and Friesen, W. V., 1971. Constants across cultures in the face and emotion. *J. Pers. Soc. Psychol.* 17, 124–9.

Elbers, L., 1982. Operating principles in repetitive babbling: a cognitive continuity approach. *Cognition* 12, 45–64.

Elbers, L. and Wijnen, F., 1992. Effort, production skill, and language learning. In C. A. Ferguson, L. Menn and C. Stoel-Gammon (eds), *Phonological Development: Models, Research, Implications,* pp. 337–68. York Press, Timonium, Maryland.

Engel, A. K., Konig, P., Kreiter, A. K. and Singer, W., 1991. Interhemispheric synchronization of oscillatory neuronal responses in cat visual cortex. *Science* 252: 1177–9.

Felleman, D. J. and Van Essen, D. C., 1991. Distributed hierarchical processing in the primate cerebral cortex. *Cereb. Cortex* 1, 1–47.

Fernel, J., 1542. *De naturali parte médicinae.* Simon de Colines, Paris.

Ferrier, D., 1873–4. The localization of function in the brain. *Proc. Roy. Soc. Lond.* 22, 228–32.

Ferrier, D., 1876a. Croonian Lecture: Experiments on the brain of monkeys (second series). *Phil. Trans. Roy. Soc. Lond.* 165, 433–88.

Ferrier, D., 1876b. *The Functions of the Brain.* Smith, Elder, London.

Fifkova, E. and Van Harreveld, A., 1977. Long-lasting morphological changes in dendritic spines of dentate granular cells following stimulation of the entorhinal area. *J. Neurocytol.* 6, 211–30.

Finger, S., 1994. *Origins of Neuroscience.* Oxford University Press, Oxford.

Flourens, M.-J.-P., 1824. *Recherches Experiméntales sur les Propriétes et les Fonctions du Système nerveux dans les Animaux Vertébrés.* J. B. Baillière, Paris.

Foley, M. G., 1954. *Galvani: Effects of Electricity on Muscular Motion.* Translation of L. Galvani, 1791, *De viribus electricitatis in motu musculari commentarius. Brundy Library, Norwalk.*

Folkman, S. and Lazarus, R. S., 1990. Coping and emotion. In N. S. Stein, B. Leventhal and T. Trabasso (eds), *Psychological and Biological Approaches to Emotion*, pp. 313–32. L. Erlbaum Associates: Hillsdale, NJ.

Foster, M., 1879. *A Textbook of Physiology*, 3rd edn. Macmillan, London.

Frankland, P. W., Cestari, V., Filipkowski, R. K., McDonald, R. J. and Silva, A. J., 1998. The dorsal hippocampus is essential for context discrimination but not for contextual conditioning. *Behav. Neurosci.* 112, 863–74.

Frey, U., Huang, Y.-Y. and Kandel, E. R., 1993. Effects of cAMP simulate a late stage of LTP in hippocampal CA1 neurons. *Science* 260, 1661–4.

Frisby, J. P., 1980. *Seeing: Illusion, Brain and Mind.* Oxford University Press, Oxford.

Fritsch, G. and Hitzig, E., 1870. Über die elektrische Erregbarkheit des Grosshirns. *Arch. Anat. Physiol. Wiss. Med. Leipzig*, 37, 300–32. See translation, 'On the electrical excitability of the cerebrum', in von Bonin, 1960, pp. 73–96.

Fuster, J. M., 1998. Linkage at the top. *Neuron* 21, 1223–4.

Gainotti, G., Silver, M. C., Daniele, A. and Giustolisi, L., 1995. Neuroanatomical correlates of category-specific semantic disorders: a critical survey. *Memory* 3, 241–64.

Galen, C., 1821a. *Hippocrates librum de alimento commentarius*, sect. III, ch. 1. In *Opera Omnia Claudii Galeni*, ed. K. G. Kühn, vol. 15, p. 257. Cnobloch, Leipzig, 1821–33.

Galen, C., 1821b. *De Symptomatum Differentis*, sect. VII. In *Opera Omnia Claudii Galeni*, ed. K. G. Kühn, vol. 7, pp. 55-6. Cnobloch, Leipzig, 1821–3.

Galen, C., 1854a. *Du Movement des muscles*, sect. I, ch. 1, trans. C. Daremberg, in *Oeuvres Anatomiques, Physiologiques et Médicales de Galen*, vol. 2, p. 323. Baillière, Paris., 1854–6.

Galen, C., 1854b. *Des Lieux affectés*, sect. III, ch. 14, trans. Daremberg, in *Oeuvres*, vol. 2, p. 579.

Galen, C., 1854c. *Utilité de Parties du Corps*, sect. VIII, ch. 6, trans. Daremberg, In *Oeuvres*, vol. 1, pp. 541–3.

Galen, C., 1854d. *Utilité de Parties des Corps*, sect. IX, ch. 14, trans. Daremberg, in *Oeuvres*, vol. 1, pp. 597f.

Galen, C., 1962. On anatomical procedures, IX. In *Galen on Anatomical Procedures*, trans. W. H. L. Duckworth, ed. M. C. Lyons and B. Towers, pp. 22–6. Cambridge: Cambridge University Press, 1962.

Galvani, L., 1791. De viribus electricitatis in motu musculari commentarius. De Bononiensi Scientiarum et Atrium Instituto atque Academia commentarii 7: 363–418; (for translation, see Foley 1954).

Gazzaniga, M. S., 1983. Right hemisphere language following brain bisection: a 20-year perspective. *Am. Psychol.* 38, 525–37.

Gazzaniga, M. S., 1995. Principles of human brain organization derived from split-brain studies. *Neuron* 14, 217–28.

Gazzaniga, M. S., 2000. *The New Cognitive Neurosciences*, 2nd edn. MIT Press, Cambridge, Mass.

Gazzaniga, M. S. and LeDoux, J. E., 1978. *The Integrated Mind*. Plenum Press, New York.

Gazzaniga, M. S., Ivry, R. B. and Mangun, G. R., 2002. *Cognitive Neuroscience: The Biology of the Mind*, 2nd edn. W. W. Norton, New York.

Geinisman, Y., de Toledo-Morell, L. and Madell, F., 1991. Induction of long term potentiation is associated with an increase in the number of axospinous synapses with segmented postsynaptic densities. *Brain Res.* 566, 77–88.

Geschwind, N., 1965. Disconnexion syndromes in animals and man. *Brain* 88, 237–94.

Glock, H.-J., 2003. *Quine and Davidson on Language, Thought and Reality*. Cambridge University Press, Cambridge.

Glynn, I., 1999. *An Anatomy of Thought*. Weidenfeld & Nicolson, London.

Goldman-Rakic, P. S., 1996. Memory: recording experience in cells and circuits: diversity in memory research. *Proc. Natl. Acad. Sci. USA* 93, 13435–7.

Gratiolet, P., 1865. *De la Physognomie et des Mouvements d' Expression*. J. Hetzel, Paris.

Gray, C. M. and Singer, W., 1989. Stimulus specific neuronal oscillations in orientation columns of cat visual cortex. *Proc. Natl. Acad. Sci. USA* 86, 1698–1702.

Gray, C. M., Koenig, P., Engel, A. K. and Singer, W., 1990. Synchronization of oscillatory responses in visual cortex: a plausible mechanism for scene segmentation. In H. Haken and M. Stadler (eds), *Synergetics of Cognition*, pp. 82–98. Springer, Berlin.

Grice, H. P. and Strawson, P. F., 1956. In defense of a dogma. *Philos. Rev.* 65, 141–58.

Gross, C. G., Bender, D. B. and Rocha-Miranda, C. E., 1969. Visual receptive field of neurons in inferotemporal cortex of the monkey. *Science* 166, 1303–6.

Guttenplan, S. (ed), 1994. *A Companion to the Philosophy of Mind*. Blackwell, Oxford.

Hacker, P. M. S., 1993. *Wittgenstein – Meaning and Mind, Part I: The Essays*. Blackwell, Oxford.

Hacker, P. M. S., 1996. *Wittgenstein's Place in Twentieth-Century Analytic Philosophy*. Blackwell, Oxford.

Hall, M., 1832. These motions independent of sensation and volition. *Proceedings of the Committee of Science, Zoological Society*, 27 Nov. 1832. In Alexander Walker, 'Documents and Dates of Modern Discoveries in the Nervous System' (1839). Facsimile reprint, Scarecrow Reprint Corp., Metuchen, NJ, 1973.

Hall, M., 1843. *New Memoir on the Nervous System*. Baillière, London.

Hall, M., 1850. *Synopsis of the Diastaltic Nervous System or the System of the spinal marrow and its reflex arcs, as the nervous agent in all the functions of ingestion and of egestion in the animal economy*. Croonian Lectures. Mallett, London.

Harris, E. W. and Cotman, C. W., 1986. Long-term potentiation of guinea-pig mossy fiber responses is not blocked by N-methyl-D-aspartate antagonists. *Neurosci. Letts* 70, 132–7.

Harris, E. W., Ganong, A. H. and Cotman, C. W., 1984. Long-term potentiation in the hippocampus involves activation of N-methyl-D-aspartate receptors. *Brain Res.* 323, 132–7.

Hauk, O., Johnsrude, I. and Pulvermuller, F., 2004. Somatotopic representation of action words in human motor and premotor cortex. *Neuron* 41, 301–7.

Heilman, K. M., 1979. Neglect and related disorders. In K. M. Heilman and E. Valint (eds), *Clinical Neuropsychology*, pp. 268–307. Oxford University Press, New York.

Helmholtz, H. von, 1871. On the relation of optics to painting. In D. Cahan (ed.), *Science and Culture: Popular and Philosophical Essays*, pp. 279–308. University of Chicago Press, Chicago and London.

Helmholtz, H. von, 1890. Die Störung der Wahrnehmung kleinster Helligkeitsunterschiede durch das Eigenlicht der Netzhaut. *Zeitschrift für Psychologie und Physiologie der Sinnesorgane*, 1, 5–17.

Helmholtz, H. von, 1894a. *Handbuch der Physiologischen Optik*. L. Vos, Leipzig. and Hamburg.

Helmholtz, H. von, 1894b. Über den Ursprung der richtigen Deutung unserer Sinneseindrucke. *Zeitschrift für Psychologie und Physiologie der Sinnesorgane*, i, 81–96. Trans. by R. M. Warren and R. P. Warren. 'The origin of the correct interpretation of our sensory impressions.' In Hemholtz, 1968, pp. 249–64.

Helmholtz, H. von, 1968. The recent progress of the theory of vision. In R. M. Warren and R. P. Warren (eds), *Helmholtz on Perception*, pp. 61–108. Wiley, New York (reprinted in translation).

Hickok, G. and Poeppel, D., 2004. Dorsal and ventral streams: a framework for understanding aspects of the functional anatomy of language. *Cognition* 92, 67–99.

Hillyard, S. A., Hink, R. F., Schwent, V. L. and Picton, T. W., 1973. Electrical signs of selective attention in the human brain. *Science* 182, 177–80.

Hornak, J., Rolls, E. T. and Wade, D., 1996. Face and voice expression identification in patients with emotional and behavioural changes following ventral frontal lobe damage. *Neuropsychology* 34, 247–61.

Hubel, D. H., 1988. *Eye, Brain and Vision*. Scientific American Library, New York.

Hubel, D. H. and Wiesel, T. N., 1959. Receptive fields of single neurons in the cat's striate cortex. *J. Physiol.* 148, 574–91.

Hubel, D. H. and Wiesel, T. N., 1962. Receptive fields, binocular interaction and functional architecture in the cat's visual cortex. *J. Physiol.* 160, 106–54.

Hubel, D. H. and Wiesel, T. N., 1968. Receptive fields and functional architecture of monkey striate cortex. *J. Physiol.* 195, 215–43.

Hubel, D. H. and Wiesel, T. N., 1977. Ferrier Lecture: Functional architecture of macaque monkey visual cortex. *Proc. Roy. Soc. Lond. B Biol. Sci.* 198: 1–59.

Hubel, D. H., Wiesel, T. N. and LeVay, S., 1975. Functional architecture of area 17 in normal and monocularly deprived macaque monkeys. *Symposium on Quantitative Biology*, vol. 40, 581–7. Cold Spring Harbor Laboratory, New York.

Indefrey, P. and Levelt, W. J. M., 2004. The spatial and temporal signatures of word production components. *Cognition* 92, 101–44.

International Symposium, 1981. *International Symposium on the Amygdala Complex*. Elsevier/North-Holland Biomedical Press, Amsterdam.

Jackson, J. H., 1863. Convulsive spasms of the right hand and arm preceding epileptic seizures. *Medical Times and Gazette* 2, 110–11.

James, W., 1890. *The Principles of Psychology*, vol. 1. Henry Holt/Dover, New York, 1950.

Julesz, B., 1960. Binocular depth perception of computer generated patterns. *Bell System Technology Journal* 39, 1125–62.

Kandel, E. R. and Wurtz, R. H., 2000. Construction of the visual image. In Kandel et al., 2000, ch. 25.

Kandel, E. R., Schwartz, J. H. and Jessel, T. M. (eds), 2000. *Principles of Neural Science*, 4th edn. McGraw-Hill, New York.

Kandel, E. R., Spencer, W. A. and Brindley, F. J., 1961. Electrophysiology of hippocampal neurons. I. Sequential invasion and synaptic organization, *J. Neurophysiol.* 24, 225–42.

Kenny, A. J. P., 1971. The homunculus fallacy. In M. Grene (ed.), *Interpretations of Life and Mind*, Routledge, London.

Killgore, W. D. S. and Yurgelun-Todd, D. A., 2004. Activation of the amygdala and anterior cingulate during nonconscious processing of sad versus happy faces. *Neuroimage* 21, 1215–23.

Kircher, T. T. J., Brammer, M. J., Williams, S. C. R. and McGuire P. K., 2000. Lexical retrieval during fluent speech production: an fMRI study. *NeuroReport* 11, 4093–6.

Kling, A. and Steklis, H. D., 1976. A neural substrate for affiliative behaviour in non-human primates. *Brain Behav. Evol.* 13, 216–38.

Kling, A., Steklis, H. D. and Deutsch, S., 1979. Radiotelemetered activity from the amygdala during social interactions in the monkey. *Exp. Neurol.* 66, 88–96.

Kluver, H. and Bucy, P. C., 1939. Preliminary analysis of functions of the temporal lobes in monkeys. *Arch. Neurol. Psychiatr.* 42, 979–1000.

Koffka, K., 1935. *Principles of Gestalt Psychology*. Harcourt, Brace, New York.

Köhler, W., 1929. *Gestalt Psychology*. Bell & Sons, London.

Köhler, W., 1947. *Gestalt Psychology: An Introduction to New Concepts in Modern Psychology*. Liveright, New York.

Köhler, W., 1969. *The Task of Gestalt Psychology*. Princeton University Press, Princeton.

Kosslyn, S. M., 1994. *Image and Brain*. MIT Press, Cambridge, Mass.

Kosslyn, S. M. and Ochsner, K. N., 1994. In search of occipital activation during visual mental imagery. *Trends Neurosci.* 17, 290–2.

Kosslyn, S. M., Pascual-Leone, A., Felician, O., Camposano, S., Kennan, J. P., Thompson, W. L., Ganis, G., Sukel, K. E. and Alpert, N. M., 1999. The role of area 17 in virtual imagery: convergent evidence from PET and rTMS. *Science* 284, 167–70.

LaBar, K. S., LeDoux, J. E., Spencer, D. D. and Phelps, E. A., 1995. Impaired fear conditioning following unilateral temporal lobectomy in humans. *J. Neurosci.* 15, 6846–55.

Lange, C. J. and James, W., 1922. *The Emotions*. Williams and Wilkins, Baltimore.

Laycock, T., 1851. *A Dissertation on the Functions of the Nervous System*. Sydenham Society, London.

Lazarus, R. S., 1982. Thoughts on the relationship between emotion and cognition. *Am. Psychol.* 37, 1019–24.

Lazarus, R. S., 1991. Cognition and motivation in emotion. *Am. Psychol.* 46, 352–67.

LeDoux, J. E., 1992a. Emotion and the amygdala. In J. P. Aggleton (ed.), *The Amygdala: A Functional Analysis*, pp. 339–51. Wiley-Liss, New York.

LeDoux, J. E., 1992b. Brain mechanisms of emotion and emotional learning. *Curr. Opin. Neurobiol.* 2, 191–7.

LeDoux, J. E., 1993a. Emotional memory: in search of systems and synapses. *Ann. New York Acad. Sci.* 702, 149–57.

LeDoux, J. E., 1993b. Emotional memory systems in the brain. *Behav. Brain Res.* 58, 69–79.

LeDoux, J. E., 1995a. Emotion: clues from the brain. *Ann. Rev. Psychol.* 46, 209–64.

LeDoux, J. E., 1995b. In search of an emotional system in the brain: leaping from fear to emotion and consciousness. In M. Gazzaniga (ed.), *The Cognitive Neurosciences*, pp. 1019–61. MIT Press, Cambridge, Mass.

LeDoux, J., 1996. Emotional networks and motor control: a fearful view. *Prog. Brain Res.* 107, 437–46.

LeDoux, J. E., 1998. *The Emotional Brain*. Simon & Schuster, London.

LeDoux, J. E., 1999. *Image and Brain*. Phoenix, London.

LeDoux, J. E., 2000. Emotion circuits in the brain. *Ann. Rev. Neurosci.* 23, 155–84.

LeDoux, J. E., Cicchetti, P., Xagoraris, A. and Romanski, I. M., 1990. The lateral amygdaloid nucleus: sensory interface of the amygdala in fear conditioning. *J. Neurosci.* 10, 1062–9.

LeVay, S., Hubel, D. H., and Wiesel, T. N. 1980. The development of ocular dominance columns in normal and visually deprived monkeys. *J. Comp. Neurol.* 191, 1–51.

Levelt, W. J. M., 1992. Accessing words in speech production: stages, processes and representations. *Cognition* 42, 1–22.

Levelt, W. J. M., 1994. The skill of speaking. In P. Bertelson, P. Eelen and G. d'Ydewalle (eds), *International Perspectives on Psychological Science*, vol. 1: *Leading Themes. Keynote Lectures XXV Int. Congr. Psychol., Brussels 1992*, pp. 89–103. Erlbaum, Hillsdale, NJ.

Levelt, W. J. M., Roelofs, A. and Meyer, A. S., 1999. A theory of lexical access in speech production. *Behav. Brain Sci.* 22, 1–75.

Levy, R. and Goldman-Rakic, P. S., 2000. Segregation of working memory functions within the dorsolateral prefrontal cortex. *Exp. Brain Res.* 133, 23–32.

Lichtheim, L., 1885. On aphasia. *Brain* 7, 433–84.

Liddell, E. G., 1960. *The Discovery of Reflexes*. Clarendon Press, Oxford.

Lømo, T., 1966. Frequency potentiation of excitatory synaptic activity in the dentate area of the hippocampal formation. *Acta Physiol. Scand.* 68, Suppl. 27.

Lynch, G., Larson, J., Kelso, S., Barrionuevo, G. and Schottler, F., 1983. Intracellular injections of EGTA block induction of hippocampal long-term potentiation. *Nature* 305, 719–21.

Magendie, F., 1822. 'Expériences sur les fonctions des Racines des Nerfs Rachidiens'. *J. Physiol. expér. path.*, Paris No. III, August, 2, 276–79. In Alexander Walker, 'Documents and Dates of Modern Discoveries in the Nervous System' (1839) with English translation. Facsimile edition 1973, pp. 87–91, ed. P. Cranefield. Scarecrow, Metuchen, NJ.

Malinow, R. and Miller, J. P., 1986. Postsynaptic hyperpolarization during conditioning reversibly blocks induction of long-term potentiation. *Nature* 320, 529–30.

Marr, D., 1971. Simple memory: a theory of archicortex. *Phil. Trans. Roy. Soc. Lond. B Biol. Sci.* 262, 23–81.

Marr, D., 1982. *Vision, a Computational Investigation into the Human Representation and Processing of Visual Information*. Freeman, San Francisco.

Martin, A., Haxby, J. V., Lalonde, F. M., Wiggs, C. L. and Ungerleider, L. G., 1995. Discrete cortical regions associated with knowledge of color and knowledge of action. *Science* 270, 102–5.

Mayford, M., Bach, M. E., Huang, Y.-Y., Wang, L., Hawkins, R. D. and Kandel, E. R., 1996. Control of memory formation through regulated expression of CaMKII transgene. *Science* 274, 1678–83.

McNaughton, B. L., Douglas, R. M. and Goddard, G. V., 1978. Synaptic enhancement in fascia dentata: cooperativity among coactive afferents. *Brain Res.* 157, 277–93.

Milner, B., 1962. Les troubles de la mémoire accompagnant les lesions hippocampiques bilaterales. In *Physiologie de l'Hippocampe, Colloques Internationaux No. 107* (C.N.R.S., Paris), pp. 257–72. English trans. in P. M. Milner and S. Glickman (eds), *Cognitive Processes and the Brain*, pp. 97–111. Van Nostrand, Princeton, NJ, 1965.

Milner, B., 1965a. Memory disturbance after bilateral hippocampal lesions. In P. M. Milner and S. E. Glickman (eds), *Cognitive Processes and the Brain*, pp. 97–111. Van Nostrand, Princeton, NJ.

Milner, B., 1965b. Visually guided maze learning in man: effects of bilateral hippocampal, bilateral frontal, and unilateral cerebral lesions. *Neuropsychologia* 3, 317–38.

Milner, B., 1972. Disorders of learning and memory after temporal-lobe lesions in man. *Clin. Neurosurg.* 19, 421–46.

Milner, B. and Taylor, L., 1972. Right hemisphere superiority in tactile pattern recognition after cerebral commissurotomy: evidence for non-verbal memory. *Neuropsychologia* 10, 1–15.

Milner, B., Corkin, S. and Teuber, H.-L., 1968. Further analysis of the hippocampal amnesic syndrome. *Neuropsychologia* 6, 215–34.

Milner, B., Squire, L. R. and Kandel, E. R., 1998. Cognitive neuroscience and the study of memory. *Neuron* 20, 445–68.

Mistichelli, D., 1709. *Trattato dell'Apoplessia*. Roma: A. de Rossi, alla Piazza di Ceri. In E. Clarke and C. D. O'Malley, *The Human Brain and Spinal Cord*, pp. 282–3. University of California Press, Berkeley, 1968.

Mora, R., Avrith, D. B., Phillips, A. G. and Rolls, E. T., 1979. Effects of satiety on self-stimulation of the orbitofrontal cortex in the rhesus monkey. *Neurosci. Lett.* 13, 141–5.

Moran, J. and Desimone, R., 1985. Selective attention gates visual processing in the extrastriate cortex. *Science* 229, 782–4.

Morris, J. S., Frith, C. D., Perrett, D. I., Rowland, D., Young, A. W., Calder, A. J. and Dolan, R. J., 1996. A differential neural response in the human amygdala to fearful and happy facial expressions. *Nature* 383, 812–15.

Morris, R. G., Anderson, E., Lynch, G. S. and Baudry, M., 1986. Selective impairment of learning and blockade of long-term potentiation by an *N*-methyl-D-aspartate receptor antagonist, AP5. *Nature* 319, 774–6.

Morton, J., 1964a. The effects of context on the visual duration threshold for words. *Brit. J. Psychol.* 55, 165–80.

Morton, J., 1964b. A model for continuous language behaviour. *Language & Speech* 7, 40–70.

Morton, J., 1969. Interaction of information in word recognition. *Psychol. Rev.* 76, 165–78.

Morton, J., 1979. Word recognition. In J. Morton and J. C. Marshall (eds), *Psycholinguistics,* vol. 2: *Structures and Processes*, pp. 107–56. Paul Elek, London.

Morton, J., 1980. The logogen model and orthographic structure. In U. Frith (ed.), *Cognitive Processes in Spelling*, pp. 117–33. Academic Press, London.

Morton, J. and Broadbent, D. E., 1967. Passive vs active recognition models, or Is your homunculus really necessary? In W. Walthen-Dunn (ed.), *Models for the Perception of Speech and Visual Form*, pp. 102–10. MIT Press, Cambridge, Mass. (Procs Symp. Boston MA, Nov 11–14 1964, Air Force Cambridge Research Labs.).

Moruzzi, G. and Magoun, H. W., 1949. Brainstem reticular formation and activation of the EEG. *Electroencephalogr. Clin. Neurophysiol.* 1, 455–73.

Mountcastle, V. B., 1957. Modality and topographic properties of single neurons of cat's somatic sensory cortex. *J. Neurophysiol.* 20, 408–34.

Mountcastle, V. B., 1976. The world around us: neural command function for selective attention. *Neurosci. Res. Prog. Bull.* 14, Suppl. 1–47.

Müller, J., 1838. *Elements of Physiology*, 2 vols, trans. of *Handbuch der Physiologie des Menschen* by W. Baly. Taylor & Walton, London, 1838, 1840.

Murphy, S. T. and Zajonc, R. B., 1993. Affect, cognition and awareness: affective priming with optimal and suboptimal stimulus exposures. *J. Pers. Soc. Psych.* 64, 723–39.

Nagel, T., 1979. What is it like to be a bat? Reprinted in his *Mortal Questions*, pp. 165–80. Cambridge University Press, Cambridge.

Nemesius, 1955. *The Nature of Man*. In Cyril of Jerusalem and Nemesius of Emesa, pp. 341–2. Trans. and ed. William Telfer. Westminster Press, Philadelphia.

Nowak, L., Bregestovski, P., Ascher, P., Herbet, A. and Prochiantz, A., 1984. Magnesium gates gluta-mate-activated channels in mouse central neurones. *Nature* 307, 462–5.

O'Keefe, J. and Dostrovsky, J., 1971. The hippocampus as a spatial map: preliminary evidence from unit activity in the freely moving rat. *Brain Res.* 34, 171–5.

O'Keefe, J. and Nadel, L., 1978. *The Hippocampus as a Cognitive Map*. Clarendon Press, Oxford.

Olmstead, J. M. D., 1944. Historical note on the Noeud Vital or respiratory center. *Bull. Hist. Med.* 16, 343–50.

Patterson, K. and Shewell, C., 1987. Speak and spell: dissociations and word–class effects. In M. Colt-heart, G. Sartori and R. Job (eds), *The Cognitive Neuropsychology of Language*, pp. 223–94. Erlbaum, London.

Pavlov, I. P., 1927. *Conditioned Reflexes*. Dover, New York.

Pechtel, C., McAvoy, T., Levitt, M., Kling, A. and Massermann, J. H., 1958. The cingulate and behavior. *J. Nerv. Ment. Dis.* 126, 148–52.

Penfield, W, 1959. The interpretive cortex: the stream of consciousness in the human brain can be electrically reactivated. *Science* 129, 1791–25.

Penfield, W. and Milner, B., 1958. Memory deficits induced by bilateral lesions in the hippocampal zone. *Am. Med. Assoc. Arch. Neurol. Psychiat.* 79, 475–97.

Penfield, W. and Rasmussen, T., 1968. *Cerebral Cortex of Man: Clinical Study of Localization and Function*. Hafner, New York.

Penfield, W. and Roberts, L., 1959. *Speech and Brain Mechanisms*. Princeton University Press, Princeton.

Perani, D., Schnur, T., Tettamanti, M., Gorno Tempini, M. L., Cappa, S. F. and Fazio, F., 1999. Word and picture matching: a PET study of semantic category effects. *Neuropsychologia* 37, 293–306.

Petersen, S. E. and Fiez, J. A., 1993. The processing of single words studied with positron emission tomography. *Annu. Rev. Neurosci.* 16, 509–30.

Petersen, S. E., Fox, P. T., Posner, M. I., Mintun, M. and Raichle, M., 1988. Positron emission tomo-graphic studies of the cortical anatomy of single-word processing. *Nature* 331, 585–9.

Petersen, S. E., Fox, P. T., Snyder, A. Z. and Raichle, M. E., 1990. Activation of extrastriate and frontal cortical areas by visual words and word-like stimuli. *Science* 249, 1041–4.

Pfluger, E. F. W., 1853. *Die sensorischen Functionen des Rückenmarks der Wirbelthiere nebst einer neuen Lehre über die Leitungsgesetze der Reflexionen*. ('The Sensory Functions of the Spinal Cord of Vertebrates, Together with a New Theory of the Laws of Transmission of Reflexes'). Hirschwald, Berlin.

Poppel, E., Held, R. and Frost, D., 1973. Residual visual function after brain wounds involving the central visual pathways in man. *Nature* 243, 295–6.

Posner, M. I., Walker, J. A., Friedrich, F. J. and Rafal, R. D., 1984. Effects of parietal injury on covert orienting of attention. *J. Neurosci.* 4, 1863–74.

Posner, M. I., Petersen, S. E., Fox, P. T. and Raichle, M. E., 1988. Localization of cognitive operations in the human brain. *Science* 240, 1627–31.

Pourfour du Petit, F., 1727. Mémoire dans lequel il est démontré que les nerfs intercostaux fournissent des rameaux qui portent des esprits dans les yeux. *Mémoires de Mathématique et de Physiologie. Histoire de l'Académie Royale des Sciences*, 1–19.

Prisko, L., 1963. Short-term memory in focal cerebral damage (Ph.D. thesis, McGill University, Montreal).

Procháska, J., 1784. *De functionibus systemis nervosi commentatio* (*Adnotationum academicarum*, Fasciculi III). W. Gale, Prague. Translated by T. Laycock as *The Principle of Physiology by John Aigustus Unzer and A Dissertation on the Functions of the Nervous System by George Prochaska*. London, Sydenham Society, 1861.

Pye-Smith, P. H., 1885. *Syllabus of a Course of Lectures on Physiology Delivered at Guy's Hospital*. Churchill, London.

Quirk, G. J., Armony, J. L., Repa, J. C., Li, X. F., LeDoux, J. E., 1996. Emotional memory: a search for sites of plasticity. *Cold Spring Harb. Symp. Quant. Biol.* 247–55.

Rahman, F., 1952. *Avicenna's Psychology*. English trans. of Kitab al-Najab, Book III, Chap VI. Oxford University Press, London.

Ramon y Cajal, S., 1904. *Histology of the Nervous System*, trans. N. Swanson and L. W. Swanson. Oxford University Press, Oxford, 1995.

Rizzo, M., Smith, V., Pokorny, J. and Damasio, A. R., 1993. Color perception profiles in central achromatopsia. *Neurology* 43, 995–1001.

Rodriguez, E., George, N., Lachaux, J. P., Martinerie, J., Renault, B. and Varela, F. J., 1999. Perception's shadow: long-distance synchronization of human brain activity. *Nature* 397, 430–3.

Roland, P. E. and Gulyas, B., 1994. Visual imagery and visual representation. *Trends Neurosci.* 17, 281–7.

Rolls, E. T., 1975. The neural basis of brain-stimulation reward. *Prog. Neurobiol.* 3, 73–160.

Rolls, E. T., 1992. Neurophysiology and functions of the primate amygdale. In J. P. Aggleton (ed.), *The Amygdala: A Functional Analysis*, ch. 5. Wiley-Liss, New York.

Rolls, E. T., 1993. The neural control of feeding in primates. In D. A. Booth (ed.), *Neurophysiology of Ingestion*, ch. 9. Pergamon, Oxford.

Rolls, E. T., 1995. A theory of emotion and consciousness and its application to understanding the neural basis of emotion. In M. S. Gazzaniga (ed.), *The Cognitive Neurosciences*, ch. 72. MIT Press, Cambridge, Mass.

Rolls. E. T., 1999. *The Brain and Emotion*. Oxford University Press, Oxford.

Rolls, E. T. and Baylis, L. L., 1994. Gustatory, olfactory, and visual convergence within the primate orbitofrontal cortex. *J. Neurosci.* 14, 5437–52.

Rolls, E. T. and Treves, A., 1998. *Neural Networks and Brain Function*. Oxford University Press, Oxford.

Rolls, E. T., Burton, M. J. and Mora, F., 1980. Neurophysiological analysis of brain-stimulation reward in the monkey. *Brain Res.* 194, 339–57.

Rolls, E. T., Critchley, H. D., Browning, A. and Hernadi, I., 1998. The neurophysiology of taste and olfaction in primates, and umami flavor. In C. Murphy (ed.), *Olfaction and Taste*, vol. 12, *Ann. New York Acad. Sci.* 855, 426–37.

Rolls, E. T., Sienkiewicz, Z. J. and Yaxley, S., 1989. Hunger modulates the responses to gustatory stimuli of single neurons in the caudolateral orbitofrontal cortex of the Macaque monkey. *Europ. J. Neurosci.* 1, 53–60.

Ryle, G., 1949. *The Concept of Mind*. Hutchinson, London.

Sakai, K. L., Hashimoto, R. and Homae, F., 2001. Sentence processing in the cerebral cortex. *Neurosci. Res.* 39, 1–10.

Sanghera, M. K., Rolls, E. T. and Roper-Hall, A., 1979. Visual responses of neurons in the dorsolateral amygdala of the alert monkey. *Exp. Neurol.* 63, 610–26.

Sartori, G., Job, R., Miozzo, M., Zago, S. and Marchiori, G., 1993. Category-specific form-knowledge deficit in a patient with herpes simplex virus encephalitis. *J. Clin. Exp. Neuropsychol.* 15, 280–99.

Scoville, W. B. and Milner, B., 1957. Loss of recent memory after bilateral hippocampal lesions. *J. Neurol. Neurosurg. Psychiat.* 20, 11–21.

Searle, J., 1997. *The Mystery of Consciousness*. Granta Books, London.

Sechenov, I. M., 1863a. *Physiologische Studier über die Hemmungs mechanismus für die Reflexthätigekeit des Rückenmarks im Gehirne des Frosches*. Hirschwald, Berlin.

Sechenov, I. M., 1863b. *Reflexes of the Brain*, trans. from the Russian by S. Belsky, ed. G. Gibbons. MIT Press, Cambridge, Mass; trans. A. A. Subkov in *Sechenov's Selected Works*. State Publishing House, Moscow and Leningrad, 1935.

Shepard, R. N. and Metzler, J., 1971. Mental rotation of three-dimensional objects. *Science* 171, 701–3.

Sherrington, C. S., 1892. Notes on the arrangement of some motor fibres in the lumbo-sacral plexus. *J. Physiol.* 13, 621–772.

Sherrington, C. S., 1897. On reciprocal innervation of antagonistic muscles: third note. *Proc. Roy. Soc. B* 60, 414–17.

Sherrington, C. S., 1900. The muscular sense. In E. A. Schafer (ed.), *Textbook of Physiology*, 2 vols., pp. 1002–5. Pentland, Edinburgh.

Sherrington, C. S., 1905a. On reciprocal innervation of antagonistic muscles: seventh note. *Proc. Roy. Soc. Lond. B* 76, 160–3.

Sherrington, C. S., 1905b. On reciprocal innervation of antagonistic muscles: eighth note. *Proc. Roy. Soc. Lond. B* 76, 269–97.

Sherrington, C. S., 1907. On reciprocal innervation of antagonistic muscles: tenth note. *Proc. Roy. Soc. B* 79, 337–49.

Sherrington, C. S., 1910. Flexion-reflex of the limb, crossed extension-reflex, and reflex stepping and standing. *J. Physiol.* 40, 28–121.

Sherrington, C. S., 1947. *The Integrative Action of the Nervous System*, 2nd edn. Cambridge University Press, Cambridge.

Sherrington, C. S., 1951. *Man on his Nature*, 2nd edn. Cambridge University Press, Cambridge.

Sherrington, C. S. and Grünbaum, A. S. F., 1902. A discussion on the motor cortex as exemplified in the Anthropoid Apes. *Brit. Med. J.*, part 2, 784–5.

Sherrington, C. S., to Fulton, J., 1937. Letter of 25 Dec. 1937. In J. P. Swazey, *Reflexes and Motor Integration: Sherrington's Concept of Integrative Action*, p. 76. Harvard University Press, Cambridge, Mass., 1969.

Sherrington, C. S., to Schäfer, E. A., 1897a. Letter of 27 Nov. 1897. In The Sharpey–Schäfer Papers in the Contemporary Medical Archives Centres, the Wellcome Institute for the History of Medicine, reference PP/ESS/B21/8.

Sidtis, J. J., 1981. The complex tone test: implications for the assessment of auditory laterality effects. *Neuropsychologia* 19, 103–11.

Singer, C. J., 1952. *Vesalius on the Human Brain.* Oxford University Press, London.

Singer, W., 1991. Response synchronization of cortical neurons: an epiphenomenon or a solution to the binding problem. *Int. Brain Res. Organ. News* 19, 6–7.

Speisman, J. C., Lazarus, R. S., Mordkoff, A. and Davison, L., 1964. Experimental reduction of stress based on ego-defense theory. *J. Abnorm. Soc. Psychol.* 68, 367–80.

Squire, L. and Kandel, E. R., 1999. *Memory: From Mind to Molecules.* Scientific American Books, New York.

Squire, L. R. and Zola-Morgan, S. 1991. The medial temporal lobe memory system. *Science* 253, 1380–6.

Stuart, A., 1739. Lecture III of the Croonian Lectures. *Proc. Roy. Soc. Lond.* 40, 36–48.

Taylor, J., 1750. *Mechanismus des Menschlichen Auges,* Erben und Schilling, Frankfurt am Main.

Thompson, R. F. and Krupa, D. J., 1994. Organization of memory traces in the mammalian brain. *Annu. Rev. Neurosci.* 17, 519–50.

Tootell, R. B. H., Rippas, J. B., Dale, A. M., Lock, R. B., Sereno, M. I., Malach, R., Brady, R. J. and Rosen, B. R., 1995. Visual motion after-effect in human cortical area M7 revealed by functional magnetic resonance imaging. *Nature* 375, 139–41.

Treisman, A. M., 1960. Contextual cues in selective listening. *Quart. J. Exp. Psychol.* 12, 242–8.

Treisman, A. M., 1961. Attention and Speech (Ph.D. dissertation, Oxford University, unpublished).

Treisman, A. M., 1969. Strategies and models of selective attention. *Psychol. Revs* 76, 282–99.

Treisman, A. M., 1986. Features and objects in visual processing. *Sci. Am.* 254 (11), 114–25.

Treisman, A. M. and Gelade, G., 1980. A feature-integration theory of attention. *Cogn. Psychol.* 12, 97–136.

Treisman, A., Sykes, M. and Gelade, G., 1977. Selective attention and stimulus integration. In S. Dornie (ed.), *Attention and Performance,* vol. 6, pp. 336–61. Erlbaum, Hillsdale, NJ.

Tsien, J. Z., Chen, D. F., Gerber, D., Tom, C., Mercer, E. H., Anderson, D. J., Mayford, M., Kandel, E. R. and Tonegawa, S., 1996a. Subregion- and cell type-restricted gene knockout in mouse brain. *Cell* 87, 1317–26.

Tsien, J. Z., Huerta, P. T. and Tonegawa, S., 1996b. The essential role of hippocampal CA1 NMDA receptor-dependent synaptic plasticity in spatial memory. *Cell* 87, 1327–38.

Ungerleider, L. G. and Mishkin, M., 1982. Two cortical visual systems. In D. J. Ingle, M. A. Goodle and R. J. W. Mansfield (eds), *Analysis of Visual Behaviour,* MIT Press, Cambridge, pp. 549–86. Mass.

Van der Heijden, A. C. H., 1992. *Selective Attention in Vision.* Routledge, London.

Van Hoesen, G. W., 1981. The differential distribution, diversity and sprouting of cortical projections to the amygdala in the rhesus monkey. In International Symposium, 1981, pp. 77–90.

Vesalius, A., 1543. *De humani corporis fabrica,* Bk. VII, Libri septum. J. Oporini, Basilae.

von Bonin, G. (ed.), 1960. *Some Papers on the Cerebral Cortex.* Thomas, Springfield, Ill.

Vulpian, A., 1866. *Leçons sur la physiologie générale et comparée du système nerveux, faites en 1864 au Musée d'Histoire Naturelle.* Gerner-Baillière, Paris.

Weinstein, E. A. and Friedland, R. P., 1977. Behavioral disorders associated with hemi-inattention. *Adv. Neurol.* 18: 51–62.

Weiskrantz, L., 1956. Behavioural changes associated with ablation of the amygdaloid complex in monkeys. *J. Comp. Physiol. Psychol.* 49, 381–91.

Weiskrantz, L., 1986. *Blindsight: A Case Study and Implications.* Oxford University Press, Oxford.

Weiskrantz, L., Barbur, J. L. and Sahraie, A., 1995. Parameters affecting conscious versus unconscious visual discrimination with damage to the visual cortex (V1). *Proc. Natl. Acad. Sci. USA* 92, 6122–6.

Weiskrantz, L., Warrington, E. K., Sanders, M. D. and Marshall, J., 1974. Visual capacity in the hemianeptic field following a restricted occipital ablation. *Brain* 97, 709–28.

Wernicke, C., 1874. *Der Aphasische Symptomenkomplex*. Cohn & Weigert. Breslau. English trans: The symptom complex of aphasia. In R. S. Cohen and M. W. Wartofsky (eds), *Boston Studies in the Philosophy of Science*, Vol. 4: *Proceeding of the Boston Colloquium of the Philosophy of Science, 1966/1968*, pp. 34–97. D. Reidel, Dordrecht.

White, A. R., 1964. *Attention*. Blackwell, Oxford.

Whytt, R., 1751a. Sensation the cause of a conservative motion in the whole or in the separated parts of animals – involuntary motion. The centre of this being the brain or spinal marrow. *An Essay on the Vital and other Involuntary Motions of Animals*, in *Works*, Edit. 1768, pp. 152, 162, 203, etc. In Alexander Walker, *Documents and dates of modern discoveries in the nervous system* (1839), pp. 112–22. Facsimile edn, Scarecrow, Metuchen, NJ, 1973.

Whytt, R., 1751b. Observations on the Sensibility and Irritability of the Parts of Man and other Animals. In *An Essay on the Vital and Involuntary Motions of Animals*. Hamilton, Balfour & Neill, Edinburgh.

Wigstrom, H. and Gustafsson, B., 1985a. Facilitation of hippocampal long-lasting potentiation by GABA antagonists. *Acta Physiol. Scand.* 125, 159–72.

Wigstrom, H. and Gustafsson, B., 1985b. On long-lasting potentiation in the hippocampus: a proposed mechanism for its dependence on coincidence pre- and postsynaptic activity. *Acta Physiol. Scand.* 123, 519–22.

Wigstrom, H., Gustafsson, B. and Huang, Y. Y., 1986a. Mode of action of excitatory amino acid receptor antagonists on hippocampal long-lasting potentiation. *Neuroscience* 17, 1105–15.

Wigstrom, H., Gustafsson, B., Huang, Y. Y. and Abraham, W. C., 1986b. Hippocampal long-term potentiation is induced by pairing single afferent volleys with intracellularly injected depolarizing current pulses. *Acta Physiol. Scand.* 126, 317–19.

Williamson, T., 2006. 'Conceptual Truths'. *Proceedings of the Aristotelian Society*, suppl. vol. 80, 1–41.

Willis, T., 1664. 'The Anatomy of the Brain and Nerves' (trans. of *Cerebri anatome*). Tercentenary Facsimile edn. ed. William Feindel, Vol. 2. McGill University Press, Montreal, 1965.

Willis, T., 1672. *De anima brutorum*. English: *Two discourses concerning the soul of brutes, which is that of the vital and sensitive of man*. Facsimile of translation by S. Pordage, 1683. Scholars' Facsimiles & Reprints, Gainesville, Fl., 1971.

Willis, T., 1683. *Cerebri anatome cui accessit nervorum descriptio et usus*, illustrated by Sir Christopher Wren. Flesher, London, ch. 10. Trans. into English by S. Pordage. Dring, Harper and Leigh, London, 1964.

Wise, R. J. S., Scott, S. K., Blank, C., Mummery, C. J., Murphy, K. and Warburton, E. A., 2001. Separate neural subsystems within 'Wernicke's area'. *Brain* 124, 83–95.

Wittgenstein, L., 1953. *Philosophical Investigations*. Blackwell, Oxford.

Wolford, G., Miller, M. B. and Gazzaniga, M., 2000. The left hemisphere's role in hypothesis formation. *J. Neurosci.* 20, 64 (1–4).

Wurtz, R. H. and Mohler, C. W., 1976. Organization of monkey superior colliculus: enhanced visual response of superficial layer cells. *J. Neurophysiol.* 39. 745–65.

Wurtz, R. H., Goldberg, M. E. and Robinson, D. L., 1980. Behavioural modulation of visual responses in the monkey: stimulus selection for attention and movement. In J. M. Sprague and A. N. Epstein (eds), *Progress in Psychobiology and Physiological Psychology*, pp. 43–83. Academic Press, New York.

Wurtz, R. H., Goldberg, M. E. and Robinson, D. L., 1982. Brain mechanisms of visual attention. *Sci. Amer.* 246, 100–7.

Yin, J. C., Del Vecchio, M., Zhou, H. and Tully, T., 1995. CREB as a memory modulator: induced expression of a dCREB2 activator isoform enhances long-term memory in *Drosophila*. Cell 81, 107–15.

Young, J. Z., 1978. *Programs of the Brain*. Oxford University Press, Oxford.

Young, M. P., 1992. Objective analysis of the topological organization of the primate cortical visual system. *Nature* 358, 152–5.

Zajonc, R. B., 1984. On the primacy of affect. *Am. Psychol.* 39, 117–24.

Zamanillo, D., Sprengel, R., Hvalby, O., Jensen, V., Burnashev, N., Rozov, A., Kaisen, K. M., Koster, H. J., Borchardt, T., Worley, P., et al., 1999. Importance of AMPA receptors for hippocampal synaptic plasticity but not for spatial learning. *Science* 284, 1805–11.

Zeki, S., 1993. *A Vision of the Brain*. Blackwell Scientific Publications, Oxford.

Zeki, S., 1999. Splendours and miseries of the brain. *Phil. Trans. Roy. Soc. Lond.* 354, 2053–65.

Index